Standards in Dementia Care

Edited by
Alistair Burns
Professor of Old Age Psychiatry
University of Manchester
Manchester
UK

on behalf of the EDCON Group:

Marcel Olde-Rikkert	Nijmegen, The Netherlands
Norman Sartorius	Geneva, Switzerland (Chair)
Jacques Selmes	Madrid, Spain (Secretary)
Gabriela Stoppe	Basel, Switzerland
Gunhild Waldemar	Copenhagen, Denmark

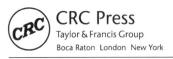

CRC Press
Taylor & Francis Group
Boca Raton London New York

CRC Press is an imprint of the
Taylor & Francis Group, an **informa** business

Contents

CARER STRESS

SERVICES

ETHICAL AND LEGAL ISSUES

Contributors

Kirsten Abelskov
Consultant
Psychogeriatric Department
Psychiatry in Århus County
Skovagervej
Risskov
Denmark

Andrew Barker
Consultant in Old Psychiatry and
Senior Policy Advisor on Older
Persons Mental Health Issues to the
Department of Health England
The Becton Centre
Barton on Sea
Hampshire
UK

Giuliano Binetti
Neurologist
Alzheimer's Unit – Memory Clinic
and NeuroBioGen Lab
IRCCS Centro S. Giovanni di Dio-
Fatebenefratelli
Brescia
Italy

Patrice Brocker
Centre Mémoire de Ressources & de
Recherche
CHU Nice
Université de Nice
Sophia Antipolis
France

Dawn Brooker
Strategic Lead for Dementia Care
Mapping
Bradford Dementia Group
School of Health Studies
University of Bradford
Bradford
UK

Errollyn Bruce
Lecturer in Dementia Studies
Bradford Dementia Group
School of Health Studies
University of Bradford
Bradford
UK

Alistair Burns
Professor of Old Age Psychiatry
University of Manchester
Division of Psychiatry
Education and Research Centre
Wythenshawe Hospital
Manchester
UK

Pasquale Calabrese
Assistant Professor of Experimental
Neurology and Neuropsychology
Faculty of Medicine
Department of Behavioural
Neurology and Neuropsychology
University Clinic
University Bochum
Bochum
Germany

Caroline Cantley
Professor of Dementia Care
Director, Dementia North
Northumbria University
Newcastle upon Tyne
UK

David Challis
Professor of Community Care
Research
PSSRU, Faculty of Medical and
Human Sciences
University of Manchester
Manchester
UK

Peter Paul De Deyn
Professor of Neurology,
Neuropsychiatrist and Director
Middelheim Memory Clinic and
Laboratory of Neurochemistry and
Behaviour
Institute Born-Bunge
University of Antwerp
Antwerp
Belgium

Wim JM Dekkers
Physician and Philosopher
Department of Ethics, Philosophy
and History of Medicine
University Medical Centre
Nijmegen
Niijmegen
The Netherlands

Murna Downs
Professor in Dementia Studies
Bradford Dementia Group
School of Health Studies
University of Bradford
Bradford
UK

Anne-Françoise Dufey
ICN Representative for EDCON
Professor and Consultant in
Geriatric Care
Haute Ecole de la Santé La Source et
Fondation Leenaards
Lausanne
Switzerland

Engin Eker
Professor of Psychiatry
Istanbul University
Cerrahpaşa Medical School
Department of Psychiatry
Division of Geriatric Psychiatry
Istanbul
Turkey

Knut Engedal
Professor of Old Age Psychiatry
Norwegian Centre for Dementia
Research
Ullevaal University Hospital
Oslo
Norway

Sebastiaan Engelborghs
Assistant Professor and Neurologist
Middelheim Memory Clinic and
Laboratory of Neurochemistry and
Behaviour
Institute Born-Bunge
University of Antwerp
Antwerp
Belgium

Sture Eriksson
Department of Geriatrics
Institution of Community Medicine
and Rehabilitation
Umeå University
Umeå
Sweden

Turan Ertan
Associate Professor of Psychiatry
Division of Geriatric Psychiatry
Department of Psychiatry
Cerrahpasa Medical School
Istanbul University
Turkey

Horácio Firmino
Consultant and Director of
Gerontopsychiatry Unit
President of Portuguese
Psychogeriatric Association
Psychiatric Clinic
Coimbra University Hospitals
Coimbra
Portugal

Susan Frade
Communications Officer
Alzheimer's Disease International
London
UK

Giovanni B Frisoni
Neurologist
LENITEM – Laboratory of
Epidemiology, Neuroimaging &
Telemedicine
IRCCS Centro S. Giovanni di Dio-
Fatebenefratelli
Brescia
Italy

Jean Georges
Executive Director
Alzheimer Europe
Luxembourg

Cristina Geroldi
Geriatrician
Alzheimer's Unit – Memory Clinic
IRCCS Centro S. Giovanni di Dio-
Fatebenefratelli
Brescia
Italy

Tomasz Hadryś
Department of Psychiatry
Medical University
Wroclaw
Poland

Cees MPM Hertogh
Nursing Home Physician
Naarderheem Center for Geriatric
Rehabilitation and Long-Term Care
Naarden
Senior Researcher in Geriatric
Medicine and Ethics
Institute for Research in Extramural
Medicine
Vrije Universiteit Medical Center
Amsterdam
The Netherlands

Kevin Hope
Senior Lecturer
School of Nursing, Midwifery and
Social Work
The University of Manchester
Manchester
UK

Jane Hughes
Lecturer in Community Care
Research
PSSRU, Faculty of Medical and
Human Sciences
University of Manchester
Manchester
UK

Andrzej Kiejna
Professor of Psychiatry
Head of the Department of
Psychiatry
Department of Psychiatry
Medical University
Wroclaw
Poland

Raymond TCM Koopmans
Professor of Nursing Home
Medicine
Department of Nursing Home
Medicine
Radboud University Nijmegen
Medical Center
Nijmegen
The Netherlands

Sylvie Lauque
Unité de Soins Aigus Alzheimer
CHU Purpan-Casselardit
Toulouse
France

Sean Lennon
Consultant Old Age Psychiatrist
Manchester Mental Health and
Social Care Trust
Wythenshawe Hospital
Manchester
UK

Carlos Augusto de Mendonça Lima
Universidade Federal do Rio de
Janeiro
Instituto de Psiquiatria
Rio de Janeiro
Brazil

Steven Luttrell
Medical Director
Consultant Physician
Camden Primary Care Trust
St Pancras Hospital
London
UK

Mary Marshall
Director, Dementia Services
Development Centre
University of Stirling
Stirling
Scotland
UK

Manuel Martín-Carrasco
Medical Director
Clinica Padre Menni
Associate Professor
University of Navarra
Pamplona
Spain

Raimundo Mateos
Professor of Psychiatry
University of Santiago de
Compostela (USC)
Coordinator of the Psychogeriatric
Unit
CHUS–University Hospital
Santiago de Compostela
Spain

Sylvie Meyer
Lecturer
Haute Ecole Santé Social de Suisse
Romande
Lausanne
Switzerland

Bère Miesen
Clinical Psycho(geronto)logist NIP
HealthCare Psychologist
Associate Professor PsychoGeriatrics
The Hague University
Consultant PsychoGeriatrics
Nursing Home WZH De Strijp-
Waterhof
The Hague
The Netherlands

Guy Nagels
Neurologist
Middelheim Memory Clinic and
Laboratory of Neurochemistry and
Behaviour
Institute Born-Bunge
University of Antwerp
Antwerp
Belgium

Marcel GM Olde Rikkert
Geriatrician
Department of Geriatrics
University Medical Centre
Nijmegen
Nijmegen
The Netherlands

Lynne Phair
Consultant Nurse for Older People
Crawley Primary Care Trust
West Sussex

Irina Pinchuk
Assistant to Faculty of Psychiatry
Donetsk Medical University
Donetsk
Ukraine

Tuula Anneli Pirttilä
Professor
Department of Neurology
University of Kuopio
Department of Neurology
Kuopio University Hospital
Hallinto
Kuopio
Finland

Rebekah Proctor
Clinical Psychologist for Older
People
Manchester Mental Health and
Social Care Trust
Wythenshawe Hospital
Manchester
UK

Philippe H Robert
Centre Mémoire de Ressources & de
Recherche
CHU Nice
Université de Nice
Sophia Antipolis
France

Rasa Ruseckiene
Gerontopsychiatrist
Gerontopsychiatric Department
Vasaros Hospital
Vilnius
Lithuania

Joanna Rymaszewska
Associate Professor
Consultant in Psychiatry
Department of Psychiatry
Medical University
Wroclaw
Poland

Manuel Sánchez-Pérez
Coordinator Psychogeriatric Unit
Sagrat Cor Hospital
Martorell, Barcelona
Coordinator Master in
Psychogeriatrics
Universitat Autònoma de Barcelona
(UAB)
Spain

Frank Schulz-Nieswandt
Professor of Social Policy
University of Cologne
Cologne
Germany

Cornel C Sieber
Professor of Medicine
Chair Internal Medicine V (Geriatric
Medicine)
Director, Institute for Biomedicine
of Aging
Friedrich-Alexander-University
Erlangen-Nürnberg
Chief Clinic II Klinikum Nürnberg
Nürnberg
Germany

Hannes B Staehelin
Professor of Geriatrics (Emeritus)
University Hospital, University of
Basel
Memory Clinic, Geriatric University
Clinic
Basel
Switzerland

Gabriela Stoppe
Professor of Psychiatry
Head of the Department of General
Psychiatry
University Psychiatric Hospitals
Basel
Switzerland

Caroline Sutcliffe
Research Associate
PSSRU, Faculty of Medical and
Human Sciences
University of Manchester
Manchester
UK

Nicoleta Tătaru
Senior Consultant Psychiatrist
Psychiatry Ambulatory Clinic
Oradea
Romania

Ingelin Testad
Hospital of Stavanger
Centre for Neuro- and Geriatric
Psychiatric Research
Stavanger
Norway

Magda Tsolaki
Neuropsychiatrist
Associate Professor of Aristotle
President of Greek Alzheimer
Association
University of Thessaloniki
Thessaloniki
Greece

Jacques Selmes Van Den Bril
Secretary General of the Alzheimer
Foundation Spain
Former President of Alzheimer
Europe
Madrid
Spain

M Vernooij-Dassen
Coordinator, Alzheimer Centre
University Medical Centre
Nijmegen
Nijmegen
The Netherlands

Gunhild Waldemar
Professor of Neurology
Memory Disorders Research Unit 6702
Department of Neurology
Rigshospitalet, Copenhagen
University Hospital
Copenhagen
Denmark

Petra Weritz-Hanf
Psychologist and Specialist for
Neurology and Psychiatry
Head of Division
Federal Ministry of Family Affairs,
Elderly
Citizens, Women and Youth (BMFSFJ)
Berlin
Germany

Anders Wimo
Associate Professor
Director, Sector of Health Economy
Stockholm Gerontology Research
Center
Stockholm
Sweden

AW Wind
Coordinator, Committee for Dutch
Dementia Guidelines for General
Practitioners
Nijmegen
The Netherlands

Orazio Zanetti
Professor of Geriatrics
Chief Geriatrician
Alzheimer's Unit – Memory Clinic
IRCCS Centro S. Giovanni di Dio-
Fatebenefratelli
Brescia
Italy

Summary of the Work of the EDCON Group

One of the main obstacles to the improvement of mental health care for the elderly is the lack of agreement about its main features among the many who should be or are participating in it. This is not all that surprising: in addition to the fact that there are many medical disciplines and various social services that must take an active role in the organization and provision of care for this group of people, aging itself adds complexity to the problems arising in connection with the diseases and impairment characterizing this period of life.

The lack of agreement about the organization of services for the elderly and about the training that is necessary to make staff deal competently with health problems in the elderly and about the stigmatisation of the elderly mentally ill led the WPA and the WHO to convene meetings involving a variety of international governmental and nongovernmental organizations with the aim of developing a consensus among them on these issues (Gustafson et al, 2003; Mendonca-Lima et al, 2003)

The consensus statements developed by these meetings were relatively easy to produce – not least because the fact that they were dealing with such a large area of discourse and involved so many organizations meant that statements had to stay on a rather general level. The statements were quoted and used in policy development but left many practitioners eager to have more specific guidance concerning the care of the elderly with specific mental disorders.

The European Dementia Consensus group (EDCON) established by the Madariaga Foundation in Brussels came into existence to respond, in part, to this need. The group is multidisciplinary and serves as a steering mechanism for the work on the development of consensus within European countries and with specific regard to dementia and related problems. Until now, the group has identified 6 areas about which it hopes to help develop consensus. These areas are: Disclosure of Diagnosis; Standards of Care; Access to Treatment; Competency; Genetic Research; Prevention of Dementia and Social Exclusion of People with Dementia

The EDCON Steering Committee selected a coordinator for the development of the texts of the consensus statements for each of these areas. As a rule, the coordinator convenes a group of experts who collaborate in the review of evidence and in the formulation of the statements. The statements are subsequently submitted to the organizations – governmental and non-governmental – that collaborate with EDCON in this project for their consideration and endorsement. The representatives of these organizations are also invited to comment on early drafts of the materials and to present evidence or views relevant to the production of the statement.

Each of the statements is accompanied by a substantial publication presenting the evidence that was considered in developing the statement. The volume edited by Professor Burns presents the material considered in the production of the consensus statement No 2, given on pages 6–7 of this volume. The texts assembled here were useful to the group that met to work on the formulation of the statement: the Steering Committee of the EDCON felt that it will be important to make this material with some additional texts available to those interested in the improvement of care for people with dementia in Europe.

It is my pleasant duty to thank members of the working group that developed the Statement 2 and the materials presented in this book on behalf of the EDCON (vide infra). Our special thanks go to Professor Burns, who has organized the consensus meetings and guided the group he convened to the successful formulation of the statement.

Norman Sartorius
Chairman of the Steering Committee of EDCON
Geneva, Switzerland

Members of EDCON

Alistair Burns, Manchester, UK
Marcel Olde-Rikkert, Nijmegen, The Netherlands
Norman Sartorius (Chair), Geneva, Switzerland
Jacques Selmes (Secretary), Madrid, Spain
Gabriela Stoppe, Basel, Switzerland
Gunhild Waldemar, Copenhagen, Denmark

References

World Health Organization (1996). Psychiatry of the Elderly – A consensus statement. WHO, Division of Mental Health and Prevention of Substance Abuse, Geneva, WHO/MNH/MND/96.7

World Health Organization (2002). Reducing Stigma and Discrimination against Older People with Mental Disorders – A Technical Consensus Statement. WHO, Department of Mental Health and Substance Dependence, Geneva, WHO/MSD/MBD/02.3

Background/introduction

chapter 1

Standards of care in dementia in Europe – a consensus

There have been significant advances in the way in which people with dementia are cared for based on increased awareness of their special needs, accumulated experience and knowledge and research. These advances have a key role to play in maximizing the quality of care which people with dementia receive in terms of identification of cognitive impairment, an understanding of causation, the benefits of better communication, avoidance of the often widespread therapeutic nihilism which surrounds dementia and a proper understanding and appreciation of end-of-life issues.

The positive benefits of providing training for staff in long-term care has been demonstrated (Proctor et al, 1999; Baltes et al, 1994). Knowledge which is provided at a basic level in terms of providing information about communication skills and facts about ageing are particularly successful when combined with an individual approach to problem behaviours: decreased dependence of residents on staff (Baltes et al, 1994) with improvement of staff morale and psychological well-being have been shown (Proctor et al, 1999). These interventions are successful, independent of their site, if the training programme is adequate. They have also been shown to be successful in reducing stress in caregivers and improving patients' quality of life. Success in specific inpatient programmes (Brodaty and Gresham, 1989) and in community settings have been demonstrated (Marriott et al, 2000). Aside from benefits in the psychological well-being of carers, delay in admission to institutional care is achieved (Mittelman et al, 1996). Use of adult day care has been shown to have a wide range of benefits on family caregivers 3 months after initiation, but with benefits continuing to occur over 1 year (Zarit et al, 1998).

Specific therapies such as reminiscence therapy and reality orientation (Spector et al, 1999) have been evaluated, the former showing relatively little promise but the latter suggesting some benefit for patients with dementia.

Provision of memory wallets (Bourgeois and Mason, 1996) and techniques to improve dressing behaviour (Beck et al, 1997), which can both be implemented in nursing homes, are also successful. The deleterious effects that medication may have on older people with dementia have been well documented, and regular review of medication by a pharmacist for older people in nursing and residential homes improves the levels of prescription without any psychological detriment to residents' mental and physical health (Furniss et al, 2000).

Effective treatments are widely available for the common symptoms of dementia, both for cognitive deficits (Tariot et al, 2000; Wilcock et al, 2000; Raskind et al, 2000) and for those non-cognitive features which can cause stress to carers and impact negatively on care, such as agitation (Teri et al, 2000). Exercise and behavioural management can also improve physical health and depression (Teri et al, 2003). Cognitive behavioural treatment of depression can yield benefits both for people with dementia and their carers (Teri et al, 1997). There is good evidence to suggest that complex and multiple interventions are more effective than simple interventions (Kennet et al, 2000). Drugs can also alleviate many of the symptoms from which older people with dementia suffer which are stressful for their carers and which detract from the quality of care provided to them (Rosenquist et al, 2000). A re-thinking of the way in which dementia is conceptualized, with a view to improving care at all levels, has been suggested (Kitwood, 1997), and has stimulated a new approach to the care and understanding of people with dementia, ennobled in the concept of Dementia Care Mapping. Much of what we regard as excellence in dementia care is based on existing good practice rather than being scientifically proven.

Implementation of standards based on current knowledge would improve care. For example, in the UK, several initiatives have been taken to address standards of care (e.g. Royal Commission on Long Term Care, 1999; Service Standards for the NHS Care of Older People, 1999), usually for older people in general but also for people with dementia. These guidelines are based on existing knowledge and represent, at one level, simply the common sense implementation of what everyone would regard as reasonable care.

There is persuasive published and anecdotal evidence that the presence and implementation of standards of care for people with dementia are variable across Europe. People with dementia come into contact with health and social services in a number of settings – in general hospitals (as medical, surgical, geriatric or orthopaedic inpatients or outpatients), in psychiatric hospitals, in primary care, in nursing and residential homes and, of course, in their own homes. The provision of care is patchy and few recognized minimum standards exist (Department of Health, 1999), carers of people with dementia are under significant stress (Donaldson et al, 1998), carer interventions can significantly reduce that stress (Brodaty and Gresham, 1989) but are currently not widely employed, staff knowledge in nursing and residential homes could be improved and lack of training impacts negatively on the quality of care provided (Proctor et al, 1999) and improvement in staff knowledge leads to improved care (Proctor et al, 1998).

In the UK, a number of Government initiatives have been launched which have potential to improve care for older people, in particular those with dementia. The Audit Commission produced a report 'Forget-Me-Not' which highlighted variability in the provision of health and social care for older people with mental health problems (Audit Commission, 2000), 'Fit for the Future' laid down minimum standards for care in nursing and residential homes (Department of Health, 1999) and the National Health Service Plan (Department of Health, 2000) plan emphasized, among other things, the need for older people with mental health problems not to be kept inappropriately in acute medical and surgical wards. The National Service Framework (NSF) for Older People (Department of Health, 2001) set an agenda for the care of older people, setting national standards of care, defining service models, outlining strategies for implementation and defining performance measures against which progress would be measured. Dementia figured highly in the National Service Framework for Older People, although it covered a whole range of health symptoms and illnesses such as stroke, falls and depression. At the level of implementation, money has been allocated to improve standards of care. Core principles of the NSF of particular relevance to dementia are:

- the need to treat individuals with dignity
- the need to have a holistic approach to care
- the need to coordinate care between health and social services
- the importance of staff training for those caring for older people.

In the rest of Europe, practice varies with regard to the care of people with dementia but they share the frustrations of the need to provide high-quality services within existing resources. The interplay between the health and social care system is highlighted by joint provision described in municipal and healthcare acts in Denmark (Abelskov, Ch. 11), Sweden (Ministry of Health and Social Affairs, 2003), Finland and Norway (Engedal, Ch. 19). National action programmes are common, such as those described in France (Robert, Ch. 5). Standardized assessment scales are often employed and descriptions of how they have been adapted to local countries are widely available, e.g. Tsolaki et al (1997) and the Cohen-Mansfield Agitation Index (Cohen-Mansfield et al, 1989). Some descriptions of services have been published, e.g. Kiejna et al (2004) and Engedal (1989).

With the evidence of advances in knowledge, the likely success of establishment and effective implementation of minimal standards and their already patchy implementation, the European Dementia Consensus Network (EDCON) developed a draft statement which it hopes will be endorsed by non-governmental organizations and governments all over Europe and possibly elsewhere.

The EDCON group proposes that the following statement should be adopted by consensus:

Standards of care for people with dementia and their carers

Bearing in mind that every person with dementia has the same right as any other person to receive the best quality health and social care and that the rights of the patient and those of the carers have to be in a dynamic balance

Aware of the fact that knowledge about the most effective practices of care is not sufficiently widely applied in European countries

Regretting that in-service training and education of different categories of staff that could significantly improve the care for people with dementia is not receiving sufficient emphasis in European countries

Cognizant also that the practices of care for people with dementia vary widely among European countries and within countries

It is therefore recommended that

1. Quality standards for the practice of care for people with dementia

should be applied in all European countries and their application should be monitored so that they can be changed when this is required for an improvement of care.

2. Quality standards should be evidence based but informed by experience and formulated respecting the need for the use of cost-effective interventions in health care. They should aim at achieving the best outcomes and maximizing the quality of life of people with dementia, of their carers and their families.

3. Standards of care provided for different types of care – e.g. home, nursing home, hospital – should be based on the same principles and developed in a manner that will allow the articulation of different types of services.

4. The partnership between patients, carers and health care staff should be expressed in an equitable distribution of tasks and in assessing the contribution of the parties.

5. Health and social services for people with dementia should be planned and evaluated with a constant awareness of the perspective of the persons with dementia and their families.

6. Care for people with dementia should be delivered in a manner that will preserve their dignity and support their carers and families.

EDCON brought together evidence and experience that might be useful in the formulation of standards by inviting a multidisciplinary expert group to present and review all aspects of dementia care. The purpose of this publication is to summarize and extend the comments and observations by this group by:

- describing the practice in dementia care across Europe in order to highlight similarities and differences
- summarizing the role of individual professions to dementia care
- documenting the major components of service provision.

We have commissioned contributions from a wide variety of individuals who have generously provided information and text at relatively short notice and EDCON thanks them for their efforts. In order to maximize the passion of each contribution, the editing style has not been prescriptive but facilitative, and so minor inconsistencies between chapters may be apparent to the experienced reader.

References

Audit Commission. Forget me not. Audit Commission, 1 Vincent Square, London SW1 2PN; available at: www.audit-commission.gov.uk

Baltes MM, Neumann EM, Zank S. Maintenance and rehabilitation of independence in old age: an intervention program for staff. *Psychol Aging* 1994; 9: 179–88.

Beck C, Heacock P, Mercer SO, et al. Improving dressing behaviour in cognitively impaired nursing home residents. *Nurs Res* 1997; 46: 126–32.

Bourgeois M, Mason LA. Memory wallet intervention in an adult day-care setting. *Behaviour Intervention* 1996; 11: 3–18.

Brodaty H, Gresham M. Effect of a training programme to reduce stress in carers of patients with dementia. *BMJ* 1989; 299: 1375–9.

Cohen-Mansfield J, Marx MS, Rosenthal AS. A description of agitation in a nursing home. *J Gerontol* 1989; 44: M77–84.

Department of Health. Fit for the Future. National required standards for residential and nursing homes for older people, 1999. Available at: www.doh.gov.uk (available by searching the publications library with the string 'Fit for the Future').

Department of Health. National Health Service Plan. 2000. Available at: www.doh.gov.uk/nhsplan/default.htm

Department of Health. National Service Framework for Older People. 2001. Available at: www.doh.gov.uk/nsf/olderpeople.htm

Donaldson C, Tarrier N, Burns A. Determinants of carer stress in Alzheimer's disease. *Int J Geriatr Psychiatry* 1998; 13: 248–56.

Engedal K. Day-care for demented patients in general nursing homes: Effects on admission to institutions and mental capacity. *Scand J Prim Health Care* 1989; 7: 161–6.

Furniss L, Burns A, Cook J, et al. Effects of a pharmacist's medication review in nursing homes. *Br J Psychiatry* 2000; 176: 563–7.

Juva K, Sulkava R, Erkinjuntti T, Valvanne J, Tilvis R. The demented elderly in the city of Helskinki: Functional capacity and placement. *Am Geriatr Soc* 1992; 40: 1146–50.

Kennet K, Burgio L, Schulz R. Interventions for in-home caregivers: A review of research 1990 to present. In: Schulz R, ed. *Handbook on dementia caregiving: Evidence-based interventions for family caregivers.* London: Springer; 2000.

Kiejna A, Rymaszewska J, Hadrys T. Organisation of mental health care for the elderly in Poland. *Eur Psychiatry* 2004; 19: 74.

Kitwood T. *Dementia reconsidered; the person comes first.* Buckingham. Open University Press; 1997.

Marriott A, Donaldson C, Tarrier N, Burns A. Effectiveness of cognitive-behavioural family intervention in reducing the burden of care in carers of patients with Alzheimer's disease. *Br J Psychiatry* 2000; 176: 557–62.

Ministry of Health and Social Affairs; *På vä mot en god demensvård.* Stockholm: Ministry of Health and Social Affairs; *Report No. DS* 2003: 47.

Mittelman MS, Ferris SH, Shirlman E, et al. A family intervention to delay nursing home placement of patients with Alzheimer disease. A randomized controlled trial. *JAMA* 1996 276(21): 1725–31.

Proctor R, Stratton-Powell H, Tarrier N, Burns A. The impact of training and support on stress among care staff in nursing and residential homes for the elderly. *J Mental Health* 1998; 7: 59–70.

Proctor R, Burns A, Stratton Powell H, et al. Behavioural management in nursing and residential homes: A randomised controlled trial. *Lancet* 1999; 354: 26–9.

Raskind MA, Pesking ER, Wessel T, et al. Galantamine in AD: A 6-month randomized, placebo-controlled trial with a 6-month extension. *Neurology* 2000; 54: 2261–8.

Rosenquist K, Tariot P, Loy R. Treatments for behavioural and psychological symptoms in Alzheimer's disease and other dementias. In: O'Brien J, Amers D, Burns A, eds. Dementia. London: Arnold; 2000: 571–602.

Royal Commission on Long-Term Care. *With Respect to Old Age: Long term care, rights and responsibilities.* A report by the Royal Commission on Long-Term Care. London: HMSO; 1999.

Service Standards For The NHS Care Of Older People. A health services accreditation publication sponsored by the Centre for Policy on Ageing. 1999. ISBN 1-901-097455.

Spector A, Orrell M, Davies S, Woods RT. Reminiscence therapy for dementia. The Cochrane Library, Issue 4. Oxford: Update Software; 1999.

Tariot P, Solomon P, Morris J, et al. A five month randomised placebo controlled trial of galantamine in Alzheimer's disease. *Neurology* 2000; 54: 2269–76.

Teri L, Logsdon RB, Uomoto J, et al. Behavioural treatment of depression in dementia patients: A controlled clinical trial. *J Gerontol Psychol Sci* 1997; 52B: 159–66.

Teri L, Logsdon RG, Peskind E, et al. Treatment of agitation in AD: A randomized, placebo-controlled clinical trial. *Neurology* 2000; 55: 1271–8.

Teri L, Gibbons L, McCurry S, et al. Exercise plus behavior management in patients with Alzheimer's disease. *JAMA* 2003: 290: 2015–22.

Tsolaki M, Fountoulakis KN, Nakopoulou E, Kazis A. Alzheimer's disease assessment scale in Greece in early demented patients and normal subjects. *Dementia and Geriatric Cognitive Disorders.* 1997; 8: 273–80.

The AM, Pasman R, Onwuteaka-Philipsen B, Ribbe M, van der Wal G. Withholding the artificial administration of fluids and food from elderly patients with dementia: Ethnographic study. *BMJ* 2002; 325: 1326.

Wilcock CK, Lilienfeld S, Gaens R. Efficacy and safety of galantamine in patients with mild to moderate Alzheimer's disease: Multicentre randomized controlled trial. *BMJ* 2000; 321: 1445–9.

Zarit SH, Stephens MA, Townsend A, Greene R. Stress reduction for family caregivers: Effects of adult day care use. *J Gerontol B Psychol Sci Soc Sci* 1998; 53: S267–77.

The Practice of Dementia Care: a European Perspective

chapter 2

The practice of person-centred dementia care: UK

Murna Downs, Dawn Brooker and Errollyn Bruce

A key development in dementia care in the UK has been the person-centred approach. The person-centred approach in dementia care is a philosophy of care that has its origins in humanism and the disability rights movement (Kitwood, 1988; Morton, 1999). The term 'person-centred' was first used in relation to people with dementia to emphasize the importance of focusing on the therapeutic potential of communication and relationships in promoting well-being and quality of life for people with dementia (Kitwood, 1988). It emphasizes the importance of focusing on the person as a human and social being rather than on the deficits and dysfunctions of the disease (Kitwood, 1993; Woods, 2001). It shares elements in common with both rehabilitative and palliative care approaches in that it seeks both to maximize retained abilities and to ensure maximum well-being and quality of life.

The person-centred approach views dementia as a biopsychosocial condition. As such, it recognizes the multiplicity of factors which affect a person's quality of life including neurological impairment, physical health, sensory ability, the individual's biography and personality and the social environment. It recognizes that little can be done to arrest neurological impairment per se. Rather, it seeks to maximize well-being by focusing on the many other dimensions that affect a person's quality of life, paying particular attention to the social environment.

A contemporary definition of person-centred dementia care describes four essential elements (Brooker, 2004):

1. Valuing people with dementia and those who care for them; promoting their citizenship rights and entitlements regardless of age or degree of cognitive impairment.

2. Treating people as individuals; recognizing that all people with dementia have a unique history and personality, physical and mental heath and social and economic resources and that these will affect their experience of living with neurological impairment.
3. Looking at the world from the perspective of the person with dementia; recognizing that each person's experience has its own psychological validity, that people with dementia act from this perspective and that empathy with this perspective has its own therapeutic potential.
4. Recognizing that all human life, including that of people with dementia, is grounded in relationships and that people with dementia need an enriched social environment which both compensates for their impairment and fosters opportunities for personal growth.

Kitwood (1997) paid particular attention to the peoples' social world and how this might be harnessed to best meet their psychological needs and, in so doing, empower and sustain them. He described the personhood of people with dementia as being undermined by a 'malignant social psychology' of care where people with dementia experience 'personal detractors', including being lied to, being treated as objects and being ignored. This malignant social psychology, he argued, is rarely created with any malicious intent; rather, it becomes woven into the culture of care. The impact of this on the well-being of people with dementia, who are already struggling to adapt to neurological impairment and to maintain their sense of self, is hypothesized as being psychologically damaging. Kitwood also used the term positive person work to describe forms of interaction that maintain personhood.

Sabat's (2001) demonstration of social positioning with respect to people with dementia lends empirical support to the manner in which interactions enhance or diminish a person's sense of self. His work also provides evidence of the way people with dementia actively cope with how they are treated. The person-centred approach is consistent with Kihlgren et al's (1994) integrity promoting care in actively seeking to foster personal growth.

The person-centred approach has been applied to understanding behavioural aspects of dementia (Kitwood, 1997; Stokes, 2000). Rather than accepting behavioural aspects as an inevitable feature of neurological impairment, a person-centred approach argues that much of what is described as 'challenging behaviour' is a rational response to an untenable situation. Taken from an understanding of, and empathy with, the perspective of the person with dementia, behaviour is viewed as a way of attempting to meet needs arising from an impoverished or unsupportive social environment. For example, people with dementia are often presented with little stimulation or opportunities for engagement in long-term care settings (Ballard et al, 2001). It is perhaps unsurprising that people seek their own stimulation by way of what is commonly labelled 'wandering' or 'disruptive vocalizations'. Common cognitive impairments in dementia such as poor learning of new information, dysphasias, dsypraxias and visuo-perceptual deficits mean that people with dementia will interpret their social and physical environments in a unique way. If these interpretations of the environment are not understood and compensated for, then the person with dementia will experience excess disability. All too often, however, this is attributed to neurological impairment rather than as a function of an unsupportive care environment (Stokes, 2000).

While most commonly associated with the UK, the person-centred approach resonates with developments in the USA around the need-driven behaviour model of dementia. As far back as 1985, Rader and colleagues used the term 'agenda behaviour' to highlight the goal-seeking that drives much of the behaviour of people with dementia. Cohen-Mansfield (2000) has provided convincing evidence that much so-called 'challenging behaviour' is a response to unmet physical or social need. She has demonstrated that incidents of physical aggression are commonly elicited by the manner of approach by care staff. Beattie and colleagues (2004) are developing the empirical basis for a non-pharmacological care approach which addresses a person's physical and psychosocial needs.

Putting person-centred care into practise is a challenge and requires adequate and appropriately arranged resources (Kitwood and Woods, 1996). In a political and economic context, where it appears that ever-increasing needs compete for a limited amount of resources, people with dementia are unlikely to ever be at the top of the list. There is a vested interest from an economic point of view in maintaining the position that people with dementia need very little in the way of skilled care interventions. There is a concern that in attempting to encourage practitioners to adopt a person-centred approach without addressing the larger organizational and economic context, we are setting them up to fail (Packer, 2000; Sheard, 2004).

One of the strategies that have facilitated the adoption of a person-centred care approach in a number of care organizations in the UK, and increasingly in other parts of the world, has been through Dementia Care Mapping (DCM) (Bradford Dementia Group, 1997; Brooker et al, 1998). Dementia Care Mapping is essentially a collaborative process with a team of care staff. It has four main components:

1 Preparing the care setting for developmental evaluation
2 Observing the experience of people with dementia of the process and effects of care
3 Sharing these observations with staff
4 In collaboration with staff, outlining short- and long-term action plans to improve the quality of experience of people with dementia in care settings.

DCM is a complex observational tool designed to be used in a series of developmental evaluations or continuous quality improvement cycles in care settings (Bradford Dementia Group, 1997; Brooker, in press; Brooker et al, 1998; Younger and Martin, 2000). As an observational tool, it measures the process and effects of care using a set of operational definitions of well-being, ill-being, positive person work and personal detractors. These observations are made by assuming the point of view of the person with dementia. Its effective use in developmental evaluation requires careful preparation of the care setting, constructive feedback to the staff and collaborative action planning (Brooker et al, 2004). In the UK, the Audit Commission (2000) recommended the use of DCM as a means of improving the quality of care in formal care settings and it has been the subject of a number of positive reports from the Commission for Health Improvement.

The tool provides a highly detailed map of the person's experience of care. The use of this information as part of developmental evaluation requires skilful handling. As such, Bradford University offers a range of courses on its use. Its basic use requires a 3-day course which covers its theoretical basis, its coding, analysis and interpretation, and preparation, feedback and action planning. Further training and accreditation is available for those who wish to lead large-scale projects outside of their own care settings. These courses are offered throughout the UK, Europe, Australia, USA and Japan. (For further information about training in its use, see www.bradford.ac.uk/acad/health/dementia.) The psychometric properties of the tool are the subject of ongoing and recently completed studies (Fossey et al, 2002; Thornton et al, 2004). The 8th edition of the tool is currently being developed.

Another approach to ensuring the implementation of a person-centred approach to dementia care has been the development of accredited education in dementia care. For example, at the University of Bradford we offer undergraduate and postgraduate degrees in dementia studies. (For further information about degree programmes, see www.bradford.ac.uk/acad/health/dementia.) Professionalizing dementia care is one approach to ensuring an adequately trained workforce, something recognized as lacking in the UK's National Service Framework for Older People (Department of Health, 2001). While there will continue to be a need for specialist secondary services such as old age psychiatry and geriatrics, the majority of people with dementia in the UK are supported by non-professional groups of staff led by nurses or social workers with little specialist training in dementia.

The implementation of a person-centred care requires more than the communication of ideas (Beck et al, 1999; Kitwood and Woods, 1996); rather, it requires the political will to ensure adequate resources for the necessary infrastructure, including appropriate supervision, induction and staffing ratios. Unlike pharmacological approaches to enhancing cognitive function or managing behaviour, person-centred approaches have no economic or business interest. Furthermore, therapeutic engagement between people with dementia and their families or staff is not generally the stuff of headline news. It is notable that the attention given to the modest gains attained by drug interventions is not equalled to that given to studies demonstrating efficacy for psychosocial interventions (e.g. Kihlgren et al, 1993; Moniz Cook et al, 1998; Teri and Uomoto, 1991).

The Department of Health's (2001) adoption of person-centred care as one of its eight standards for services for older people serves both to highlight the concept and to potentially dilute its full meaning. In using the language of 'person-centred care', it firmly establishes it as central to policy and practice. In focusing almost exclusively on the need for individualized care and autonomy, however, it neglects the emphasis on the therapeutic potential within the interpersonal and social dimension of people's lives (Brooker, 2004; Kitwood, 1997; McCormack, 2004; Nolan et al, 2004; Zgola, 1999). It is essential that the full meaning of the approach be embraced by policy to ensure that the necessary adjustments and reforms are made to health and social care practice to achieve the potential of a person-centred approach in dementia care.

References

Audit Commission. *Forget me not: Mental health services for older people*. London; 2000. www.audit-commission.gov.uk.

Ballard C, Fossey J, Chithramohan R, et al. Quality of care in private sector and NHS facilities for people with dementia: cross sectional survey. *Br Med J* 2001; **323**: 426–7.

Beattie ERA, Algase DL, Song J. Behavioural symptoms of dementia: Their measurement and intervention. *Aging Ment Health* 2004; **8**: 109–116.

Beck C, Ortigara A, Mercer S, Shue V. Enabling and empowering certified nursing assistants for quality dementia care. *Int J Geriatr Psychiatry* 1999; **14**: 197–211.

Bradford Dementia Group. *Evaluating dementia care: The DCM Method*, 7th Edition. University of Bradford; 1997.

Brooker D. What is person-centred care for people with dementia? *Rev Clin Gerontol* 2004; **13**: 212–22.

Brooker D. Dementia care mapping: A review of the research literature. *Gerontologist* (in press).

Brooker D, Foster N, Banner A, Payne M, Jackson L. The efficacy of dementia care mapping as an audit tool: report of a 3-year British NHS evaluation. *Aging Ment Health* 1998; **2**: 60–70.

Brooker D, Edwards P, Benson S, eds. *DCM: Experience and insights into practice*. London: Hawker Publications; 2004.

Cohen-Mansfield J. Approaches to the management of disruptive behaviours. In: Powell Lawton M, Rubinstein RL, eds. *Interventions in dementia care: Toward improving quality of life*. London: Springer Publications; 2000.

Department of Health. *National service framework for older people*. London: Department of Health; 2001. Crown Copyright. www.doh.gov.uk/nsf

Fossey J, Lee L, Ballard C. Dementia care mapping as a research tool for measuring quality of life in care settings: psychometric properties. *Int J Geriatr Psychiatry* 2002; **17**: 1064–70.

Kihlgren M, Kuremyr D, Norberg A, et al. Nurse–patient interaction after training in integrity-promoting care at a long term ward: analysis of video-recorded morning care sessions. *Int J Nurs Stud* 1993; **30**: 1–13.

Kihlgren M, Hallgren A, Norberg A, Karlsson I. Integrity promoting care of demented patients: Patterns of interaction during morning care. *Int J Aging Hum Dev* 1994; **39**: 303–19.

Kitwood T. The technical, the personal, and the framing of dementia. *Social Behaviour* 1988; **3**: 161–79.

Kitwood T. Discover the person, not the disease. *J Dementia Care* 1993; **Nov/Dec**: 16–17.

Kitwood T. *Dementia reconsidered: the person comes first*. Buckingham: Open University Press; 1997.

Kitwood T, Woods RT. *Training and development strategy for dementia care in residential settings*. Bradford: University of Bradford; 1996.

McCormack B. Person-centredness in gerontological nursing: An overview of the literature. *Int J Older People Nurs* 2004; **13**: 31–8.

Moniz-Cook ED, Agar S, Gibson G, Win T, Wang M. A preliminary study of the effects of early intervention with people with dementia and their families in a memory clinic. *Aging Ment Health* 1998; **2**: 166–75.

Morton I. *Person-centred approaches to dementia care*. Bicester: Speechmark Publishing Limited; 1999.

Nolan MR, Davies S, Brown J, Keady J, Nolan M. Beyond 'person-centred' care: a new vision for gerontological nursing. *Int J Older People Nurs* 2004; **13**: 45–53.

Packer T. Does person-centred care exist? *J Dementia Care* 2000; 8: 19–21.

Rader J, Doan J, Schwab M. How to decrease wandering, a form of agenda behavior. *Geriatr Nurs* 1985; 6: 196–9.

Sabat S. *The experience of Alzheimer's disease: Life through a tangled veil.* Oxford: Blackwell; 2001.

Sheard D. Person centred care: the emperor's new clothes? *J Dementia Care* 2004; 12: 22–4.

Stokes G. *Challenging behaviour in dementia: A person-centred approach.* Bicester: Speechmark Publishing; 2000.

Teri L, Uomoto J. Reducing excess disability in dementia: Training caregivers top manage depression. *Clin Gerontol* 1991; 10: 49–63.

Thornton A, Hatton C, Tatham A. Dementia care mapping reconsidered: exploring the reliability and validity of the observational tool. *Int J Geriatr Psychiatry* 2004; 19: 718–26.

Woods RT. Discovering the person with Alzheimer's disease: Cognitive, emotional and behavioural aspects. *Aging Ment Health* 2001; 5: 7–16.

Younger D, Martin G. Dementia care mapping: An approach to quality audit of services for people with dementia in two health districts. *J Adv Nurs* 2000; 32: 1206–12.

Zgola JM. *Care that works: A relationship approach to persons with dementia.* Baltimore, MD: Johns Hopkins University Press; 1999.

chapter 3

The practice of dementia care: Italy

Orazio Zanetti, Giuliano Binetti, Cristina Geroldi and Giovanni B Frisoni

Impairment of cognitive function represents one of the more prevalent causes of disability in the elderly, affecting about 10% of people older than 65, and 25–50% of those aged 85 and over, in the general population, and 50–80% of the subjects living in nursing homes (Evans et al, 1989; Rocca et al, 1986).

Imprecise definitions and incomplete differential diagnoses have led to the underdiagnosis, misdiagnosis or overdiagnosis of the dementia syndrome in many clinical settings. Inappropriate management of patients affected by dementia can increase mortality and morbidity, determine worse quality of life for patients and caregivers, and increase healthcare expenditures. In the last 20 years, different health services have been designed to diagnose dementia more accurately and to improve the care of patients. Aims (diagnostic evaluation, treatment/referral, case management, research, training and continuing education, rehabilitation programmes, special programmes of care), target subjects (outpatients, inpatients, nursing home residents), organization and costs of these services are specific.

In June 1991 the first Italian ward (called the 'Alzheimer's Unit') specifically devoted to research and care for demented patients was built up in Brescia (Italy) thanks to the convergence of feelings between the Fatebenefratelli Institution of Brescia and the Health Government of the Lombardy Region.

Since that time, in our institution, about 7000 patients have been evaluated with a multidimensional approach as inpatients and more than 27 000 as outpatients. From the beginning, our work has been inspired mainly by two aims:

1 To deliver an holistic approach – addressing biological, psychological and social aspects – for patients and their families along the wide variability of the disease course from its appearance until the later stages of

dementia, overcoming the traditional dichotomous approach which separates diagnosis (a neurologist's task) from behavioural disturbances management (a psychiatrist's task), and from the complex clinical and ethical problems of the more advanced phase of the disease (a geriatrician's task).

2 The search for significant outcomes of each procedure adopted for the diagnosis, the staging and the therapeutical – pharmacological and non-pharmacological – interventions.

These aims are still alive and constitute the basis of our daily work of research and care with people affected by cognitive impairment and their caregivers. The holistic approach, nourished by the evidence-based geriatric multidimensional culture, has led to a deeper understanding of the wide range of the biological and clinical aspects of Alzheimer's disease. The assessment procedure for Alzheimer's disease (AD) and related disorders that has been evaluated and validated in-depth in our Memory Clinic is now widely adopted (Trabucchi, 2002) in different settings in our country – i.e. nursing home, hospital and home care – and permits cross-cultural comparisons. Genetical susceptibility, determinants of caregiver burden and clinical questions regarding the determinants of disability, the clinical and neuropsychological profile and the neurobehavioural problems of the demented patient have been comprehensively addressed.

The Alzhemer's Unit consists in a 40-bed ward for inpatients, a day hospital service for 15 outpatients, and an outpatient clinic. The early staff consisted of two full-time neurologists, two full-time geriatricians, one full-time neuropsychologist, six full-time medical fellows, 12 full-time nurses, one full-time social worker, two full-time physical therapists, 6 full-time occupational therapists, 16 full-time hospital attendants and 4 full-time and 2 part-time biologists. Patients were referred to the outpatient clinic by their family doctors or by other specialists (mainly neurologists, geriatricians or psychiatrists) for a preadmission visit. Only a small number (about 20%) of patients observed in the outpatient clinic needing accurate diagnostic evaluation, or hospital care and rehabilitation, were admitted to the inpatient clinic or to the day hospital.

During their stay in the ward, patients undergo a complete clinical evaluation, including:

- comprehensive personal and family history, collected partially from the patients, and mainly from the patients' relatives by a medical fellow

- neurological and somatic examination performed by a neurologist and a geriatrician, respectively
- routine laboratory tests and instrumental examination
- brain neuroimaging – computed tomography (CT) and magnetic resonance imaging (MRI) scans
- clinical neuropsychological testing.

Furthermore, they undergo pharmacological and non-pharmacologic interventions such as cognitive rehabilitation, formal or informal occupational therapy and physical rehabilitation.

In 1995, following our Alzheimer's Unit experience, the Lombardy Region launched an enterprise called the 'Alzheimer Project', with the institution of 20-bed special care units (SCUs) for patients with severe cognitive impairment and relevant behavioural disturbances in 60 nursing homes. These SCUs proved their efficacy in reducing physical and pharmacological restraints and in improving the quality of life of the demented patients.

In 1996 the Alzheimer Center of Brescia was recognized by the National Health Ministry as the first National Research Center specifically devoted to research for AD and related disorders whose aim is to provide sound and 'evidence-based' guidelines for the management of dementia in our country. In this same year, we studied the early typology of our patients by describing 196 consecutive patients with cognitive impairment admitted to the in-patient ward of the Alzheimer's Unit between 1 June and 31 December 1996. The most frequent cause of admission was the first diagnosis of a cognitive disturbance, followed by therapy of behavioural disturbances; a quarter of patients were admitted because of imbalance of somatic diseases or needing physical rehabilitation, whereas only about 6% were again admitted to the ward to undergo follow-up of cognitive disturbance. The great majority of subjects came from home; only a minority came from a nursing home. On the contrary, on discharge, 10% of patients were institutionalized.

On admission, less than one-third of the patients had a diagnosis of cognitive disturbance confirmed after complete assessment. About half of the patients were admitted to the ward without a cognitive diagnosis or diagnostic hypothesis, and about a quarter had an aspecific diagnosis of cognitive disturbance (e.g. 'cognitive impairment', 'senile psycho-organic disturbance', 'atherosclerotic dementia'), or a diagnostic definition that was not confirmed after the assessment. Therefore, the diagnostic definition of the cognitive disturbances appeared to have great importance, and has been one of the primary skills of our Memory Clinic since its foundation. We defined outcomes as changes of clinical status and perception of quality of life during the stay in the ward, evaluated in four domains: global cognition, physical function, behaviour and complaint of somatic symptoms (marker of well-being and subjective physical health). Global cognitive status, basic activities of daily living, physical function, behavioural disturbances and subjective physical health (spontaneously reported and evoked somatic pain and discomfort) improved in the whole sample. In particular, demented patients improved 1.5 points on the MMSE score; about 5 points on the Barthel index; about 2.5 points on the Tinetti Scale, reducing the risk of fall; 20 points on the NPI scale, with reduction of behavioural disturbances and reaching of easier management of patients at home or in the nursing home.

After a stay of about 30 days, all patients received a diagnostic definition of cognitive impairment. The relevance of diagnosis should be underlined for a number of reasons: first, reversible dementias exist, but patients affected by these forms can recover only if reversibility of disease is recognized; secondly, misdiagnosis of non-reversible dementia can lead to inappropriate management of demented patients, increasing their mortality and morbidity, and worsening their quality of life; finally, we think that a precise and correct diagnosis is a patient's right, even if the patient's disease is a non-reversible form of dementia and resolutive treatments are lacking. Furthermore, patients showed sensible and clinically evident improvement in all of the considered domains. The achievement of these results justifies the role of our Alzheimer's Unit. Patients with a correct diagnosis of cognitive impairment can be treated with specific interventions, determining positive outcomes in physical and daily functions. About half of the patients were diagnosed as affected by Alzheimer's dementia (Table 3.1), about another quarter by vascular dementia or vascular cognitive impairment and about 10% were affected by other forms of dementia. In Table 3.1 the proportion of diagnoses formulated at the Alzheimer's Unit in the year 2000 (4 years after) is also reported, showing the appearance of the mild cognitive impairment (MCI) diagnosis.

Due to the increased awareness of the needs of demented patients, the National Health Service in September 2000 started the so-called 'Cronos project'. This consisted of the foundation of about 500 outpatient clinics (UVA, Alzheimer Evaluation Unit), whose main aim was the assessment of demented patients and the free delivery of cholinesterase inhibitor drugs for patients with probable mild to moderate AD (MMSE 10–26). This wide

Table 3.1 Distribution of diagnoses in 196 and 501 patients seen at the Alzheimer's Unit–Memory Clinic of Brescia in the years 1996 and 2000, respectively

Diagnosis	Proportion (%)	
	1996	2000
Probable or possible AD	50.3	37.4
Probable or possible VaD, or SVD	23.8	15.6
VCI – vMCI		14.4
FTD or Pick's disease	4.2	6.6
slowly progressive aphasia	1.1	
MCI (Mayo Clinic)	–	9.2
Parkinson dementia	2.1	1.4
Dementia with Lewy body (probable + possible DLB)	1.1	1.8
Alcohol-induced persisting dementia	0.5	–
Creutzfeldt–Jakob's disease	0.5	–
Other dementias[a]	3.2	4.5
Reversible dementia	6.9	9.0
Other neurological or somatic diseases without dementia[b]	6.3	–

AD = Alzheimer's disease; VaD = vascular dementia; FTD = frontotemporal dementia; SVD = subcortical vascular dementia; VCI = vascular cognitive impairment; vMCI = mild cognitive impairment of vascular type.

[a] Other dementias include progressive supranuclear palsy, cerebral tumour, luetic dementia, paraneoplastic dementia and Huntington's disease.
[b] Other neurological or somatic diseases without dementia include Parkinson's disease, multiple system atrophy, previous neurosurgical intervention for cerebral tumour, subjective memory disturbance, Wernicke's encephalitis, subdural haematoma, and ventriculoperitoneal shunt for normal pressure hydrocephalus, post-traumatic extrapyramidal syndrome.

network of facilities contributed to the increased quality of care for patients with cognitive impairment in Italy. In the meantime, the characteristics of our patients (mainly in the outpatient section) are progressively changing, with severity of symptoms at the first observation being significantly lower in the last few years.

Now our work with patients and their families ranges from the challenging diagnostic (and therapeutical) problem of MCI (Frisoni et al, 2002) to the genetic evaluation of some forms of cognitive impairment (Alberici et al, 2004), and to the definition of the impact of the vascular damage component in the determinism of cognitive impairment (Geroldi et al, 2003). Moreover, we are trying to define a more positively oriented approach for structural neuroimaging (Frisoni et al, 2003), seeking evidence on an imaging procedure that may have some specific additional diagnostic information (examples are medial temporal or focal atrophy and vascular changes). Finally, the limited efficacy of the available anticholinesterase drugs has fuelled non-pharmacological interventions (Zanetti et al, 2002; Oriani et al, 2003) which are now coming of age; unpublished data from our Alzheimer's Unit–Memory Clinic suggest a synergic role of cognitive rehabilitation with cholinesterase inhibitor drugs.

As to our second main aim – the search for significant outcomes – we are still looking for an answer. It has been claimed that 'dementia is a particularly postmodern condition' signalling that 'some communities believe that modern technologically oriented society support value systems that should be challenged and modified' (Whitehouse, 2001). Surely, the search for significant outcomes needs to confront itself with the cultural, ethical and economic aspects of our postmodern society. Only from a wide debate among the different members of our society will emerge a new horizon about caring, quality of life and the role of technology in the care of our members affected by devasting diseases such as Alzheimer's disease. But this will be our own future landscape.

Acknowledgements

This shortly resumed story could not have been written without the valuable contribution of Brother Marco Fabello, Professor Marco Trabucchi, Angelo Bianchetti and a long list of many other health workers.

References

Alberici A, Gobbo C, Panzacchi A, et al. Frontotemporal dementia: Impact of P301L tau mutation on a healthy carrier. *J Neurol Neurosurg Psychiatry* 2004; 75: 1607–10.

Evans DA, Funkenstein HH, Albert MS, et al. Prevalence of Alzheimer's disease in a community population of older persons. *JAMA* 1989; 262: 2551–6.

Frisoni GB, Galluzzi S, Bresciani L, Zanetti O, Geroldi C. Mild cognitive impairment with subcortical vascular features: Clinical characteristics and outcome. *J Neurol* 2002; 249: 1423–32.

Frisoni GB, Scheltens P, Galluzzi S, et al. Neuroimaging tools to rate regional atrophy, subcortical cerebrovascular disease, and regional cerebral blood flow and metabolism: consensus paper of the EADC. *J Neurol Neurosurg Psychiatry* 2003; 74: 1371–81.

Geroldi C, Galluzzi S, Testa C, Zanetti O, Frisoni GB. Validation study of a CT-based weighted rating scale for subcortical ischemic vascular disease in patients with mild cognitive deterioration. *Eur Neurol* 2003; **49**: 193–209.

Oriani M, Moniz-Cook E, Binetti G, et al. An electronic memory aid to support prospective memory in patients in the early stages of Alzheimer's disease: A pilot study. *Aging Ment Health* 2003; **7**: 22–7.

Rocca W, Amaducci L, Schoenberg BS. Epidemiology of clinically diagnosed Alzheimer's disease. *Ann Neurol* **19**: 1986; 415–24.

Trabucchi M, ed. Le demenze (Dementias). *UTET periodici*, 3rd edn., 2002.

Whitehouse PJ. The end of Alzheimer's disease. *Alzheimer Dis Assoc Disord* 2001; **15**: 59–62.

Zanetti O, Oriani M, Geroldi C, et al. Predictors of cognitive improvement after reality orientation in Alzheimer's disease. *Age Ageing* 2002; **31**: 193–6.

chapter 4

The practice of dementia care: Spain

Raimundo Mateos, Manuel Sánchez-Pérez and Manuel Martín-Carrasco

Important aspects of the Spanish National Health System for dementia care

The Spanish population has increasingly aged over the last few years. 17% of its 41 million inhabitants are older than 65, which reaches 25% in some provinces.

The Spanish political organization comprises 17 autonomous communities with extremely different sociodemographical, economic and cultural characteristics. State (general) laws guarantee every citizen free and universal access to all health services, but each autonomous community's laws and rules determine healthcare services organization, set their objectives and award budgets. Therefore, it is widely known that there are remarkable differences in healthcare resources among the different autonomous communities, especially in the psychogeriatrics field and, to be precise, in relation to dementia care.

Apart from the care they receive from the National Health Service, dementia patients and their natural/main carers benefit from Social Services and, in some communities, from a combined public social and healthcare system ('Sociosanitario'). This is a hybrid system which tries to alleviate the noticeable coordination difficulties between both large service systems as well as restraining the unlikely to be maintained increase in public expenditure.

Private caring services are a good complement in this field; this is still a marginal practise in most communities although a growing one, especially in the area of Social Services (i.e. day hospitals and nursing homes, etc.).

Some examples of dementia care

The Sociosanitario patterns, born to alleviate the above-mentioned limitations, also show important differences in practice, as we will show by means of the Catalonian and Galician model.

Table 4.1 Public health care resources for patients suffering from cognitive and behavioural disorders

- Long-term hospital confinement
- Medium-term hospital confinement
- Home care
- Day hospital
- Dementia diagnostic and treatment units

In 1986 the autonomous Catalonian Government started the programme 'Vida als Anys', addressed at people suffering from chronic pathologies, most of them (80%) being old people. From the very beginning, this program counted with the necessary funds to support a series of services assigned to its specific goals (Servei Català de la Salut, 2004).

The Sociosanitario resources in Cataluña (Table 4.1) take in more than 30% of patients suffering from dementia, which reaches 50% if we take into account all the patients admitted to old people's homes. People suffering from dementia who are being cared for in those centres are usually at an advanced stage of the disease (Reisberg's GDS: 6–7) (Servei Català de la Salut, 2004). Public health care given to patients suffering from dementia is included in the 2000–2005 Dementia Care Plan.

One's experience shows that long-term Sociosanitario units bring together many patients with serious cognitive impairment, which are an important necessity of nursing attention and socially troubling; on the contrary, 'psychogeriatrics health-care units' (mid-term ones) group together some patients suffering from a similarly evolved dementia but showing more behavioural problems and having more family support. In both cases the level of dependency to carry out basic activities of daily living is a high one. In practise, this justifies the fact that many Sociosanitario centres end up creating specific areas for dementia patients within their 'long-term care units'.

Sociosanitario boarding facilities, unlike hospitals or welfare institutions, can pay attention to somatic and mental problems provided that they are not acute ones.

Dementia home care in the public social and healthcare field provides primary health care with its own qualified support (or with hospital or welfare workers). The patient's profile is that of a person suffering from a moderate/serious dementia with other related disorders (active or inactive ones), who is quite dependent from a functional point of view, but living at home in charge of his family. The intervention of the home care team is delimited by time, depending on the objectives agreed with the primary healthcare professionals who, in short, are ultimately responsible for the patient at home. The receiver of this type of assistance must fulfil a series of basic conditions, which are as follows:

- the patient's somatic and behavioural set of symptoms can be managed at home
- this kind of help is accepted by the patient and his family
- there is one or more carers who are able to take liability for the patient's basic care.

In 1996 the Sociosanitario 'PASOS' (Subdirección Xeral do Programa de Atención Sociosanitaria, 1999) was created in Galicia. One of its biggest achievements was the creation of the Psychogeriatrics Advisory Committee (1999), composed of some representatives of the different professional and user's sectors, who made a thorough revision of dementia care in this community; consequently, it developed a care plan. It also carried out a series of support and training activities for those relatives taking care of this type of patient (Subdirección Xeral do Programa de Atención Sociosanitaria, 2003). But, unlike the comparable Catalonian programme, the Galician example does not have any specific budget to implement its goals and lacks the competence to organize a network of services. Its objective is the functional coordination of the previously existing social and healthcare resources, which might explain the restricted impact the above-mentioned initiatives have had on everyday care of dementia patients. The difficulty of coordinating health care and social services is a recurrent topic in professional and media debates. As for dementia care, it has been explicitly recognized by its main protagonists within the framework of the last Congress of the 'Sociedade Galega de Xerontoloxía e Xeriatría' (Galician Gerontology and Geriatrics Society) in 2004.

Public opinion and social and healthcare resources

Over the last few years, media interest on dementia-related topics and, at the same time, the rate of social concern about this pathology, almost unknown a decade ago, has quickly grown.

The review of all the available epidemiological research has led us, on the one hand, to estimate a high prevalence of dementia among people older than 65, even though there may be a noticeable degree of variation between different towns and/or methodological discrepancy among all the research carried out (Del Barrio et al, 2005); on the other hand, it has made it possible to know the relationship between cognitive impairment and other pathologies (Mateos et al, 2000).

Although the family is still the main source of social support for these patients, the evolution of demography and the woman's social and working role is questioning its continuity. The fact that there are a series of validations of internationally accepted instruments to measure the carer's burden (Martín Carrasco et al, 1996) or these patients' and their carers' necessities (Mateos et al, 2004) will make the analysis of these topics easier. They are important not only from a scientific point of view but also for the organization of care.

Good examples to take into account

Coordination among the different services has been achieved, especially in some restricted geographical areas that are provided with high economic resources and are administratively autonomous.

The consolidation of the Spanish Psychogeriatrics Society, federated with the International Psychogeriatrics Association, contributes increasing leadership in the development of psychiatric assistance to old people. Its yearly congresses, courses and publications are milestones along its development. Among them one must remark the journal *Revista de Psicogeriatría*, which is the official means of expression of the above-mentioned society, as well as the second edition of the *National Consensus on Dementia* (elaborated together with the Spanish Society of Psychiatry).

There are a number of psychogeriatrics units that follow the internationally accepted principles which must rule psychiatric assistance to old people, having fully dedicated multidisciplinary teams with a community philosophy (Martín-Carrasco et al, 1991; Mateos et al, 1994; Sánchez-Pérez, 2002).

Likewise, there are some good examples of modern nursing homes that have respite care programmes (SEGG, 1995) as well as home care programmes (SEEG, 1997).

The two main associations of Alzheimer patients' families carry out an important work of social concern and mutual support, and have an increasing impact on society.

Several universities offer postgraduate courses in gerontology. The Autonomous University of Barcelona is the only one carrying out master and postgraduate courses in psychogeriatrics in Spain, and is currently holding its seventh course (Sánchez-Pérez, 2003).

Autonomous governments – first in Catalonia and then in Galicia, Cantabria and Asturias – have created psychogeriatrics advisory committees assigned to reach a consensus philosophy for the coordination of resources as well as for the development of operating protocols and therapeutic strategies for dementia patients (Servei Català de la Salut, 1988; Psycho-geriatrics Advisory Committee, 1999).

Deficiencies

But there are important deficiencies which must be overcome, among which the following ones must be stressed:

- There is still scarce coordination between primary health care and specialized care and between the three mainly involved medical specialties (psychiatry, neurology and geriatrics) and health care services as a whole and social services.
- Old people's homes are not always officially approved from a professional point of view. There is shortage of basic resources such as posts in residences, day hospitals and home care. There is also shortage of specialized centres having specific programmes for dementia care which carry out not only the diagnostic but also continuous assistance to dementia patients, consistently with WPA and WHO recommendations (WHO, 1997).
- Training on geriatrics and psychogeriatrics is not consolidated enough in the pregraduate courses of most medicine faculties around the country. Many professionals, especially in the fields of primary health care and community social services, lack training programmes in those areas (Mateos, 2000).
- Relatives' critical situation has not been appropriately recognized by society and they still suffer from important legal loopholes about their working status or the economic impact of the illness (Martín Carrasco et al, 2002).

This unsatisfactory situation led the Spanish Parliament in 1997 to ask the Government for the development of a National Plan on Alzheimer's disease, an initiative which has not yet been fixed.

References

Comisión Asesora en materia de Psicoxeriatria [Psychogeriatrics Advisory Committee]. *Plan Galego de atención ó enfermo de Alzheimer e outras demencias [Galician plan for the assistance to those patients suffering from Alzheimer and other types of dementia].* Santiago de Compostela: Xunta de Galicia; 1999.

Del Barrio JL, de Pedro-Cuesta J, Boix R, et al. Dementia, stroke and Parkinson's disease in Spanish populations: a review of door-to-door prevalence surveys. *Neuroepidemiology* 2005; 24(4): 179–188.

Martín-Carrasco M, Abad R, Nadal S. Instituciones intermedias en el tratamiento de las demencias y otros trastornos psiquiátricos en la vejez: El Centro de Día Psicogeriátrico [Intermediate institutions for the treatment of dementia and other psychiatric disorders in old age: The Psychogeriatric Day Hospital]. *Revista Española de Geriatria y Gerontologia* 1991; 26: 39–45.

Martín-Carrasco M, Salvadó I, Nadal S, et al. Adaptación para nuestro medio de la Escala de Sobrecarga del Cuidador (caregiver burden interview) de Zarit [Adaptation to our environment of Zarít's caregiver burden interview]. *Revista de Gerontologia* 1996; 6: 338–46.

Martin Carrasco M, Ballesteros RJ, Ibarra GN, et al. Alzheimer's caregiver burden and psychological distress. A neglected association in the assessment of dementias. *Actas Esp Psiquiatr* 2002; 30: 201–6.

Mateos R. Formación específica en Psicogeriatría: necesidades y situación actual [Psychogeriatrics-specific training: current necessities and situation. *Informaciones Psiquiátricas* [Papers on Psychiatry] 2000; 162: 335–40.

Mateos R, Camba MT, Gomez R, Landeira P. La Unidad de Psicogeriatría del Area de Salud. Un dispositivo asistencial novedoso en la red de Salud Mental de Galicia [Psychogeriatry unit of health care area. An innovative assistencial device within the Galician mental-health network]. In: Saúde Mental e Sociedade. Proceedings of II Congreso da Asociación Galega de Saúde Mental, Santiago de Compostela; 1994; 259–75.

Mateos R, Droux A, Páramo M, et al. The Galicia Study of Mental Health of the Elderly II: The use of the Galician DIS. *Int J Meth Psychiatric Res* 2000; 9: 174–82.

Mateos R, Ybarzábal M, García MJ, Amboage MT, Fraguela I. The Spanish CANE. Validation Study and Utility in Epidemiological Surveys. In: Orrell M, Hancock G, eds. *Needs assessment in older people: The Camberwell Assessment of Need for the Elderly.* London: Gaskell; 2004.

Sánchez-Pérez M. Asistencia sociosanitaria en Salud Mental: evaluación de una experiencia [Public health care for mental health: assessment of an experience]. *Informaciones Psiquiátricas* 2002; 167: 95–103. Proceedings of VI Jornadas de Actualización en Psicogeriatría, Martorell; May 2001.

Sánchez-Pérez M. Training in geriatric psychiatry in Spain. *Int Psychogeriatr* 2003; 15: 77.

Servei Català de la Salut. *The Working Groups of the Psychogeriatric-Advisory Council: Cognitive and behavioural disorders in social health care* (bilingual document). Pla de Salut, Quadern No. 10. Barcelona: Bayer; 1988.

Servei Català de la Salut. *L'atenció Sociosanitària a Catalunya. Vida als Anys [Public health care in Cataluña. Life in old age]* 2003: 17–18.

SEGG, Sociedad Española de Geriatría y Gerontología. In: Rodríguez P, ed. *Residencias para Personas Mayores. Manual de Orientación [Old people's homes. Guidance handbook].* Madrid: SG Editores; 1995.

SEGG, Sociedad Española de Geriatría y Gerontología. In: Rodríguez P, Valdivieso C, eds. *El Servicio de Ayuda a Domicilio. Programación del Servicio. Manual de Formación para Auxiliares [Homecare service: its planning. Training handbook for clinical assistants].* Madrid: Fundación Caja Madrid & SEGG; 1997.

Sociedade Galega de Xerontoloxía e Xeriatría. *Coordinación de Servicios Socias e Sanitarios: unha necesidade, un reto [Social and health care services coordination: one need, one challenge]*. XVI Congreso. Santiago de Compostela, 5–6 November 2004. Available at URL: http://www.usc.es/congxero.

Subdirección Xeral do Programa de Atención Sociosanitaria. *Plan Estratégico [Public healthcare programme's bureau. Business plan]*. Santiago de Compostela: Xunta de Galicia.

Subdirección Xeral do Programa de Atención Sociosanitaria. *Preguntas arredor do Alzheimer [Questions about Alzheimer]*. Santiago de Compostela: Xunta de Galicia; 2003.

WHO. *Organization of care in psychiatry of the elderly: a technical consensus statement.* (Doc:WHO/MSA/MNH/MND/97.3). 1997 Geneva: World Health Organization. (Spanish translation: OMS y WPA. Declaraciones de Consenso de la OMS y WPA sobre Psiquiatría Geriátrica (Declaraciones de Lausanne). *Revista de Psicogeriatría* 2002; 2: 6–21.

chapter 5

The practice of dementia care: France

Philippe H Robert and Patrice Brocker

Alzheimer's disease (AD) and other related dementias are characterized by neuropsychological and neurological deficits associated with behaviour problems. Symptomatic treatments are most efficient in the early stages of disease. A prompt diagnosis and early initiation of treatment are crucial for optimal results. However, AD has often been underrecognized and therefore undertreated in the primary care setting in France. Behavioural disturbances are also important manifestations, because they are associated with caregiver distress, thus increasing the likelihood of institutionalization, and may be associated with more rapid cognitive decline.

This chapter aims to briefly describe and comment on the present state of diagnosis and treatment of dementia within the French National Health System.

Dementia has become a major healthcare challenge due to the increasing longevity of the population. Table 5.1 gives information on the percentage of elderly persons in France.

Table 5.1 Percentage of elderly persons compared to the total French population (1999 Census)

	Percent of the total population		
	Total	*Male*	*Female*
65–69 years	4.4	4.2	4.6
70–74 years	4.2	3.8	4.6
75–79 years	3.5	2.9	4.1
80–84 years	2.2	1.7	2.8
85–89 years	1.1	0.7	1.5
90–94 years	0.6	0.3	0.9
> 95 years	0.2	1.1	0.3

Table 5.2 Percentage of persons older than 60 years living in institution (1999 Census)

Age	Percent living in institution
60–64 years	1.7
65–69 years	1.8
70–74 years	2.6
75–79 years	4.7
80–84 years	9.8
85–89 years	19.6
90 years and over	36.0

It is estimated that approximately 400 000 persons older than 75 years suffer from dementia. About 61% of them live at home, but these rates vary according to the age of subjects in proportion to the general population (Table 5.2).

At a national level, dementia care needs to be planned and developed globally as well as with a specific strategy, starting with prevention, including pharmacological, non-pharmacological treatments and social workers' intervention. In October 2001, the French Ministry of Health publicly announced an action programme for elderly persons suffering from AD or related disorders. On April 2002, an official letter was published developing this programme in six main points:

- early identification of the first clinical symptoms
- organizing a diagnostic network
- preserving the dignity of the individual
- supporting and helping the ill and their families
- Improving the quality of accommodation
- promoting medical studies and clinical research.

The following aspects have already been implemented:

- Increasing the number of courses in teaching programmes for the medical students, general practitioners, neurologists, psychiatrists and geriatricians for both a specific task and an overall knowledge acquisition of various disease aspects.
- Development of two types of consultations with different population ranges (Table 5.3). There are approximately 160 proximity memory

Table 5.3 Proximity memory consultations and CMRR (Research and Resource Memory Centres) missions

Roles and objectives of proximity memory consultations:

- Recognizing memory disorders and diagnosis of a dementia syndrome
- Reassuring patients with memory disorders, not presenting a dementia syndrome, and proposing a follow-up
- Identifying complex situations justifying CMRR intervention
- Organizing a personalized individual care programme
- Patient follow-up working beside physicians (general practitioners, neurologists, psychiatrists) and social workers
- Participation in the training of involved professionals

Roles and objectives of CMRR (these centres can only be found in a university hospital setting):

- Be in charge of memory consultations for a specific geographical area
- Be a last resort for difficult cases for memory consultations and difficulties encountered by specialists
- Developing research
- Providing university training
- Heading a regional and/or intraregional plan of action, working along with memory consultations
- Approaching and treating ethical questions

consultations in France today. The second type consists of the development of Research and Resource Memory Centres (CMRR; Figure 5.1), having additional objectives, particularly organizing the network of memory consultations.

- Beginning the development of dementia special care units.
- Development of specific clinical research programmes such as early evaluation of cognitive and behavioural tools: for example, demonstration of the efficiency of information programmes for patients and families must be underlined because this measure has not been frequently adopted in France.

This long-term action programme, which was established between health professionals and patient/family associations, is very constructive since it presents the stages to be followed in a specific order. However, it has not been fully developed due to lack of resources. In fact, in France and perhaps

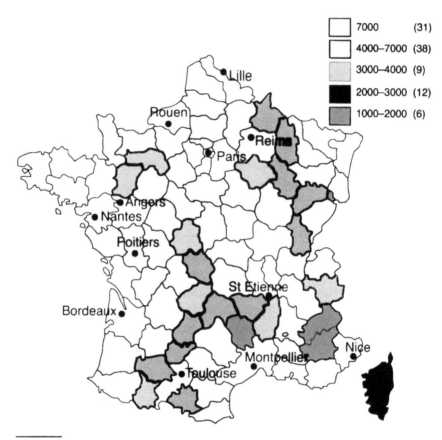

☐	7000	(31)
☐	4000–7000	(38)
☐	3000–4000	(9)
■	2000–3000	(12)
▨	1000–2000	(6)

Figure 5.1 *Total estimation of the number if Alzheimer patients in France (patients older than 75 years – 10 years follow-up of the PAQUID cohort & 1999 INSEE Census) and localization of CMRR (Research and Resources Memory Centre).*

in other countries also, this type of long-term programme is not supported by politicians, who mostly have short-term objectives. However, it is evident that professionals are ready to collaborate in limiting healthcare costs and providing evaluation methods to pursue this type of programme, which is so important in AD and other dementia treatments.

Further reading

Circulaire du 16 avril 2002 relative à la mise en oeuvre du programme d'actions pour les personnes souffrant de la maladie d'Alzheimer ou de maladies apparentées. Circulaire No DHO5/02/DGS/SD5D/DGA5/SD2C/DSS/1A/2002/222 (texte non paru au journal officiel) Grille de classement: SP3 31 – Renvoi à : SP 4 431 ; AS 3 35 ; SS 554
Livre blanc de la Gériatrie Française, Fondation nationale de Gérontologie, Paris, 2004-08-29.
Rapport d'activités des CMRR du Sud de la France, Rapport interne CHO 2004.

chapter 6

Practice of dementia care: Romania

Nicoleta Tătaru

To the social, economic and medical problems that old age brings to society, one may also add a continuing increase in the proportion of old people in the general population.

In our country, around 12–14% of the general population are over 65, compared with Northwest Europe, where 14–16% is over 65. Care of the elderly requires a strong contribution from old age psychiatry, which becomes a basic discipline for all the socio-medical providers and a specialty for physicians and health workers who devote themselves to the care of the elderly (WHO, 1996).

As in all countries in this part of the world, geriatric psychiatry is still not strongly represented: only in some countries is old age psychiatry a recognized specialty. In Romania, old age psychiatry has been a recognized subspeciality of psychiatry since 2001. The number of professionals working in the field is still too low to satisfy the needs of care of the elderly with mental disorders. Scientific organizations such as the Romanian Alzheimer Society (1996) and Romanian Association of Geriatric Psychiatry (1999) try to improve this situation by organizing postgraduate courses for young doctors and psychiatrists to be able to provide much better care of the elderly. There is a postgraduate 1-year course organized in Bucharest for a diploma in psychogeriatrics for psychiatrists, geriatricians and medical residents (Tătaru et al, 2002). Part of the educational programme includes summer courses on geriatric psychiatry, organized in Romania, for psychiatrists of all Eastern European countries.

General practitioners and community nurses should also be involved in the care of the elderly (Jolley and Arie, 1992). In this regard, we have initiated an educational programme which includes courses for family doctors who are involved in the primary care of dementia.

In most developing countries there is no specific organization and most of these countries have no policies and programmes to care for the elderly with mental disorders. This is the reason that the World Health Organization, in collaboration with the World Psychiatric Association and other European and international psychiatry associations, has produced four consensus statements and technical documents to provide a basic guide for all those involved in the field of mental health for older people: i.e. to provide much better care of the elderly (WHO, 1996, 1997, 1998, 2002).

Mental health policy and development

In Romania there are 908 psychiatrists for 21.8 million people (4.16 per 100 000 population) who work in the public health sector; some of us also work in private ambulatory clinics. There are also psychologists and social workers working in the mental health care system.

Mental health services

In Romania most of the psychiatric services are provided by hospitals and outpatient services attached to the Ministry of Health. There are no private psychiatric hospitals.

In the last few years, in most countries the psychiatric services have been more and more orientated towards the community. The special needs of mentally ill people were not always recognized and respected by the generic services.

The Mental Health Law appeared in Romania in August 2002. This is the first step towards the reform of mental health services and care systems for mentally ill patients. In the next section, the forms of specific mental health services existing in Romania are listed, along with the care standards for people with mental disorders (Mental Health Law, 2002).

In Romania only recently we have tried to add to the traditional system of active psychiatric hospital care, the community mental health care services. We started by reducing fundamentally the number of beds, but unfortunately without ensuring care programmes and services in the community for these patients. A great number of long-stay psychiatric wards were transferred to the social services.

Stigma remains, maybe more than in developed countries, a major obstacle to ensuring access to good care for the elderly mentally ill patients.

Stigma against the mentally ill leads to the development of negative attitudes, including that against professionals and services in terms of poor-quality treatment and care and inadequate funding at both national and local levels (WHO, 2002). In most developed and developing countries, a dementia diagnosis may be used to exclude individuals from some forms of care (nursing homes, inpatient units, emergency resuscitation). Action against stigma and discrimination of older people with mental disorders should be a major component of all levels of a health and social care programme.

Inpatient services

People with acute or chronic mental disorders – also with dementia – are treated in:

- psychiatric hospitals for acute mental disorders
- day hospitals
- long-stay accommodation/continuing hospital care
- psychiatric wards in general hospitals (where psychiatric hospitals do not exist)
- the Consultation-Liaison Psychiatry Department in the University General Hospital
- psychiatric departments in geriatric hospitals
- sheltered homes for schizophrenic patients – founded by non-governmental organizations (NGOs).

These services are in most, but not in all, districts.

In developed countries, mentally ill people have begun to be treated in general hospitals in consultation-liaison psychiatry departments as a new way of integrating care for patients with physical/psychiatric co-morbidity (Lipsitt, 2003). In Romania and other developing countries, we have traditionally treated the mentally ill in general or geriatric hospitals, as there was insufficient psychiatric hospitals for financial reasons.

Older people with dementia and no behavioural disorders or significant physical disabilities are also admitted to nursing homes and other social services for long-stay units organized by the state, NGOs or churches. The cooperation between social and medical services is difficult, because they are separate organizations.

Psychogeriatric services will need to retain a proportion of their long-stay beds for rehabilitation and treatment of elderly people with functional illness and demented people with behavioural problems (Wattis, 1994).

Outpatient units

In Romania there are some outpatient services, but only in a few districts, because there is still a severe lack of resources:

* Outpatient or community assessment units – day care centres, some of them especially for dementia (Bucureşti, Brasov, Cluj, Iaşi, Sibiu, Timişoara, Nehoiu, Galati).
* Primary care/residential care.
* Hostel respite care (Oradea).
* Community mental health centre for older people, organized in Oradea in 1996 by the Foundation 'Worrying about grandparents'. The centre is a link between the patients and their families, GPs, and hospitals for acutely or chronically mentally ill people (Tǎtaru 1997, 2003).
* The Memory centre Bucureşti was opened in 2000 within the 'Prof. Dr. Alexandru Obregia' University Hospital in Bucharest by the Romanian Alzheimer Society. The Memory Centre is a modern ambulatory facility for diagnosis and intervention (Tǎtaru, 2003).
* Community and social support services (organized by NGOs and churches in almost all districts).
* Clubs for elderly.

Day programmes contribute to reducing stigma and discrimination against people with mental disorders by reducing isolation and increasing their abilities to face daily life.

Community Care Centre for the Third Age. Organized in Oradea in 1996 by an NGO (the Foundation 'Worrying about grandparents', the first one in Romania), this centre comprises:

* a day care centre that is able to accommodate 40 mobile patients
* a respite hostel with 28 beds that provides temporary care for the elderly with or without family, with or without mental disorders
* residential medical and social care for old people who are unable to leave their homes.

Its main objectives are

* keeping the elderly in their own homes for as long as possible, while at the same time minimizing the cost of caring for them
* granting patients autonomy, so that they can live and die with dignity in their own homes

- restoring patients' self-esteem so that they feel they are an asset to the social group they belong to.

Memory Centre Bucharest. Opened in 2000 inside 'Prof. Dr. Alexandru Obregia' University Hospital in Bucharest, this modern ambulatory facility for diagnosis and intervention has, as its *main goals*, early diagnosis of memory disorders with various aetiologies in adults and the elderly, early diagnosis of dementia and the differential diagnosis of affective disorders in the elderly.

Its other activities include elaboration of therapeutic strategies for cognitive and affective disorders in the elderly, assistance of the families of the sufferers with dementia, promotion of clinical research, professional education for early detection of cognitive disorders, psychoeducation, counselling and psychotherapy.

Its responsibilities include discovering the nature of the problems of the patients and their families, preliminary evaluation of the seriousness of the medical problems of the patient who is asking, preliminary evaluation of the family resources for caring, presenting the services offered by the Memory Centre, referral to specialists and consultations schedule, counselling and education.

Its geographical distribution is 70% in urban areas (Bucureşti, Călăraşi, Olteniţa, Galaţi, Suceava, Iaşi, Focşani, Tîrgu-Mureş, Timişoara, Cîmpina) and 30% in rural areas.

It offers family and patient assistance, by providing information about the community services that the Romanian Alzheimer Society can offer, psychoeducation for patients and their families, counselling for patients and families, supportive psychotherapies (individual, group, support groups), patient's follow-up and periodical evaluation of the stage of the disease.

Residential care

In 2003 a programme for residential care and follow-up of all patients began, including the elderly with mental disorders and dementia (Health Department, 2003). It provided medical treatment and also domiciliary services, including home helps, meals-on-wheels and help for the handicapped and the elderly to remain at home.

There is also some financial support from the Labour Department and Social Protection as compensation for families or caregivers of the chronically ill with handicaps (including those with dementia), who are treated at their home. The Romanian Alzheimer Society organized training courses for nurses to be able to care for demented patients at home.

In our country there does not exist an intermediate stage between home care support and the nursing home, which provides sheltered accommodation for elderly people or those with less severe dementia and behavioural disorders (Lovestone and Gauthier, 2001).

Most of our people with dementia who have a family are treated at home. It is difficult for families to place them in a long-stay unit, not only because of attitudes, shame and feeling of guilt but also because patients who have families or relatives are not admitted to the state nursing homes. The role of NGOs and churches in the system of community care for the elderly is increasing in our country as in many developing countries, but it is still very limited.

Patients with dementia who have behavioural disturbances, psychotic symptoms or agitation require admission to a psychiatric hospital for acute or chronic illness, both the ones who live in nursing homes and the ones who live in their own homes.

The extension of outreach services of nursing homes and residential homes in conjunction with day-care centres, day hospitals and residence care could be a valuable alternative to the high degree of institutionalization of Romanian elderly people with or without mental disorders (Tătaru, 2003; Tudose, 2001).

One of the key theoretical issues for the future development of community services is likely to be the distinction between care and treatment.

Mental health programmes

The national programme for elderly care is a project that for the time being lacks financial support.

The Romanian Alzheimer Society, together with the police in Bucharest, has initiated the project 'Bratara' to prevent the straying of demented patients, wandering behaviour and other behavioural and psychological symptoms of dementia (BPSD).

The aim of any mental health intervention for older adults is to preserve, enhance and give them back personal autonomy and self-esteem if it is possible, permitting them to live and die with dignity in their own homes (Tătaru, 1997).

Conclusions and future needs

- Today in Romania, as regards care of mentally ill people, we are trying to change the focus of mental services from the classical psychiatric hospitals towards community care services.
- The elderly with chronic mental disorders, as well as those with dementia, are taken care of in both psychiatric long-stay hospitals and by social services, which are inadequately trained to care for these patients, being without professional staff qualified in geriatric psychiatry or in social work. Most dementia patients are still in the care of their families, if they have one.
- It is a pity, but we do not have either a clear picture of all services for elderly care or epidemiological studies in this field.
- In spite of the endeavour of professionals specializing in the teaching and educational programme, there are still only a few psychogeriatric services and less special care services for dementia patients.
- The national programme for elderly care is a project that, for the time being, lacks financial support.
- Stigma remains an obstacle to ensuring access to good care for the mentally ill patient. Work against stigmatization should become one of our most important activities.
- We should improve the quality standards concerning the mentally ill elderly and their health by developing a community psychiatric network by geographical catchment area, involving the community, carers and users in the care, and involving the Government and local authorities in mental health care.

In Romania, as in all former communist countries, there are economic problems, and we need national fundraising to support the national psychiatric organizations, services and educational and training programmes.

References

Health Department /318 – Standards for residence care. *Monitorul oficial al Romaniei,* XV, Nr. 255, April 2003.

Jolley D, Arie T. Developments in psychogeriatric services. In: Arie T, ed. *Recent advances in psychogeriatrics,* 2nd Edn. London: Churchill Livingstone; 1992: 117–35.

Lipsitt DR. Psychiatry and the general hospital in an age of uncertainty. *World Psychiatry* 2003; 2: 87–92.

Lovestone S, Gauthier S. *Management of dementia.* London: Martin Dunitz; 2001: 109–19.

Mental Health Law. *Monitorul oficial al Romaniei,* XIV, Nr. 589, 8 August 2002.

Tătaru N. Project for the development of an ambulatory and semi-ambulatory centre for the Third Age. *Dementia and Geriatric Cognitive Disorders* 1997; 8: 128–131.

Tătaru N. Mental health services for the elderly in Central and Eastern European countries. *IPA Regional European Meeting,* April 2003, Geneva, Switzerland.

Tătaru N, Dicker A, Tudose C. The old age psychiatry in Eastern Europe countries. *The 30th Symposium of EAGP,* 14–16 November 2002, Padova, Italy.

Tudose C. *Dementele, o provocare pentru medicul de familie.* Bucuresti: Infomedica; 2001: 98–103.

Wattis JP. The pattern of psychogeriatric services. In: Copeland JRM, Abou-Saleh MT, Blazer DG, eds. *Principles and practice of geriatric psychiatry.* Chichester: John Wiley; 1994: 779–883.

WHO. World Health Organization – Division on Mental Health and Prevention of Substance Abuse. *Psychiatry of the elderly – A consensus statement.* Geneva; 1996.

WHO. World Health Organization – Division on Mental Health and Prevention of Substance Abuse, and World Psychiatric Association. *Program on mental health, organization of care in psychiatry of the elderly – A technical consensus statement.* Geneva; 1997.

WHO. World Health Organization – Department of Mental Health and World Psychiatric Association. *Education in psychiatry of the elderly – A technical consensus statement.* Geneva; 1998.

WHO. World Health Organization – Division on Mental Health and Prevention of Substance Abuse and World Psychiatric Association. *Management of mental and brain disorders – Reducing stigma and discrimination against older people with mental disorders, A technical consensus statement.* Geneva; 2002.

chapter 7

The practice of dementia care: Poland

Andrzej Kiejna, Joanna Rymaszewska and Tomasz Hadryś

In Poland, as in many other European countries, the ageing of the population is posing new challenges for the organization of medical care, including psychiatric care, as well as for scientific research and standardization of treatment philosophy.

The demography of Poland

According to the National Census conducted in 2002, Poland at that time had 38 230 100 inhabitants (51.6% women). The population over age 65 amounted to 4 852 600 persons, which was 12.7% of the whole population (7.9% of them women and 4.8% of them men).

Figure 7.1 presents the age structure of the Polish population as of the 2002 Census. There are two visible demographic peaks: the first is caused by the so-called baby boom after the Second World War, while the second represents a temporary upsurge in the number of births after the political and economic transformation of Poland that began in 1989.

Over the 12 years preceding the 2002 Census, the average life expectancy for both men and women over 45 years of age and over 60 years of age has been prolonged by an average of 2 years (Statistical Bulletin of the Ministry of Health 2002). Although the total size of the Polish population has shown only small fluctuations within a range of 500 000 inhabitants, and is generally constant, the number of older persons grew steadily during this same 12-year period (from 4 903 000 in 1990 to 5 749 000 in 2002) (Statistical Yearbooks 2000 and 2001). The 2002 Census found more than 109 000 people over the age of 90 living in Poland, including 1541 centenarians. Of these, 79% were women, and more than two-thirds of them live in cities (Polish National Census 2002).

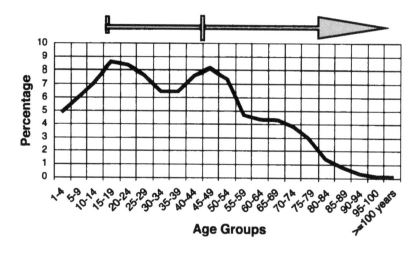

Figure 7.1 *Age structure of the Polish population in 2002.*
(from the Statistical Bulletin of the Ministry of Health 2002)

The epidemiology of dementia in Poland

There have been several studies carried out on the prevalence of dementia in Poland, but they have covered only selected areas (small cities, a borough of a larger city or a rural district). The results have been diverse, due to the use of different methods and criteria for dementia syndromes. The reported rate for dementia has ranged from 5.7% to 10.1%, while for Alzheimer's disease the reported percentages fall between 2.3% and 3.5%. It is currently estimated that there are about 200 000 Polish citizens with Alzheimer's disease. If the 10% figure for the distribution of all dementia syndromes is assumed to be correct, some degree of dementia occurred in 2002 in more than 485 000 people in Poland over the age of 65. Even though all drugs known to be effective can be obtained in Poland, their availability is limited by financial considerations, since they are inadequately covered by the state health insurance programme. Some indication of the level of proper diagnosis, classification and treatment of dementia syndromes is given by the fact that only 10–15% of dementia patients are correctly diagnosed and treated (Bilikiewicz, 2004). The diagnosis of 'psychoorganic syndrome' is still often encountered, though this diagnosis means nothing more than to say, 'Here is an older person with cognitive deficits, as one might expect in someone of this age.'

Table 7.1 Total and first-time patients treated with a diagnosis in the range F00–F09 in outpatient clinics (without reference to age) and hospital care (age 65 and older) per 100 000 inhabitants (from the Polish National Census 2002)

Year	Outpatient clinics		Hospital care (age 65 and older)	
	Total treated	First-time admissions	Total treated	First-time admissions
1997	170.2	40.6	139.4	84.1
1998	207.7	51.8	150.4	91.3
2002	410.2	105.6	223.6	135.6

On the basis of the *Statistical Yearbook* (Institute of Psychiatry and Neurology, 2002), the only statistical data on this subject available in Poland, 14.6% of persons with an ICD-10 diagnosis in the range from F00 to F09 were in outpatient psychiatric care in 2002: 9.4% of these patients were in day-care facilities, while 14.5% were hospitalized, including 10.4% with a diagnosis of psychotic disturbances (F03, F05, F06). A comparison of the rates of occurrence and morbidity for disorders in class F00–F09 during the period 1997–2002 (Table 7.1) shows a significant 38% increase in the number of persons over the age of 65 confined to psychiatric hospitals, and an about 60% increase in the number of those in outpatient psychiatric care (without reference to age).

Given the demographic data and the foregoing morbidity indices, the changes are extremely worrisome, and decisive steps will have to be made to adjust the organization and financing of psychiatric treatment.

Old age psychiatry services

According to official data from the Institute of Psychiatry and Neurology, as of 31 December 2002 there were:

- 4 officially registered day hospitals serving elderly patients, offering an average of 14 places/unit (mean length of stay: 65 days)
- 15 inpatient geriatric psychiatry departments, offering an average of 28 beds/unit (mean length of stay: 41 days)
- 6 closed long-term care geriatric psychiatry wards, offering an average of 39 beds/unit (mean length of stay: 191 days).

There were only 486 beds in geriatric psychiatry inpatient departments, which accounted for 1.6% of all psychiatric beds.

The number of outpatient clinics for elderly psychiatric patients is known to have been rising since 1997; however, no reliable data are available. Various kinds of both public and private part-time old age psychiatry services have been developed, offering day care centers for the elderly. Again, these services are not officially registered by the Institute of Psychiatry and Neurology. Some data are probably collected in National Health Fund registers, but these are not publicly available. Various kinds of information regarding facilities for demented persons are presented on website services for medical professionals (doctors and psychologists). The number of outpatient clinics for old age psychiatry is quite large (96), but they are unevenly distributed over Poland – concentrated mainly in the capital region (26%).

Reform of mental health services in Poland

In the course of the last decade, two important legal enactments pertaining to psychiatry have been issued:

- the Mental Health Act (MHA, 1994).
- the National Health Care Programme (NHCP) for the years 1996–2005, specifying the target network of public mental health services. The NHCP was developed in cooperation with experts from the WHO.

The development of a community-based model of mental health care is an important part of this programme. However, NHCP has no direct references to old age psychiatry. It is stressed that geriatric inpatient psychiatry wards should be established.

Reform of social insurance

The reform of the public health insurance system in Poland initiated in 1999 changed the model of financing healthcare services, making it independent of the state budget, and creating 17 regional health insurance agencies. As a consequence of these reforms, the accessibility of mental health services worsened significantly, while the number of hospitalizations and the rate of bed use rose. Due to the inadequacies of the system, the National Health Fund was introduced in 2003, replacing the previous system. The health insurance premium was raised from 7.5% to 7.75%, which is 3.9% of the GDP (gross domestic product). Unfortunately, this reform has so far had no positive impact on psychiatric health care for the elderly in Poland.

Quality assurance

The Institute of Psychiatry and Neurology in Warsaw is the main unit responsible for:

- monitoring the realization of the Mental Health Act and the NHCP in Poland
- evaluating the functioning of mental health services in Poland
- gathering and publishing all statistical data describing mental and neuro-logical disorders in Poland (*Statistical Yearbooks*).

Research and science

The Institute of Psychiatry and Neurology in Warsaw was established in 1951, and since then has served as a scientific and organizational unit monitoring mental health care in Poland. It is also a WHO collaborative centre. There are several leading university-based old age psychiatry centres in Poland working in different fields of geriatric psychiatry (from genetics, aetiology and pharmacotherapy to psychopathology and diagnostics). These include:

1 the Institute of Pharmacology at the Polish Academy of Sciences in Cracow
2 the Institute of Immunology and Experimental Therapy at the Polish Academy of Sciences in Wroclaw
3 the Department of Degenerative Disorders at the Central Clinical Hospital of the Ministry of Internal Affairs in Warsaw
4 the Department of Neurology of the Jagiellonian University's Collegium Medicum in Cracow
5 the Department of Developmental Psychiatry and Old Age Psychoses at the Medical University of Gdansk
6 the Department of Old Age Neurology at the Silesian Medical University in Katowice
7 the Department of Old Age Psychiatry and Psychoses at the Medical University of Lodz
8 the Psychogeriatric Ward, Institute of Psychiatry and Neurology in Warsaw
9 the Research Unit of Old Age Psychiatry Unit in the Department of Psychiatry at the Wroclaw Medical University.

In addition to the active research centres, there are a number of organizations involved with the issues of mental health in later life. These include:

- scientific associations (the Old Age Psychiatry and Alzheimer's Disease Section of the Polish Psychiatric Association, the Alzheimer's Disease Section of the Polish Neurological Association and, finally, the newly founded Polish Association of Geriatric Psychiatry)
- organizations for families and patients (the Polish Alzheimer Foundation, the Polish Aid Society for Persons with Alzheimer's Disease, etc.).

Their role and involvement is both extremely important and very obvious. Scientific conferences and educational workshops are organized each year. In addition to information bulletins, there is now a scientific periodical, the *Polish Journal of Geriatric Psychiatry*.

Despite the progress, however, the lack of coordination or an integrated approach to research and administration in the field of old age psychiatry is still evident in Poland. There is a strong need for improvement in this respect. In view of the data and the demographic forecasts, there will soon be a major increase in the number of cases of age-related illnesses. Thus, action plans should take into account the working assumptions of the European Dementia Care Standard.

References

Bilikiewicz A. Current situation of geriatric psychiatry in Poland. *Psychogeriatr Pol* 2004; **1**: 1–6.

Statistical Yearbooks. Warsaw: Institute of Psychiatry and Neurology; 1997–2002.

Kiejna A, Rymaszewska J, eds. *Epidemiology of psychiatric disorders*. Kraków: Biblioteka Psychiatrii Polskiej; 2003..

Kiejna A, Rymaszewska J, Hadryś T. Organization of mental health care for the elderly in Poland. *Eur Psychiatry* 2004; **19**: 74.

Polish National Census. Results of 2002 National Census published on the website of Polish Official Statistics: http://www.stat.gov.pl/english/index.htm

Statistical Bulletin of the Ministry of Health. Warsaw; 2002

chapter 8

The practice of dementia care: Greece

Magda Tsolaki

Greece, as all Western countries is experiencing a demographically driven increase in the size and proportion of its elderly population. It is well known that such demographic changes are dramatically increasing the importance of dementia disorders, among them the most frequent is Alzheimer's disease (AD). Indeed, the prevalence of AD is also age-related in Greece (Tsolaki et al, 1999a), as in other countries (Ritchie and Kildea, 1995).

Currently, 14 memory clinics cover the densely populated nation of Greece. In Athens, there are two memory outpatients clinics in the university neurological department and one in the university psychiatric department; two other outpatients clinics are in general hospitals and one in a private centre. In Pireus, there is one clinic that works in the neurology department and one in the psychiatry department. In Thessaloniki, there are seven outpatients clinics (three in university neurological departments, one in the psychogeriatric department, two in the neurological departments in general hospitals and one in the geriatrician department). In Chania, there is one clinic that works in a psychiatry department. In Patras and Ioannina, there is one clinic in the neurological department. These centres offer not only diagnostic and pharmaceutical help to patients living in those cities but also to patients living in rural areas, who have to travel more than 50 or 100 km to reach such a centre.

The first Thessaloniki Memory Clinic is an outpatient facility of the 3rd University Department of Neurology (Head: Aristides Kazis). Since opening in 1990, over 2000 patients have been referred by physicians with different specialties from Larissa and Volos (Central Greece) to Alexandroupolis (Eastern Greece).

Assessment and diagnosis

It is well known all around the world that the earlier the diagnosis of dementia can be made, the better and more effectively comprehensive treatment can begin. Our centre advocates a simple step-by-step approach for detection of dementia and differential diagnosis.

First, a neuropsychologist or a neuropsychiatrist screens patients for possible dementia or depression by taking a detailed medical history (including information of spouses/relatives) by performing a physical, psychiatric and neurological examination (neurologist) and by examining each patient's cognitive and affective function using standardized screening such as the mini mental state examination or MMSE (Fountoulakis et al, 1994) and Geriatric Depression Scale (Fountoulakis et al, 1999). If the patient has only mild cognitive problems, we follow a multidimensional diagnostic procedure. When the diagnosis of mild cognitive impairment or dementia is certain, neuroradiologists perform magnetic resonance imaging (MRI) and routine blood examinations. During the second visit, we use a long neuropsychological examination that gives us the opportunity for the differential diagnosis of the dementia. We use Cambridge cognitive examination of the elderly or CAMCOG (Tsolaki et al, 1996), functional cognitive assessment scale or FUCAS (Kounti et al, 1999), Cornell and Hamilton Scale for Depression Neuropsychiatric Inventory, UPDRS for the extrapyramidal symptoms and signs (Fahn and Elton, 1987). If the patient fulfils the criteria for inclusion in different international studies, then we use the Alzheimer's disease assessment scale (ADAS) (Tsolaki et al, 1997) or other required scales. We do lumbar puncture to measure tau protein and beta amyloid levels. We also use nootropics or ginkgo biloba for treatment and neurorehabilitation programmes. Last year we started the DESCRIPA study, a study which is funded by the European Commission. If the patient has dementia, we start cholinesterase inhibitors, art therapy, reminiscence and supporting groups.

Management of dementia

If the patient has dementia, we start with cholinesterase inhibitors, art therapy, exercise programs, reminiscence and supporting groups. If the patient has mild or very mild dementia or mild cognitive impairment we suggest neurorehabilitation programs such as exercises of memory, attention and language. We also use nootropics or ginko biloba for treatment and rehabilitation programs for patients with mild cognitive impairment.

In addition to the efforts of early detection of dementia, our memory clinic in Thessaloniki is in close collaboration with Greek Alzheimer's Disease and Related Disorders Association (GADRDA) and offers a comprehensive management programme. The memory clinic provides the clinical setting for medical and psychological services as well as the medication therapy. Until September 1996 we used only nootropics and neuroleptics with antidepressants for behavioural and psychological symptoms of dementia, but when tacrine became available in the Greek market, we started therapy with tacrine, and, then, since February 1998 with donepezil, March 1999 with rivastigmine, September 2001 with galantamine and February 2003 with memantine. We now have great experience with these drugs in our centre.

The Greek Alzheimer's Disease and Related Disorders Association is an organizing and professional counselling centre with a staff of thirteen health professionals. It offers supporting groups; seminars for caregivers and professionals; memory, language and attention exercises for patients in early-stage disease; music therapy for all-stages patients; speech therapy; and physiotherapy in 3-day centres provided to GADRDA by the church.

All these programmes are free for all patients and caregivers. GADRDA translated and published the *Alzheimer's Europe Manual for Caregivers* and the *Children's Brochure* which all families who are members of this Association can read. It publishes a Newsletter, entitled *Communication*, every 3 months. It has organized three National Conferences about Alzheimer disease and related disorders and one in collaboration with Alzheimer Europe, and proceedings of all these conferences are available in Greek. Recently, in January 2005, we published a book with 693 pages about dementia. Families are required to contribute only a small fee of 30 euros every year and can have all the above material and services free.

The most favourable programme of GADRDA is our educational programme every Tuesday morning. The Charissio for Old People Home of Thessaloniki Church offers a Hall for this programme. Over 60 people – patients, caregivers or professionals – attend this programme every week. The Municipality of Thessaloniki gave us the opportunity to have also a very good hall in the centre of our city, at the Central Library, where we do another educational program for 100 health professionals every Friday afternoon.

Patients in the early stage of dementia can participate in the cognitive neurorehabilitation programme, which aims at the intense stimulation of the brain through the enhancement of attentional processes (selective, sustained and divided) and parameters of executive function. A scientific team (neurologist, psychologists, radiologist and psychiatrist) and the caregivers work with the patient for 5 months. The patients are in preclinical or early stage of Alzheimer's disease: they have insight, and they are free from behavioural symptoms.

They come to our day centre, once a week for 2 hours, where they have to do paper and pencil visual tasks, under the guidance of psychologists. As soon as they complete the task, they have to find their faults alone or with the help of the psychologist. When they leave the day centre, they take with them the task of the week as homework. They have to deal with it for half an hour every day for the rest of the week, under the surveillance of the trained caregiver. Preliminary results show an impressive improvement in cognitive flexibility, which is transferred to real-life daily activities (Tsantali et al, 2003).

There is also a programme of cognitive neuropsychological rehabilitation of memory and language disorders in patients with primary Alzheimer's disease which intends to ameliorate the quality of life of patients and their caregivers. The steps of this programme are:

1. Clinical and neuropsychological assessment, using a cognitive and language battery, for people who complain of memory problems.
2. A 1-hour individual programme three times per week for learning memory strategies, in order to maintain patients' intact information.
3. Reorganization of the semantic memory or relearning rules of reorganization.
4. Home exercises in order to become familiar with the matrix of the seasons and to go deeper into it.

Our main aim is to transfer the training abilities and knowledge to everyday life and to keep the patient in self-service conditions at home.

Patients in the moderate stage of dementia can take part in art therapy, where they are encouraged to express feelings and creativity through painting. This programme is based on scientific research which believes in the existence of strong emotions, even in advanced stages of dementia. The art becomes a symbolic language of their inner emotions and helps them bridge the internal with the external reality. We tend to move patients in certain directions –

- they become more aware of all of their senses

- they learn to accept responsibility for what they do, including accepting the consequences of their actions
- they move from outside support towards increasing internal support
- they are able to ask for and get help from others
- they move towards increased awareness of themselves
- they gradually assume ownership of their experience
- their creativity and self-esteem are regenerated
- they develop skills and acquire values that will allow them to satisfy their needs without violating the rights of others.

Patients can also participate in the reminiscence programme. Reminiscence therapy is a group intervention that involves people with moderate and severe dementia. The reminiscence therapy aims at the improvement of their social life, the emotional and the interpersonal relationship between patients and their caregivers. The aim of the therapy is achieved through recalling pleasant memories, giving sensual stimuli that accompany the memories, discussing present events, the dynamic of the group and the interaction between the people of the group. The expected result of the therapy is to improve self-esteem and self-respect and to gain emotional balance. At the same time, it is attempting to improve the education of the caregivers in communicational skills, in behavioural skills, to improve their ability to work with the patient and to enhance their own quality of life. We try through multisensory stimulation to help them remember pleasant moments from their past and to regain self-respect.

There is also a gymnastic group for patients and caregivers, three times a week. A physiotherapy programme is provided for our patients, once a week.

Patients and caregivers have the opportunity, once a month, to meet together with other patients and caregivers at the 'Alzheimer Café', where they find a way for social communication and education about the disease. Modelled on a network of such cafés pioneered in the Netherlands, the Alzheimer Café in Greece is designed to provide a monthly hosting time and space for people with dementia and/of their family and friends, to be together in a safe, welcoming environment, in the company of other carers, volunteers and health professionals, for the purposes of emotional support, education and social interaction. A typical evening at the café starts with an informal chat. A presentation by a professional then follows, combined with a relaxed interview with a willing family member who has hands-on, real experience of the subject being discussed. The evening continues with further social interaction and refreshments and the opportunity to informally chat to the guest speakers. The evening is enhanced further by live music or other entertainment.

Caregivers can participate in counselling programmes, for individual psychotherapy or support groups, in order to improve their emotional health, and their communication with the patient. All programmes are carried out by trained cognitive and clinical psychologists.

We are now ready to start a day centre in collaboration with the Municipality of Thessaloniki. We are also preparing, in collaboration with the Ministry of Health, an Alzheimer centre with three units, one day centre, one mobile unit and a nursing home, where patients in the late stages of disease will have the care they need.

Research activities

Research activities are an integral part of the Thessaloniki and Athens University memory clinics. The focus of studies range from validation of useful scales (MMSE, GDS, ADAS, BNS Zarit, FRSSD etc) and development of new assessment instruments (for example FUCAS) to examination of cerebrospinal fluid (CSF) for determination of beta-amyloid and tau protein levels and MRI. Our centre is a member of the European Alzheimer Disease Consortium and takes part in the ICTUS and DESCRIPA studies. Unfortunately, as yet, we have no facilities for cliniconeuropathological correlations and genetics. We are ready to organize a brain bank and are in collaboration with the University of Zurich and Department of Biology of Aristotle Univeristy of Thessaloniki for genetics. We try to have some collaboration with the Institute of Cyprus and we dream also of an Alzheimer's Institute in Greece, where we can work on all dimensions of dementia.

Another area of considerable interest is CSF tau protein levels in patients with dementia and demented patients under medication (Tsolaki et al, 1999b).

An exercise programme in patients with Alzheimer's disease is a project supported by the European Commission (Grant No. SOC 97 201421 05F03) (Mouzakuidis et al, 1999). We now run a programme of exercises three times a week.

During the last 2 years, our memory clinic has also offered about 100 patients the opportunity to participate in trials examining new pharmacotherapeutic interventions such as cholinesterase inhibitors. We now participate in the ICTUS study, which is funded by the European Commission.

Education and Training

Every year, since 1995, about 120 students of the department of psychology have attended a course on neuropsychological assessment of elderly people. Students of the medical school have also had the opportunity to attend seminars and conferences on dementia (excluding a 2-hour lesson on dementia and a 2-hour examination of patients with dementia of different types). In May 2004, we organized a full day programme on Alzheimer's disease, which about 600 students attended.

Almost every month, members of our memory clinic, in collaboration with members of other memory clinics, visit one city – Kalamata, Volos, Chania, Alexandroupolis, Athens or Xanthi – in our country where there are no facilities for patients with dementia and educate physicians and other professionals about dementia. There are now branches of the Greek Alzheimer's Disease and Related Disorders Association in 16 other cities and some other cities are almost ready to start their activities.

Summary

The specific aims of our memory clinic are:

1. The diagnosis of dementia.
2. The management of dementia, pharmaceutical and non-pharmaceutical.
3. The collaboration, with the Greek Alzheimer's Disease and Related Disorders Association, to providing advice to patients, caregivers and health professionals.
4. The collaboration, with the Greek Alzheimer's Disease and Related Disorders Association, the European Commission, the Ministry of Health and the Ministry of Education, to create community and social services.
5. Research on epidemiological aspects of AD in Greece: prevalence, incidence, outcome and institutionalization.
6. Train and teach healthcare professionals and organize awareness campaigns to help promote the public's awareness of dementia and the impact of the disease on society.

References

Fahn S, Elton RL, and members of the UPDRS Development Committee. In: Fahn S, Marsden CD, Calne DB, Goldstein M, (eds). *Recent developments in Parkinson's disease*. Florham Park, NJ: Macillian Healthcare Information; 1987: 153.

Fountoulakis KN, Tsolaki M, Chantzi H, Kazis A. Mini Mental State Examination (MMSE). A validation study in demented patients from the elderly Greek population. *Egephalos* [Greek Journal] 1994; 31: 93–102.

Fountoulakis KN, Tsolaki M, Iacovides A, et al. The validation of the short form of the Geriatric Depression Scale (GDS) in Greece. *Aging Clin Exper Res* 1999; 11: 367–72.

Kounti F, Tsolaki M, Kazis A, Evklides A. FUCAS – Functional-Cognitive Assessment Scale: a new scale to predict early dementia. A meeting of minds. *Care and Science in Dementia, 9th Alzheimer Europe Meeting, 20th Anniversary Conference*, Alzheimer's Disease Society, London, 30 June to 2 July, 1999.

Mouzakuidis C, Tsolaki M, Theodorakis J, Efremidou E, Kampitsis C. Exercise program in patients with Alzheimer's disease. *Alzheimer's Dis Rel Disord* 1999; 90: 781–5.

Ritchie K, Kildea D. Is senile dementia 'age-related' or 'ageing related' – evidence from meta-analysis of dementia prevalence in the oldest old. *Lancet* 1995; 346: 931–4.

Tsantali E, Tsolaki M, Efklides A, Kiosseoglou G. Memory and language exercises and their effects in the first stages of the probable Alzheimer's disease. *First Conference of Brain Aging*, 6–8 October, 2003: 43.

Tsolaki M, Fountoulakis KN, Chantzi H, Kazis A. The Cambridge Cognitive Examination for the elderly (CAMCOG). A validation study in demented patients from the elderly Greek population. *Egephalos* [Greek journal] 1996; 33: 57–75.

Tsolaki M, Fountoulakis KN, Nakopoulou E, Kazis A. Alzheimer's disease Assessment Scale: The validation of the scale in Greece in early demented patients and normal subjects. *Dementia Geriatr Cognitive Disord* 1997; 8: 273–80.

Tsolaki M, Fountoulakis C, Pavlopoulos I, Chatzi E, Kazis A. Prevalence and incidence of Alzheimer's disease and other dementing disorders in Pylea, Greece. *Am J Alzheimer's Dis* 1999a; 14: 138–48.

Tsolaki M, Sakka P, Chatzizisi O, et al. CSF tau protein levels before and after tacrine therapy in patients with dementia of Alzheimer's type. *Alzheimer's Dis Rel Disord* 1999b; 85: 741–5.

chapter 9

The practice of dementia care: Switzerland

Carlos Augusto de Mendonça Lima

Demography and Alzheimer's disease in Switzerland

As with other developed countries, the Swiss population is characterized by a low fertility rate and a high life expectancy. These two factors explain why this country has now an important number of old people: people over 65 years old (about 1 115 000) represented more than 15.5% of all the population in 2000. This number is expected to grow significantly in the following years: until 2035, the number of old people will grow by 56–73%. By this same year, 25% of the Swiss population will be aged over 65 years old. The number of people over 80 years old is also quite important: 4.2% of the total population in 2000, which is expected to reach more than 8% of the total population in 2060 (Office Fédéral de la Statistique website).

The distribution of this old population is quite different among the cantons. Basel city has 20.09% of its population over 65 years old, whereas the canton of Zoug has only 10.95%. The high concentration of old people in urban areas is also another characteristic of the ageing population in the country (d'Epinay et al, 1998). In 2000, 43.8% of women and 15.5% of men over 65 years old were living alone (Office Fédéral de la Statistique website).

These factors have several consequences for the country (Office Fédéral de la Statistique website):

- the number of people living with a retirement pension is increasing more quickly than the number of people in the labour market
- with the decrease in the number of young people, there is a high risk of a significant lack of employees
- the increase in the number of old people contributes to the increase in the cost of the health system

- the increase in the number of old people influences the results of elections in the country (by 2010, 50% of electors in the country will be aged over 50 years old).

At the moment, there are about 89 000 persons in Switzerland with a dementia. Each year, there are 21 000 new cases. By 2020, it is expected that the number of cases will grow to 113 000 (25% more than in 2004). A total of 28 000 patients with dementia are not recognized and cared for; 32 000 patients don't have the diagnosis, despite the fact that their general practitioner suspects the disease. This means that 60 000 patients and their respective caregivers live with the symptoms and consequences of the dementia but they don't know the cause of the problem. Only 25% of patients receive a specific drug for Alzheimer's disease and only 14% benefits from a non-pharmaceutical therapy. Of those 53 400 patients living at home, 23 000 patients need sporadic help, 25 100 need everyday support, and 5300 are completely dependent; 28 000 patients living at home don't receive any professional support, whereas 25 400 patients receive some help from the community health care facility but only 9800 patients are recognized as suffering with a dementia. In Switzerland, there is the possibility of receiving care at a day centre, 1000 patients per day (when there are 53 400 living at home); 35 600 patients with dementia live in a nursing home, where only 6100 patients are recognized as having a dementia (Association Alzheimer Suisse, 2004).

Mental health policy and mental health programmes

Considering the important gap between the healthcare needs of the population with Alzheimer's disease and the offer of care for that population, Stuckelberger and Hopflinger (2000) the authors of the National Research Programme 32, the most important research ever made in the country concerning old people, recommended:

- offering support and counselling sections with experts to relatives in order to calm their fears about the disease and to plan care duties in an adequate way
- creating a wide range of services for the relief of the relatives
- increasing the number of special places for patients with dementia in day centres

- offering a care's benefit or tax reduction for whoever regularly cares for an elderly sick or disabled person at home.

These recommendations are just a small part of an ideal strategy to improve the offer and the quality of care for people with Alzheimer's disease. Three other components should be considered in a global strategy:

- the development of a national policy for mental health
- the creation of a specific health programme for those affected by Alzheimer's disease
- the development of standards of care.

According to WHO:

'A mental health policy describes the values, objectives and strategies of the governments to reduce the mental health burden and to improve mental health. They describe a vision that helps to establish a blueprint for the prevention and treatment of mental illness, the rehabilitation of people with mental disorders, and the promotion of mental health in the community. Policies specify the <u>standards</u> that need to be applied across all programmes and services, linking them all with a common vision, objectives and purpose. Without this overall coordination, programmes and services are likely to be inefficient and fragmented' (WHO, 2001a).

Besides the importance of a mental health policy, such a document was not available in 32.73% of the countries of the WHO Region Europe in 2001 (WHO, 2001b): Switzerland was one of them. One of the reasons to explain the absence of this document is the fact that Switzerland is a confederation with a degree of autonomy at the canton level. Each canton has the possibility of defining its priorities in terms of healthcare needs and organizing the resources and services to satisfy the healthcare needs of its population. Since the publication of the WHO document (WHO, 2001b), an important effort has been made in the country to produce this policy (Politique Nationale Suisse de la Santé, 2000). All sectors concerned by mental health problems are being consulted in an important effort to create a policy that is as representative of the population needs as possible.

WHO has also defined a mental health programme as

An organized aggregate of activities directed towards the attainment of specified objectives and targets, at national level, consistent with those of the national health policy and strategy. It should set out clearly the requirements in terms of health workers, physical facilities, technology, equipment and supplies, information and intercommunication, the methods of monitoring and evaluation, the timetable of activities, and the ways of ensuring correlation between its various elements and related programmes (WHO, 1994).

According to this definition we can imagine that, after creating a mental health policy, Swiss health authorities could decide to develop some specific programmes and actions to prevent some disorders and to treat, care and rehabilitate people affected by these disorders. It is too early to say now if national programmes will be launched inspired by the national mental health policy, if each canton will be free to define the programmes according to their needs or even if authorities at the national or canton level will adopt some programmes.

Standards in mental health care

If a mental health policy should define standards, it is necessary to know what standards are and why they are useful.

It is a goal of all governments to offer the best mental health care for their respective population but also to control the increasing costs that this health care represents. They need to know if services are doing what they should be doing and doing it in an acceptable way. Mental health care is becoming progressively more expensive, especially in the case of Alzheimer's disease. The criteria for the diagnosis have become more and more precise: a high technology in terms of imaging, for example, was created, the organization of professionals in specific services was proposed to identify the disease as early as possible (such as memory clinics) to care for the affected persons and support their caregivers, new specific drugs were produced and an enormous effort in terms of research have consumed a significant part of the limited resources for research in mental health in these last 15 years.

As these resources are limited, we must now look more carefully at the community needs for services and set priorities based on those needs. Otherwise, it is a high priority to reduce the number of patients with Alzheimer's disease that are excluded from the care system just because they are not properly identified: these are the roles of a mental health policy and a mental health programme. But at the same time, we must do better with what we have, which means we must organize and manage more carefully and continually evaluate how we are doing. For that, we need standards against which to measure our performance. Standards assist us to define the meaning of quality as it relates to healthcare delivery and to help professionals to justify the effectiveness and efficiency of what they do (Heidemann, 1993).

According to Donabedian (1982), standards are professionally developed expressions of the range of acceptable variations from a norm or criterion. For Bertolote (1993), standards define the boundary between acceptable and unacceptable care and place some aspects of guidelines in specific context. They are usually established by authorities through a process of adapting guidelines to national priorities. This process takes into account local technical, economic, social, cultural and political conditions.

Requirements which must be in place prior to developing standards are the following:

- The *belief* that standards are desirable and useful.
- The *will* and knowledge to develop standards.
- The *resources* for developing the standards and subsequently implementing and maintaining them.
- The ability to *promote* the standards once they are established and to educate potential users in how to meet them.
- The *recognition* that standards must be 'tailor-made' if they are to serve well the specific constituency for which they are intended.
- Someone must take responsibility for the development of standards. This might be government agencies or groups of healthcare providers or healthcare facilities, or a combination of those groups.

For Donabedian (1982), there are different types of standards. *Categorical* or *monotonic* standards are used for elements of which 'the more we have the better or the less we have the better'. By contrast, *inflected* standards are useful for those phenomena which have their most desirable value at some maximum or minimum point, on either side of which the valuation placed upon them is less. But we also can define the types of standards by what they are directed towards: structure (things we use), process (what we do) or outcome (the results of what we do with the things we have) (Bertolote, 1993). The majority of standards focus on:

- The organization and management of healthcare and the resulting care: they tend to address the ability of the healthcare facility to deliver quality care or service.

- Clinical practice: they describe the precise nature of what should be delivered. They are used to guide those professionals in the ideal ways to carry out their patient care responsibilities given certain sets of circumstances and patient diagnoses.

Standards are first and foremost based on some form of collective judgement settled in a consensus and consultation. The precise consultation procedures and methods to arrive at consensus can vary, and appropriate procedures and methods should be clearly defined. The best and most effective standards are those which have involved peer judgements by people who set standards for themselves and very often reflect the authors' values (Heidemann, 1993).

Governments can also play an important role in the process of setting standards. As they have the responsibility to look after the collective public good, they may quite legitimately play a role in determining what national standards for health care might be in terms of the quantity of health care to be made available, the organization of services, equity of what care is available and accessibility to the care of all members of the population, etc. Governments have an important role to play not only in establishing the standards for the delivery of health care but also the contribution from the public tax purse to the financial support of the standards which have been established for health care (Heidemann, 1993).

Standards are dynamic in nature and should change to reflect the changes in the collective judgement about their object or values placed on it. Within health care, standards change constantly to reflect the changing nature of health care itself, as reflected in technology, professional practice, economic conditions, consumer expectation, treatment modalities and life expectancies (Heidemann, 1993). Thus, after setting standards, it is necessary to decide how they will be evaluated as regards their relevance and, if they are no longer satisfactory, how they should be revised (Heidemann, 1993).

Diagnoses and care of Alzheimer's disease: A consensus for Switzerland

Taking into account the important impact that Alzheimer's disease has on the Swiss population, the high number of patients underdiagnosed and undertreated and the existence of several associations, institutions and professionals dedicated to this disease, it became necessary to create an institution that was able to put all these efforts together in an interdisciplinary way. So, in 1998 the Swiss Forum Alzheimer was created, whose goals are to list and discuss present problems related to the disease, to find strategies to solve them and to assure the promotion of necessary research (Alzheimer Forum Schweiz, website).

There are five commissions working in the different fields of epidemiology, diagnoses and therapy, social aspects, health economy and public relationship/education on the disease. A first document was created and published as result of a consensus meeting held at Interlaken on 17–18 October 1998 which produced a statement called *Diagnoses and care of Alzheimer's disease: A consensus for Switzerland* (Alzheimer Forum Schweiz, 1999).

This document, written by 34 authorities, concerned the research and care of Alzheimer's disease around the country. It considered a number of different topics, including:

1. *Diagnoses of Alzheimer's disease*
   - Guidelines for the initial assessment
   - Guidelines for the screening of dementia
   - Guidelines to define the intensity of the dementia
   - Interdisciplinary assessment

2. *Care of Alzheimer's disease*
   - The treatment made by the general practionner
   - Specific therapeutic measures

In Switzerland this statement has become the best reference on the matter, and corresponds to what was defined before as a clinical standard. The purpose was not to control the cost of care but to increase the quality of diagnoses and treatment, offering useful tools to those concerned.

Unfortunately, there was no procedure defined to measure the use of these guidelines and their impact on the improvement of the quality of diagnoses and care of Alzheimer's disease. We regret that there is no provision to update the document to the most recent advances of clinical and research findings.

Conclusions

Donabedian (1995) said that there is much we do not know about standards and much we have to learn, but our limited knowledge base should not prevent our exploration of the development and use of standards if their use will potentially result in an improvement in healthcare delivery.

Practice and clinical standards are not without controversy. Some professionals consider them too restrictive and that it is difficult to exercise their best judgement when treating an individual patient. Besides these arguments, they also agree that something less restrictive is still of value to practice.

Step by step, Switzerland is adopting documents which will offer to those affected by Alzheimer's disease the best advice on what is acceptable and what is not for the care of people affected by the disease and its associated cost. It is urgent to increase, in Switzerland, the competence of all professionals to recognize the disease at the first stages and to help them to care for patients and to support their caregivers. The future will show the outcome of these measures.

References

Alzheimer Forum Schweiz. Diagnostik und Therapie der Alzheimer-Krankheit. *Schweizerische Aerztezeitung* 1999; 80: 843–51.

Association Alzheimer Suisse. *Vivre avec la maladie d'Alzheimer en Suisse. Les chiffres-clés 2. La prise en charge actuelle.* Bern: AAS; 2004. http://www.alz.ch/f/html/alzheimer+24.html

Alzheimer Forum Schweiz. http://www.alzheimerforum.ch/f/links/institut.htm

Bertolote JM. Quality assurance in mental health care. In: Sartorius N, de Girolamo G, Andrews G, Allen German G, Eisenberg L, eds. *Treatment of mental disorders: a review of effectiveness.* Washington: WHO and American Psychiatric Press; 1993: 443–61.

d'Epinay Ch L, Brunner M, Albano G. *Atlas Suisse de la population âgée.* Lausanne: Réalités Sociales âge et Société; 1998: 110–13.

Donabedian A. *Explorations in quality assessment and monitoring: Volume II. The criteria and standards of quality.* Ann Arbor, Michigan: Health Administration Press; 1982: 8–9.

Donabedian A. *Explorations in quality assessment and monitoring: Volume III. The methods and findings of quality assessment and monitoring. An illustrated analysis.* Ann Arbor, Michigan: Health Administration Press; 1985: 450.

Heidemann EG. *The contemporary use of standards in health care. WHO/SHS/DHS/93.2.* Geneva: WHO; 1993.

Office Fédéral de la Statistique. Population: Vue d'ensemble – faits, évolutions, interactions. http://www.bfs.admin.ch/bfs/portal/fr/index/infothek/lexikon/bienvenue_login/blank/zugang_lexikon.topic.1.html

Politique Nationale Suisse de la Santé. *Politique nationale suisse pour la santé psychique.* http://www.nationalegesundheit.ch/main/Show$Id=1245.html

Stuckelberger A, Hopflinger F. Ageing in Switzerland at the dawn of the XXIst century. *National Research Program on Ageing (NRP32).* Bern: Swiss National Science Foundation and Gerontological Economic Research Organization; 2000: 37–8.

World Health Organization. *Quality assurance in mental health care. Check-lists & Glossaries, Volume 1.* Geneva: WHO; 1994.

World Health Organization. *Mental health policy project. Policy and service guidance package. Executive summary.* Geneva: WHO; 2001a.

World Health Organization. *Atlas. Mental health resources in the world 2001.* Geneva: WHO; 2001b.

.

chapter 10

The practice of dementia care: Germany

Pasquale Calabrese

Epidemiology and carers' profile

Recent sociodemographic data are based on an actual survey, which was guided by a special task force aimed to evaluate the present situation of elderly people living in Germany as regards age structure, resource allocations and health-related social services, with a special focus on dementia. According to this survey, the diagnostic pathways to identify, treat and allocate patients with dementia are still to be coordinated.

Actual prevalence estimates in Germany indicate a total amount of 1.2 million elderly people suffering from dementia. In most cases, first contact with primary care physicians is only established when dementia-related behavioural disturbances have already caused substantial distress to caregivers. Most of the German elderly with dementia are cared for by younger family members within their homes (60%). There is a clear predominance of spouses (60%) and daughters/sons (30%) caring for demented individuals. The majority of carers are women (nearly 60%); the mean age of carers is about 60 years. In most of the cases, the carers had taken the initiative to have their relative diagnosed. According to a recent comparative evaluation across several European countries, in half of the cases the mean time that elapses between carers realizing that 'something is wrong' and the confirmation of the diagnosis of dementia is longer than 1 year.

Referrals

The first symptoms which draw the attention of the family are loss of memory and psychobehavioural changes. Most of the early dementia cases are seen by general practitioners. However, although general practicioners present a unique setting for identification of high-risk patients, their detection rate varies considerably, since there is no strict application of guidelines although such have been developed by different medical associations. This explains why there is still a significant time-lag until patients are referred to specialized institutions, although referral to psychiatric services in the early stages of dementia is an important step in the process of care. Neurologists and/or psychiatrists in private practice are thus only rarely involved at first contact, and are mostly consulted to exclude treatable and/or reversible causes of dementia in those cases where aggravating conditions are obvious. In these cases patients are mainly referred to hospitals with internal medicine or psychiatric hospitals, depending on symptom preponderance. Although they are well equipped, neurological departments are only a second-line option for referral at the present. The two most relevant and widely used codes are senile and presenile organic psychotic conditions which mainly features senile dementia, simple type and other cerebral degenerations which consists mainly of Alzheimer's disease. The relevant hospital activity diagnostic clinical diagnoses in patients with dementia are senile and presenile organic psychotic conditions and other degenerative and hereditary disorders of the central nervous system.

However, since the lengths of stay in general hospitals have significantly decreased due to budgetary restrictions, there is a growing pressure towards long-term care facilities.

Care services

For those people with mild dementia who are still able to live on their own, there are some different forms of community-based ambulant care services which provide a limited amount of time for help and assistance (personal hygiene, preparing meals, medication). Additionally, there are also professional care services that are funded on a private basis.

Some psychiatric hospitals with gerontopsychiatric units offer 'day clinics' where people with dementia who are still cared by relatives have the possibility to be involved in some group activities. This model of assistance is further supplemented by some other, community-funded institutions (e.g. the Red Cross) as well as some local Alzheimer societies. They are a substantial source, offering temporary respite for relatives and allowing them some time off.

There are different services for those patients who are not cared for by relatives and thus have no possibility of living in their own homes:

- Assisted living settings (i.e. complexes consisting of private rooms or apartments, offering help in cooking, housekeeping and shopping). Since assisted living is not fully covered by social security, this model can only be an option for an individual with a solid financial background.
- Residential care and nursing homes. They are principally open to everyone and basically funded by moneys accrued thoroughout one's working life. Since the costs of this kind of long-term inpatient care in many cases exceed by far the individual pension (social security), this alternative tends to pauperize elderly patients directly and also to consume estates, since owner-occupied housing is incorporated into the means testing process. The medical supervision in these institutions is provided by external physicians, in most cases by general practitioners.

The quality of these long-term care settings may differ significantly. Some institutions offer a differential care setting with specialized Alzheimer wards run by skilled professional nurses. However, most residential care and nursing homes have mixed settings with patients with different medical conditions cared for by only partly specialized staff. Although the number of individuals with a dementia in nursing homes amounts to 50%, many institutions still lack adequate dementia-adjusted architectural designs as well as qualified staff (Table 10.1).

Table 10.1 Care services

	Description	Funding
Extramural model		
Nachbarschaftshilfe (Neighbourhood care)	Informal visits by non-professionals assisting elderly people (shopping, etc.) with basically preserved autonomy	Privately organized
Sozialstation (Social service)	Living in their own homes.	Funded through social service budgets
Private Pflegedienste (Private hospital services)	Assistance offered by for-profit companies with a differential care package.	Organized by for-profit companies
Betreuungsgruppen (Care groups)	Weekly meetings in 'social clubs' (1–2 hours per week) providing activities with demented patients to alleviate caregiver burden	Organized by non-profit associations (e.g. local Alzheimer societies)

Table 10.1 continued

	Description	Funding
Intramural models		
Institutional Care		
Daily care (without beds)		
• Tagespflege (daycare)	Outpatient service (from Monday to Friday) offering pick-up service, meals, group activities as well as dispensing of medication	Funded through social service budgets
• Tageskliniken (day-clinics)	Specialized units that are adjuncted to psychiatric hospitals, offering special diagnostic work-up (memory clinic) as well as a day-care facility.	Reimbursed through National Health Service and private insurances
24 hour care settings		
• Pflegeheime (nursing homes)	Classical nursing home structure for long-term care.	Reimbursed through National Health Service and private insurances
• Gerontopsychiatrische Wohngruppen (gerontopsychiatric supported housing)	Intermediate form of care as a compromise between support at home and institutional care, with a 24-hour supervision.	Reimbursed through National Health Service and private insurances, and/or funded through social service budgets
• Gerontopsychiatrische Kliniken (gerontopsychiatric hospitals)	Specialized units adjuncted to psychiatric hospitals, offering diagnostic as well as curative possibilities for an intermediate time period for patients referred from long-term care units and/or patients to be allocated to long-term care	Reimbursed through National Health Service and private insurances
• Kurzzeitpflege (short-term care units)	Specialized inpatient units offering respite care periods allowing some time off for caregivers	Reimbursed through National Health Service and private insurances.

Prescriptions, reimbursements and general costs

In Germany, cholinesterase inhibitors (donepezil, rivastigmine and galant-amine) as well as memantine are approved to treat Alzheimer dementia. They are reimbursed by the National Health Service and private health insurances. Unfortunately, these medications are only prescribed to roughly

6% of the patients in need. An estimate of the costs to treat patients with a diagnosis of probable Alzheimer's disease has been calculated by Schulenburg et al (1998). These authors differentiated between patients with an Mini Mental State (MMS) score above and below 15 points. The average costs per patient per year were thus estimated to be between 11 500 and 24 500 euros for MMS <15 and between 5000 and 7600 euros for MMS >15.

Problems to be solved

Although dementia and other psychiatric illnesses are common in older people there are still many structural problems to be solved. First, there is still a lack of common sense regarding which diagnostic path has to be taken, once dementia is suspected. Secondly, once dementia has been recognized, there are still problems in allocating individual patients to the different health services on the basis of their individual needs. Thirdly, although there are some pharmacological options which have been proven to delay the disease progression as well as related behavioural disturbances, most individuals with dementia are still non-medicated. Facing these deficiencies, the German government has funded a research project Network of Competence (Kompetenz-Netzwerk-Demenz) to enhance diagnostic predictivity and accuracy as well as communication between the different medical disciplines engaged in the treatment of dementia. This is performed by 'vertical' as well as 'horizontal' projects that are aimed at enhancing different levels of dementia research (from molecular to clinical medicine) and clinical communication between neurologists, psychiatrists, general practitioners and psychologists.

References

Schulenburg JM, Schulenburg I, Horn R et al. (1998) Cost of treatments and care of Alzheimer's disease in Germany. In: A Wimo, B Jönnson, G Karlsson & B Winblad (Eds.): *Health Economics in Dementia*. 1998; J Wiley & Sons; pp218–230.

chapter 11

The practice of dementia care: Denmark

Kirsten Abelskov

The first legislation of direct relevance to dementia care in Denmark was the Act on Social Service, passed in 1933. At that time, there was a focus on the care of frail elderly people in Denmark. According to the latest Act on Social Service, the municipal authorities or the county authority shall ascertain whether any relative or other person is in a position to safeguard the interests of the individual, and if not, the county authorities (the institution is called the state-county) should be requested to appoint a legal guardian under the Legal Guardianship Act §67, Act on Social Service 2002 (Consolidation Act on Social Services No. 755, www.sm.dk/english).

There are 276 'kommuner' municipals and 16 'amter' counties in Denmark. From the beginning of the 1980s, the options for the care of elderly people changed. The focus of caring changed from nursing homes to the peoples' own homes. At the same time, the numbers of nursing home beds have been reduced from 40 000 to 27 000, and the sheltered apartments from 5500 to 3900 (www.sm.dk/netpublikationer). No new nursing homes have been established in the last 16 years and the reduction is still continuing. The old homes have been changed to 'nursing apartments' and to two-room flats with a kitchen. The kitchen gives the nursing home rooms status as a flat, which grants the possibility for the municipals to sell them to a private contractor. This has caused a substantial waiting time to get one of the few flats in a nursing care centre (former nursing home) with a flexible amount of help from the community nurses, as one can only move into these flats on the 1st of the month. The citizens' right to choose private or public help is underlined with a new law, the Act on Free Options (Lovforslag, 2004). The whole system is still financed by taxes and almost free for older people. To ensure that only the necessary care is given, the municipals have officers (nurses or occupational therapists) who assess the person and decide how much help they can be offered. The whole system is bureaucratic, with much delay of decision of the amount of public help. The elderly receive a list of what help they can expect to get. The list is often one or two pages, listed after the time the help was decided. It is not easy to get an overview for old and frail people, not even for care staff.

Twenty-five per cent of the 800 000 elderly people in Denmark over the age of 65 receive some degree of this free help and 13 800 get at least 20 hours a week (www.sm.dk.netpublikationer).

Furthermore, legislation on preventative home visits to those over the age of 75 was passed some years ago, as a result of a controlled study from 1984 (Hendriksen et al, 1984) which proved that home visits reduced the need for hospitalization and also reduced the death rate. The municipals have to contact all elderly people over 75 and this is often done by a letter as the elderly have to accept if they want to participate.

What does a person with dementia do to get help and care? The general practitioners (GPs) are central. They can refer to either a memory clinic or the psychogeriatric department. There are memory clinics at Denmark's three university hospitals in Copenhagen, Aarhus and Odense. The memory clinics concentrate on assessment for people with mild dementia and the younger demented patients. Nearly all counties have psychogeriatric departments. Most patients suffer from moderate to severe dementia and the cause of referral is often behavioural and psychological problems. The psychogeriatric departments have beds, but work mostly at home and assessment and treatment in the patient's own home in collaboration with the patient's GP and the municipal nurses. The team that works in the patient's own home are a nurse, a gerontopsychologist and/or a psychogeriatrician. The psychogeriatrician and the psychologist work flexibly both in the wards and with outpatients. The first visit after referral is often done by a nurse and a psychogeriatrician or a gerontopsychologist.

The social ministry arrange educational programmes for municipal nurses. Currently, there are more than 800 of these so-called dementia coordinators. The coordinators work in the communities and advise other nurses and social workers about patients with dementia. Often they ask for a psychogeriatric evaluation from the local psychogeriatric department, and when the system works (which is not all the time), these individuals coordinate between the patients and their families, GPs, municipality nursing staff, psychogeriatric departments and others.

Patients with dementia can be referred to a day-care centre, up to 5 days a week. The spouse carer can be referred to some well-functioning groups with special interests such as literature, music, foreign languages and so on, while the staff take care of the patient in their own home. There are only a few places where a night-care bed is possible, but sometimes it is a help for the family that the community nursing care system can offer accommodation where a patient can stay 3 weeks or more.

Private organizations can offer their help to families for a person with dementia. The Red Cross, church organizations, and private old age organizations have groups of people who are willing to stay some hours a week with the family. People in these groups can take a short course that highlights how to take care of a demented person.

Staff in the community nursing system are, in general, very knowledgeable about dementia. To be a registered nurse takes 3½ years of education and practical work, a 'health and social' assistant takes 3 years and has less training and there is a grade of 'health and social' helper with 14 months of training.

Even though Denmark is a small country, there are many differences in the care given in the many community nursing systems. One of the differences is the use of medication. There have been several investigations in the last 12 years of the use of medication, the first being in 1992. In all counties, the registration of the use of medication was done in two nursing homes and one specialized nursing home for psychogeriatric patients (Tybjerg and Gulmann, 1992). Kitty El-Kholy, Professor Marianne Scroll and colleagues in 1994 investigated some nursing homes in Copenhagen, and Libeth Soerensen (2001) looked at the medication in nursing homes in Northern Jutland county. Legal doctors who have an obligation to control nursing care centres investigated the use of psychopharmacological treatment in 35 nursing homes in West Sealand. Lars Larsen and Inga Petersen reported on 32 nursing care centres in Aarhus Municipal, Aarhus County (Figure 11.1).

In Aarhus County, attention is paid to education for community staff. In cases with severe behavioural problems, the Cohen–Mansfield Scale is used to assess the patient's Cohen-Mansfield Agitation Inventory (CMAI) (Cohen-Mansfield et al, 1989). The scale is modified as follows: the scale is done in every shift, day, evening and night, 3 days in a row. The score is changed

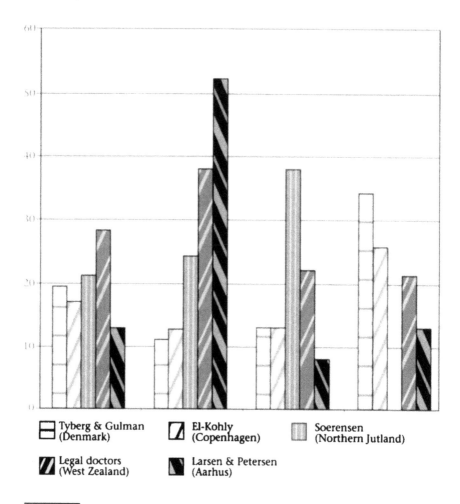

Figure 11.1 *Differences in medication treatment in the community nursing systems in Denmark.*

from 1–7 to 0–6 to do a computer registration of the scoring. And we have added a caregiver burden scale of 5 items. In this way we assess demented people who would score 5–7 on the original CMAI.

The results of the modified CMAI scoring is shown on one sheet. The score of the patient on all 29 items is on the left side. Then a graphic illustration of the scoring, daytime in blue, evening in red and night time in a yellow colour, and in the middle the name of the items 1–29 in the clusters:

1. Physical aggressive: hitting, kicking, grabbing, pushing, throwing things, biting, scratching, spitting, hurting self or others, tearing things, physical sexual advances.
2. Physical non-aggressive: pace, inappropriate dress or disrobing, trying to get to a different place, intentional falling, eating and drinking inappropriate substances, handling things inappropriately, hiding things, hoarding things, performing repetitious mannerisms, general restlessness.
3. Verbal aggressive: screaming, making verbal sexual advances, cursing or verbal aggression.
4. Verbal non-aggressive: repetitive sentences or questions, strange noises, complaining, negativism, constant unwarranted request for attention or help.

The right graphics is the caregiver burden, and the score is to the left side.

Adding the caregiver's burden scale has highlighted the relation between the patients and their carer. Often it is not the patient who has the problem but the carers (Figure 11.2). This case was an 81-year-old vascular demented man referred with a great wish from the staff to give antipsychotic medication because of his aggressive behaviour. What the scale shows is that the staff had the problem, not the patient. The treatment was supervising the staff group, and 3 months later there were no problems with the patient (Figure 11.3). He did not get any medication.

In Aarhus County there has for a long time been an awareness that knowledge and good care of patients gives higher quality care for the demented patient than giving unnecessary medication.

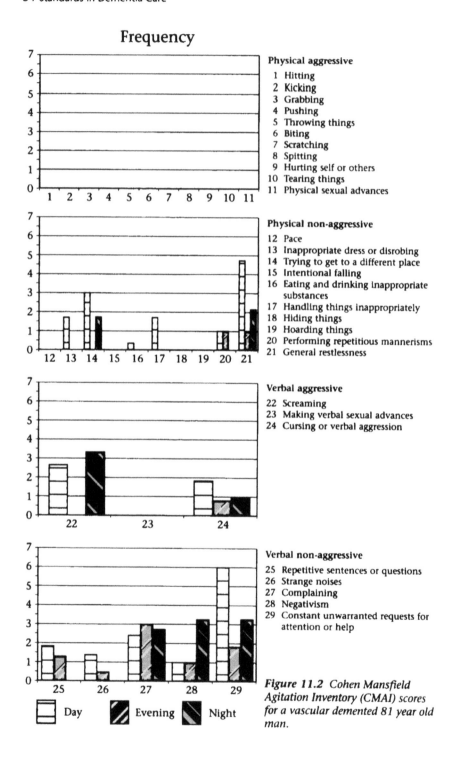

Frequency

Physical aggressive

1 Hitting
2 Kicking
3 Grabbing
4 Pushing
5 Throwing things
6 Biting
7 Scratching
8 Spitting
9 Hurting self or others
10 Tearing things
11 Physical sexual advances

Physical non-aggressive

12 Pace
13 Inappropriate dress or disrobing
14 Trying to get to a different place
15 Intentional falling
16 Eating and drinking inappropriate substances
17 Handling things inappropriately
18 Hiding things
19 Hoarding things
20 Performing repetitious mannerisms
21 General restlessness

Verbal aggressive

22 Screaming
23 Making verbal sexual advances
24 Cursing or verbal aggression

Verbal non-aggressive

25 Repetitive sentences or questions
26 Strange noises
27 Complaining
28 Negativism
29 Constant unwarranted requests for attention or help

☐ Day   ▨ Evening   ◩ Night

Figure 11.2 Cohen Mansfield Agitation Inventory (CMAI) scores for a vascular demented 81 year old man.

Caregiver burden

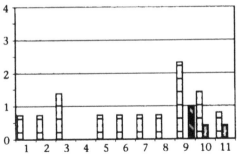

Physical aggressive

1 Hitting
2 Kicking
3 Grabbing
4 Pushing
5 Throwing things
6 Biting
7 Scratching
8 Spitting
9 Hurting self or others
10 Tearing things
11 Physical sexual advances

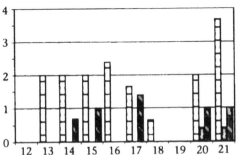

Physical non-aggressive

12 Pace
13 Inappropriate dress or disrobing
14 Trying to get to a different place
15 Intentional falling
16 Eating and drinking inappropriate
   substances
17 Handling things inappropriately
18 Hiding things
19 Hoarding things
20 Performing repetitious mannerisms
21 General restlessness

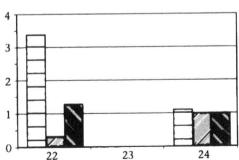

Verbal aggressive

22 Screaming
23 Making verbal sexual advances
24 Cursing or verbal aggression

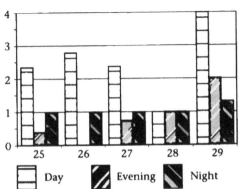

Verbal non-aggressive

25 Repetitive sentences or questions
26 Strange noises
27 Complaining
28 Negativism
29 Constant unwarranted requests for
   attention or help

☐ Day   ▨ Evening   ◪ Night

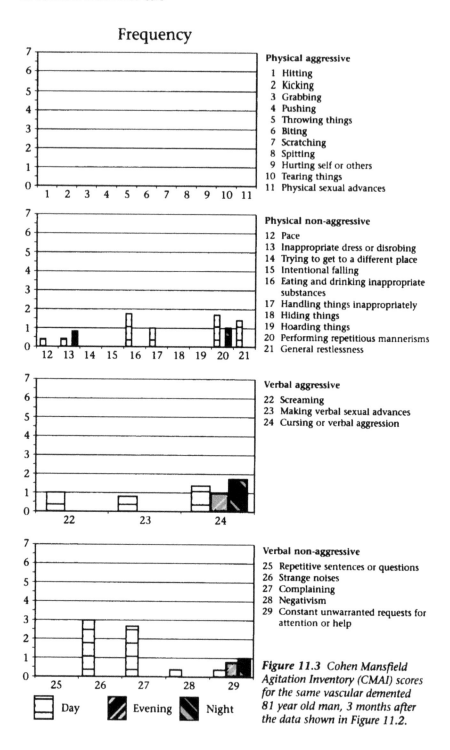

Frequency

Physical aggressive

1 Hitting
2 Kicking
3 Grabbing
4 Pushing
5 Throwing things
6 Biting
7 Scratching
8 Spitting
9 Hurting self or others
10 Tearing things
11 Physical sexual advances

Physical non-aggressive

12 Pace
13 Inappropriate dress or disrobing
14 Trying to get to a different place
15 Intentional falling
16 Eating and drinking inappropriate
   substances
17 Handling things inappropriately
18 Hiding things
19 Hoarding things
20 Performing repetitious mannerisms
21 General restlessness

Verbal aggressive

22 Screaming
23 Making verbal sexual advances
24 Cursing or verbal aggression

Verbal non-aggressive

25 Repetitive sentences or questions
26 Strange noises
27 Complaining
28 Negativism
29 Constant unwarranted requests for
   attention or help

☐ Day   ▨ Evening   ◩ Night

Figure 11.3 Cohen Mansfield Agitation Inventory (CMAI) scores for the same vascular demented 81 year old man, 3 months after the data shown in Figure 11.2.

Caregiver burden

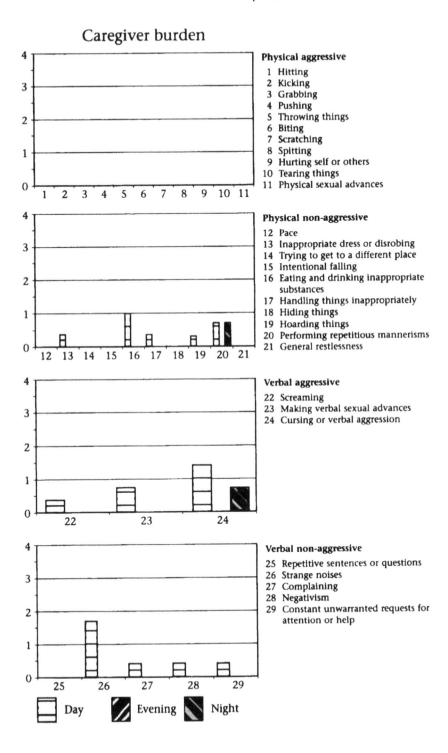

Physical aggressive

1 Hitting
2 Kicking
3 Grabbing
4 Pushing
5 Throwing things
6 Biting
7 Scratching
8 Spitting
9 Hurting self or others
10 Tearing things
11 Physical sexual advances

Physical non-aggressive

12 Pace
13 Inappropriate dress or disrobing
14 Trying to get to a different place
15 Intentional falling
16 Eating and drinking inappropriate substances
17 Handling things inappropriately
18 Hiding things
19 Hoarding things
20 Performing repetitious mannerisms
21 General restlessness

Verbal aggressive

22 Screaming
23 Making verbal sexual advances
24 Cursing or verbal aggression

Verbal non-aggressive

25 Repetitive sentences or questions
26 Strange noises
27 Complaining
28 Negativism
29 Constant unwarranted requests for attention or help

☐ Day   ▨ Evening   ◨ Night

References

Cohen-Mansfield J, Marx MS, Rosenthal AS. A description of agitation in a nursing home. *J Gerontol* 1989; **44**: M77–84.

Hendriksen C, Lund E, Stromgard E. Consequences of assessments and intervention among elderly people: a three year randomised controlled study. *BMJ* 1984; 289: 1522–4.

Larsen L, Petersen II. *Gerontologi og Samfund 2004* in press.

Soerensen L. *Psychiatric morbidity and use of psychotropics in Danish nursing homes.* Aarhus University Press; 2001.

Lovforslag om frit valg 27.5. 2004.

Tybjerg J, Gulmann NC. Brug af psykopharmaka på kommunale plejehjem. *UGL* 1992; 154: 3125–9.

West Zealand legal doctors' study at http://www.elidk/upload/brug-af-medicin-paa-plejehjem.pdf

chapter 12

The practice of dementia care: Finland

Tuula Anneli Pirttilä

Finnish health care and social welfare system

All residents in Finland are by law guaranteed access to social welfare and health care. Finland's 448 municipalities are in charge of the tax-based funding of social welfare and health services for all their inhabitants. Most of these social welfare and healthcare services are statutory, meaning that there are laws that require the municipalities to provide the services in question. The municipalities may provide services as part of their own operations, through membership of a joint municipal board or by purchasing services from other municipalities or private providers.

Public healthcare services comprise primary healthcare and specialized hospital care. Municipalities are required to provide medical care for local residents. This includes medical examination and treatment, and also medical rehabilitation. Medical care can be provided at health centres as non-institutional care or in health centre wards, or in the form of home nursing. Primary health care is provided by municipal health centres. Health centres have many branches and wards for bed care. Municipalities are responsible for arranging specialized hospital care for their residents. To this end, Finland is divided into 20 hospital districts and, in addition, the semi-autonomous province of Ahvenanmaa forms its own such district. Each municipality therefore belongs to a particular hospital district, each of which contains a central and regional hospital. Of the central hospitals, five are university hospitals that provide specialized levels of treatment. Each hospital district organizes and provides specialized hospital care for the population in its area.

The Social Welfare Act states that it is the duty of municipalities to provide general social welfare services, which include social work, home help services, housing services, institutional care, family care and support for informal care. A personal service plan is drawn up for each disabled person to clarify the services and support he or she requires. Officials of the municipality together with the client and his or her carer or relatives prepare the plan. The service plan is designed to improve clients' autonomy and their possibilities to influence their situation. Other services include transportation services, home modifications and assistive devices to improve home care.

Special forms of financial support include pensioners' care allowance and support for informal care. Pensioners' care allowance is intended to make it possible for pension recipients with an illness or disability to live at home, as well as to promote home care and to reimburse pension recipients for extra costs caused by illness or disability. Support for informal care is a form of care payment and support service provided for those looking after an old, disabled or ill person at home. What it actually comprises is set down in a care and service plan drawn up for the person concerned.

Dementia care

Dementia care is provided as part of the general health care and social welfare system. According to the statistics of the National Research and Development Centre for Welfare and Health (STAKES), the number of residents over 65 years old in 2001 was 786 771 (15.1% of all residents), of whom 13.5% used home-help services, 3.3% lived in old people's houses, and 1.5% in long-term institutional health care. It is well known that people with cognitive impairment make up a large proportion of those needing institutional care or intense home support. The estimated number of cognitively impaired individuals in Finland varies from 100 000 to 150 000. The use of social services and health care of dementia patients was evaluated by STAKES in 1995. The evaluation was based on the Finnish national Care Register, which includes information on all inpatient activities, the use of nursing homes and supported home care. According to the survey, the prevalence of dementia in the residents over 65 years old was 6.3%, whereas previous population-based studies have shown that the prevalence of moderate and severe dementia is 8.5% in Finland (Juva et al. 1992, Koivisto 1995). It is notable that the causal diagnosis of dementia was lacking in the majority. The STAKES survey showed that 24% dementia patients were in long-term wards, 32% lived in old people's homes, 4% in service housing, 9% used interval hospital care and 27% received home-help and home-care services. Altogether, 46% of the clients in old peoples' homes, 22% of those living in service housing and 58%

of the patients in long-term wards, had a diagnosis of dementia. Approximately 14% of the clients receiving home-care services had dementia.

The Subcommittee of Ministry of Social Affairs and Health gave a statement in 1996 that cognitively impaired residents need a wide range of services in different levels of the healthcare system. They emphasized early diagnosis, rehabilitation and caregiver support to improve home care of dementia patients. In 2000 The Finnish Alzheimer Society made a postal survey on the state of the care for cognitively impaired individuals in Finland. Altogether, 67% of representatives of the municipalities responded. Only 12% of the municipalities had a separate dementia care strategy, but 60% had some type of suggestions, particularly for dementia care, included in their general elderly care strategy. Over half (60%) estimated that knowledge and skills of the staff were good. Most of the municipalities considered that outpatient services were adequate and 75% answered that diagnostic services were adequate. Half of the municipalities estimated that early dementia counselling was well organized, whereas there is lack of early educational courses and psychoeducational adaptation programmes for dementia patients and their caregivers.

There are no official treatment guidelines for patients with memory disorders and dementia in Finland. However, the consensus statement of Finnish dementia experts for examination of patients with memory disorders was published in 1996 in a Finnish medical journal. The basic clinical examination of the patients and necessary laboratory tests are performed by general practioners in primary care centres. In many regions there are also dementia nurses and coordinators who are also specially trained to perform a short cognitive test battery (CERAD). Translation of the original CERAD battery was carried on by the dementia experts after the initiative of Finnish Alzheimer's Research Society. The translation was finished in 1999 and, since then, the use of CERAD battery has increasingly been adopted in many different settings. Finnish CERAD is currently distributed by the Finnish Alzheimer's Research Society. The patients with a possible progressive dementing disease should be referred to a specialist for further diagnostic evaluation. It is estimated that the number of new dementia cases is 10 000–15 000, and less than half of cognitively impaired patients are adequately examined and receive a causal diagnosis. However, the access of diagnostic services differs regionally.

Some hospitals have established special memory polyclinics, but mainly patients are examined in departments of neurology or geriatrics. There are also private memory clinics in large cities. Further evaluation of patients with a possible dementing disease includes imaging, brain computed tomography (CT) or magnetic resonance imaging (MRI), depending on the resources, and neuropsychological tests, or at least the CERAD battery, if not done already. Another initiative carried out by the Finnish Alzheimer's Research Society was the translation of the instruments for the assessment of activities of daily living (ADCS-ADL), neuropsychiatric symptoms (NPI) and severity of the disease (CDR and GDS-FAST). These scales are variably used and they are distributed by pharmaceutical companies.

Alzheimer drugs (acetylcholine esterase inhibitors and memantine) are reimbursed by the Social Insurance Institution of Finland (KELA). The requirements for the reimbursement are that the patient has dementia that is mainly caused by Alzheimer's disease and that the diagnosis is performed by a neurologist or geriatrician. There are no limitations, according to the severity of the dementia. It is estimated that 15–20% of all Alzheimer patients are currently using these drugs. The treatment is started by the specialist but the GPs are in charge of the long-term follow-up as well as the overall medical care of the patients. There are psychogeriatric facilities in some hospitals, but primary care centres mainly provide behavioural management services.

At the beginning of the 1990s, the Finnish Alzheimer Society organized a dementia counsellor project that was funded by Finland's Slot Machine Association (RAY). As a result of this initiative, there is a dementia counsellor in each hospital district and many municipalities have their own trained counsellors. Still, the availability of continuing counselling for families is rare, and there are still considerable regional differences in the availability of counselling. Other rehabilitation services are sparse. Psychoeducational adaptation courses are organized mainly for patients under 65 years old. Physiotherapy and occupational therapy are not commonly provided for dementia patients.

Many primary care centres provide day-care services and intermittent hospital services to support home care but they are not specially organized for demented individuals and therefore caregivers are unwilling to make use of these services.

Special training programmes of dementia care for nurses have been organized in many polytechnic institutes in Finland. However, there are no guidelines on the substance and quality of these programmes. Currently, there are no special training programmes for doctors but there are plans for dementia subspecialty training. Many primary care centres have established special dementia care units and there has been a rapid growth in the number of private dementia care units during recent years. However, the quality of these units varies greatly, and currently there is no official quality control system.

Social and healthcare services provided by voluntary associations supplement those arranged by municipalities and offer an alternative to them. The associations provide various forms of services aimed mainly at supporting home care, such as counselling, support groups for demented individuals and their caregivers, personal assistants for dementia patients, evening care and rehabilitative day-care services. However, these services are lacking in small rural communities, since the associations are concentrated in urban areas.

References

Juva K, Sulkava R, Erkinjuntti T, Valvanne J, Tilvis R. The demented elderly in the city of Helsinki: Functional capacity and placement. *J Am Geriatr Soc* 1992; 40:1146–50.

Koivisto K. Population-based dementia screening in the city of Kuopio, Eastern Finland. Evaluation of screening methods, prevalence of dementia and dementia subtypes. *University of Kuopio, Series of Reports, Department of Neurology No. 33*, Kuopio, 1995.

chapter 13

The practice of dementia care: Lithuania

Rasa Ruseckiene

Present situation and problems

Every year, in Lithuania, the number of elderly people who suffer from diverse mental diseases increases. According to the latest statistical data presented by the Psychiatric Health Centre, there are 955 000 people of pensionable age, i.e. women over 65 years old and men over 62 years old. According to the statistical data presented by the European Union, 20% of the elderly people who are over 65 have mental disorders. In Lithuania, no such epidemiological surveys have been made, but (on the grounds of the statistical data used by the other countries) it can be expected that in Vilnius there are 20 000 elderly people who suffer from mental illnesses and approximately 10% (i.e. 2000 people) of them need constant nursing, treatment and supervision because of their serious condition. During recent years, the number of people who are suffering from Alzheimer's disease is increasing. Despite treatment, people are incapable of taking care of themselves and being self-dependent; therefore, almost every patient is given invalid status.

The main problems which elderly people with mental disorders face are supervision, further residence and treatment. These problems are especially urgent for patients who have no relatives and family. The present number of psychiatric inpatient departments in Lithuania is insufficient in order to ensure skilled medical aid as well as to satisfy the needs of the patients. Today, in Lithuania, there are only a few psychiatric hospitals (asylums) in bigger cities to render psychiatric assistance for elderly people (Vilnius Psychiatric Hospital and Vasaros Clinical Hospital in Vilnius, Ziegzdriu Psychiatric Hospital in Kaunas and the Psychiatric Hospital in Siauliai) but they are insufficient for the present needs. The biggest shortage of inpatient departments is felt for male patients, because very often they are treated in the same departments as people with acute mental disorders because the existing gerontopsychiatric departments provide only medicines and nursing.

Because of historical circumstances in Lithuania, it is commonly accepted that elderly people are cared for by their children at home or live alone, whereas, it is common worldwide practice for elderly people with mental disorders to live and undergo a treatment in specialized accommodation. Also, not enough attention is paid to the patient's family members: their emotional condition and their quality of life.

Working family members encounter huge problems when their close relatives suddenly fall ill not only with somatic disease but also with mental disease. It is a huge problem when one of the family members who behaves in unexpected ways and cannot take care of himself is home alone without supervision. Furthermore, the lack of information and knowledge (in this case of children) makes this problem even more serious. In Lithuania, people usually try to solve this problem by hospitalizing relatives with mental disorders to the inpatient departments; unfortunately, this solution is temporary. Nowadays, the prevalent opinion in our country is that elderly patients are useless in our society and therefore should be put into psycho-neurologic boarding houses and isolated from normal life. The lack of specialized services (communal and inpatient departments), specialists and professionals (doctors, gerontopsychiatrists, therapists, psychotherapists who work with elderly patients) make such a patient incapable of adapting himself and unwelcome in the society.

The lack of specialized treatment – institutions where elderly people with mental disorders can undergo treatment, specialized boarding houses and day-care inpatient departments where such patients can get diverse professional aid and supervision – constrain to turn society's and foreign specialist's attention to the present gerontopsychiatric situation in Lithuania (Table 13.1).

What means are taken in order to solve this problem?

In consultation with foreign specialists, different reforms are taking place in the Vasaros Clinic Hospital, which is situated in Vilnius. Measures are being taken in order to integrate patients who suffer from mental diseases back into society and ensure their quality of life and to create community-orientated services as well as change the opinion on the variety of services that should be provided.

Table 13.1 The number of residents in Lithuania according to sex and age at the beginning of the year

Age groups	Total		Male		Female	
	2003	*2004*	*2003*	*2004*	*2003*	*2004*
60–64	183654	180355	77156	75678	106498	104677
65–69	165572	165388	65259	64937	100313	100451
70–74	146131	144178	53194	52591	92937	91587
75–79	105892	110546	31979	34105	73913	76441
80+	92090	97789	24783	26047	67307	71742

In Vilnius, a few years ago after reconstruction and renovation, the gerontopsychiatric department, which started its work in 1994, was reopened. During these years, distinctive treatment traditions have formed. The gerontopsychiatric department as well as other projects in the Vasaros Clinical Hospital are supported by the international organization 'Geneva's Initiative in Psychiatry' and financed by the Dutch Ministry of Foreign Affairs (MATRA project). Consultants such as Professor Robin Jacoby, the therapist Carolina Buttholf and nurses from Oxford are constantly visiting Vasaros Clinical Hospital to share their knowledge with hospital personnel and to teach them how to work with gerontopsychiatric patients; moreover, new services are being introduced, together with the new methods of working and personnel training. Moreover, in the Vasaros Clinical Psychiatric Hospital, educational function is being realized: doctors are being assisted by externs and patients receive consultations from the personnel of Vilnius University Psychiatric Hospital.

In its architectural layout, the gerontopsychiatric department is different from other departments. The department is divided into two sections, which are used for different purposes. In one section, medical aid for the patients with acute mental illnesses is provided, whereas, in the other section, medical aid is provided for the patients who are ill with less severe mental diseases. They are more self-dependent and, therefore, need less tending.

The department has 20 beds for female patients and 10 beds for male patients. The department admits patients not only from Vilnius but also from throughout Lithuania. Following our foreign consultants' recommendations, wards were named after flowers in order to help patients to orient in the department and remember their ward as well as to exercise their cognitive functions. The department staff consists of three psychiatrists, a social worker, a psychologist, a rehabilitologist, a neurologist and nursing personnel; if necessary, doctors of other specialities can come in to consult the patients. During staff meetings the state of each patient is discussed and an integrated and individual cure and nursing plan is assigned for the particular patient. The department has two activity rooms where patients come every day to take exercise. Also, using music and art therapy, the memory and self-sufficiency of patients are being trained. The newest medicines, which have less side-effects and effectively eliminate the symptoms of the illness, are used. In the department, patients with different mental disorders (organic, depressive or severe mental illnesses) are treated and the diagnosis of dementia is carried out. Subject to the origin of the mental disorders, an optimal treatment is chosen. The effectiveness of the treatment is strengthened by the skilled help of clinical psychologists and psychotherapists, i.e. patients are treated not only with the medicines but also viva voce, helping them to form a new point of view to their problems; moreover, a lot of attention is paid to their relatives. The social worker helps to solve the social and daily problems that the patients encounter. Most attention is paid to their activities and the rehabilitation of their social skills. Therefore, a kitchen, where patients will be able to cook their favourite meals, is being installed. Afternoon meetings are arranged during which patients read and discuss the press together and share their experiences and worries. On the second floor, a laundry, where patients will be able to wash their clothes, is being installed. This will help them not to lose everyday skills. Patients who were discharged are not forgotten; they are visited by social workers and once a month they come to a meeting where they have the opportunity to discuss their problems and share their joys and worries. Close collaboration with specialists from regional psychiatric health centres, if necessary, ensures further aid to the patient. In the gerontopsychiatric department, as well as in the whole hospital, the staff strictly confine themselves to the principles of confidential information and medical etiquette.

The future plan is to extend the service of aid for the gerontopsychiatric patients by creating social services that will help to ensure the supervision of the patients at home. Specially trained nurses will visit patients, observe their state, help to do the daily household work and, if necessary, will recommend the help of a psychiatrist or any other specialist.

chapter 14

The practice of dementia care: Portugal

Horácio Firmino

The distribution of the elderly population in Portugal is not homogeneous, reflecting the socioeconomic diversities of each region. At this time 17% of the Portuguese population lives to over 65 years old. The largest percentage of population over 65 years old resides in the centre and south of the country. According to a study of the National Institute of Statistics (2002) the population over 65 years old has doubled in the last 40 years, so that in about 30% of families there is at least one elderly person and around half of these are composed by elders.

The increase of this elderly population has led to the development of social politics to guarantee an ageing with quality of life, using such new solutions as home support and day centres for beyond the nurses' home and to maintain the elderly in their own residences. Integrated residential support was one of the answers created from a former decision of the Health Ministry and Work and Solidarity Ministry No. 407/98 (15 May 1998), with the objective of establishing orientation that enabled an articulated intervention between the remits of health and social action, taking into account the physical, mental and social transitory or permanent situation of the dependency of the elderly. In this way, they tried to find a global integrated answer to the needs of this population that face such dependency within a sociofamilial context, by giving them greater autonomy and by satisfying their needs, within an integrated nursing, medical care and social support system.

Since the 1960s, the mental health problems of older individuals have been given more attention and social interest due to the growing number of the older people in the population. Because of this increase, relatively rare situations such as dementia have become more frequent. The suffering caused by these disorders, not only to patients themselves but also to their families, imposes urgent medical action, which goes from early diagnosis to possible therapeutics and even prevention.

In psychiatry and neurology, there was an urge to give answers to these problems, delving deeper into the scientific basis and creating technical specialities. In fact there was an awareness that mental diseases at this stage have their own characteristics and that the ways of possible intervention are quite specific, but most physicians and even psychiatrists/neurologists were unprepared to undertake such an action. From 1978 there have been in our country several initiatives in this domain, with the creation of psychogeriatrics consultations in psychiatric hospitals and university hospitals and dementia consultations/memory clinics at Neurological Services.

In a study in 2003 organized by the Mental Health Work Group on the Ageing (subordinated to the Mental Health Director (Health Minister)), the object was to evaluate specifically from answers given by psychiatric units in the country regarding patients over 65 years old (Situação Assistencial às Pessoas Idosas 2004). The study concluded that in a majority of those units it already exist specific consults for this population, and in only two of the public psychiatric hospitals were there departments of psychogeriatrics (Figure 14.1). However, the majority of these answers (except those of the two psychogeriatrics units) were supplied by a limited number of psychiatrists, who said that only a short percentage of their work time was dedicated to patients over 65 years old.

At the present moment in Portugal there are no epidemiological studies on the prevalence or incidence of Alzheimer's disease (AD). However, a study of

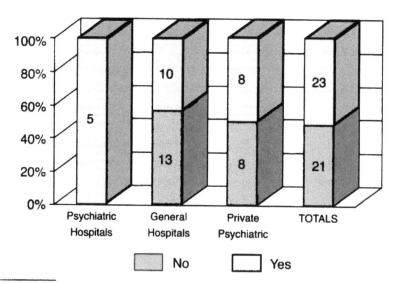

Figure 14.1 Psychiatric services with specific geriatric psychiatry consultation.

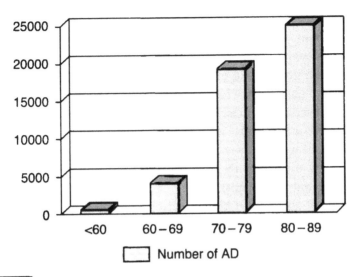

Figure 14.2 Estimated dementia (Alzheimer's disease) of the Portugese population.

Garcia et al (1994) estimated that in Portugal there are around 50 000 patients with AD, the majority being over 70 years old (Figure 14.2).

In our country, until 2003 there was no available information concerning the origin of the patients, methodology of the evaluation and the use of instruments/tests used in the consultations and of the use of and efficacy of specific drugs. For this reason we (the Portuguese Psychogeriatric Association) decided to organize an inquiry among the different professionals – psychiatrists and neurologists – who treat patients with dementia (Firmino et al, 2003).

In this study, general practitioners and internal medicine are the most frequent filters for this disease (near 70%), but the majority of these patients, when they are referred to a specialist, are in a moderate or moderate to severe stage of progression of the disease. Usually, each evaluation of this patient had an interval between bimonthly and quarterly.

Neuropsychological tests are used in most consultations to make the diagnosis and/or to evaluate the course of the disease, but like almost all other countries, the most commonly used method is the Folstein Mental State Examination (MMSE) and in some cases Clock Draw Design. All of the responders consider it important to teach and explain about AD to the caregivers and the majority say it is important to explain the course of the disease, and usually to promote this kind of information.

Almost all the responders consider treatment as long as effective using guidelines of other countries, with acetylcolinesterase inhibitors or NMDA.

Reflecting on these results, we consider that we have much to develop in our organization and in the practical clinic to improve the needs of Alzheimer's patients.

In reality, within the field of psychiatry in Portugal, there are only two psychogeriatric units, with hospitalization, consultation and home support and with connection to primary care, with a multidisciplinary team. In this team there are psychiatrists, neurologists, psychologists, social assistants, occupational therapists, nurses and with the support of internal medicine. In other hospitals, there are only specific consultants with a few technicians, generally with only psychiatrists.

In neurology, especially at the university hospitals and central hospitals (not in all), there are some memory clinics or dementia consultations (with neurologists and neuropsychologists). In both, we have verified that a significant percentage of technicians work in care with patients with dementia; they dedicate part of their time to the diagnosis and accompaniment of these patients without the support of other professionals, which thus limits the intervention they are able to dispense, resulting in a wide range in diagnosis and prescription of drugs and to subsequent re-evaluation of the outcome as revealed in the course of the evolution of the illness. In the politics of support for the patients with Alzheimer's disease, a growing worry has existed by the authorities within the area of social support: namely, the financial support to dependants (although modest) and the financial support to caregivers, should they need their own residencies, and the necessary income needed for the nursing homes subsidised by social security. However, the patient and family should bear a significant part of the costs of this illness – i.e. when patients need to go into a nursing home – given the shortage of subsidized state-owned, ONEST – and for the specific drugs needed for this illness such as AChEI and NMDA. Barely 50% of the price of these medicines are supported by the state and it is obligatory that they be prescribed by psychiatrists or neurologists. Given the elevated price of these drugs, only a small number of these patients have the means to acquire them. The economy of the Portuguese population is one of the minnows of Europe, and this patients' group lives with extremely low pensions, and so it is very hard for them to buy such drugs. The social security system in Portugal has been tentative in giving answer to some of the problems of the ageing and of Alzheimer's disease. There continue to exist, in our opinion, an assembly of gaps, in the scope of treatment, in the answers it gives to those who are sick, namely in the knowledge of the illness, lateness in referral to specialists and in the accessibility of specific and efficient drugs.

The Portuguese Psychogeriatric Association presented an Educational Formative Programme to the Portuguese Medical Board in order to create a subspecialty of psychogeriatrics after specialization in psychiatry.

We are working with the Mental Health Director (who was subordinated to the Health Minister) to improve organizational issues concerning ageing people, namely in order to increase psychogeriatrics departments in the central and university hospitals and to develop different educational programmes in primary care.

References

Envelhecimento em Portugal (Aging at Portugal): situação demográfica e socioeconomica recente das pessoas idosas, INE, 2002

Firmino H, Falcão D, Marques L, et al. Current trends on clinical evaluation of Alzheimer's patients in Portugal. Poster presented at IPA Congress, Chicago; 2003.

Garcia C, Costa C, Guerreiro M, et al. Estimativa da prevalência da demência e da Doença de Alzheimer em Portugal. *Acta Médica* 1994; 7: 487–91.

O silêncio da memória: o (des) conhecimento da doença de Alzheimer em Portugal. *Associação Portuguesa de Familiares e Amigos do Doente de Alzheimer*; 2004.

Situação Assistencial às Pessoas Idosas: Inquérito Nacional. Mental Health Work Group in the Aging (subordinated to the Mental Health Director (Health Minister)). Paper presented at IPA Regional Meeting, Chile; 2004.

chapter 15

The practice of dementia care: Turkey

Engin Eker and Turan Ertan

The total population of Turkey is 70 781 568. A rapid increase in the elderly population in Turkey has been observed in the last 10 years. The proportion of the population over 65 years old in Turkey was 4.3% in 1990. Despite the Organization for Economic Cooperation and Development's (OECD)'s projection indicating that 7.7% of the population will be over 65 by 2020, the results published by the Directorate of Population Registry showed that this rate is already 8% in 2003. In fact, ageing in Turkey is clearly going to be a reason to force goverment to think more seriously about problems of the elderly in the next decades.

Turkish culture has traditionally emphasized paternal authority and family loyalty, and children are typically expected to care for their parents, even if they are demented. Relative caregivers of demented patients do not want to place their patients in nursing homes. In Turkey, demented patients are cared for mostly by their spouses or by their eldest daughter in their homes.

On the other hand, Turkey has no good-quality services for demented patients. There is drastic shortage of specific centres for demented patients with behavioural and psychological symptoms. The estimated number of patients with Alzheimer's disease (AD) is 250 000 in Turkey. Currently, most of the patients remain undiagnosed or are not even considered as suffering from a disease such as dementia. Their dementias are still perceived as the natural consequence of ageing, especially in rural areas. Today, institutions for the elderly in Turkey are directed by different organizations, including:

1. government institutions organized as elderly homes or elderly care and rehabilitation centres
2. local authorities (municipalities)
3. non-profit associations

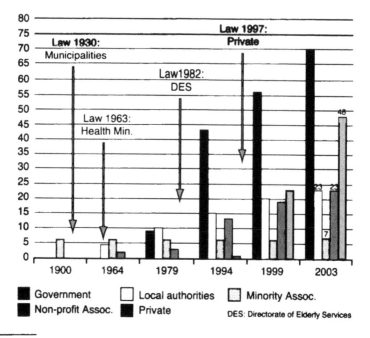

Figure 15.1 *Number of the institutions for the elderly in Turkey.*
Presented the 11th Congress of IPA, 2003, Chicago by Turan Ertan: Psychogeriatrics in Turkey.

4. minority associations
5. private institutions.

Figure 15.1 shows the historical development of institutions for the elderly in Turkey. The first law in Turkey left the responsibility to local authorities in 1930. Despite this law, in the 43 years between 1900 and 1943, no new institutions were established. In the following years, elderly care became a part of the government politics, probably as a result of immigration to big cities beginning in the late 1940s. The new law in 1963 gave some of the responsibility to the Health Ministry. The period between the 1960s until late 1980s is not a period of effort in this field by the government. We observe a dramatic increase in government institutions in the last 20 years following the organization of the Directorate of Social Services and Child Protection with the new law in 1982. Following the new law, in 1997, permitting private investment in the field, a remarkable number of private elderly homes have emerged in the last 10 years (Directorate of Social Services and Child Protection, 2003).

Distribution of bed capacity 2003

- **Number of beds per institution:**
  Government: 130
  Local authority: 107
  Minority association: 139
  Non-profit association: 75
  Private: 34

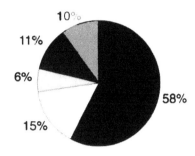

- **Care & rehabilitation centres:**
  Government: 55%
  Local authority: 13%
  Minority association: 66%
  Non-profit association: 8%
  Private: 25%

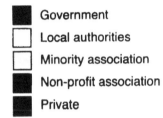

Figure 15.2 *Capacity distribution of elderly homes in Turkey.*
Presented the 11th Congress of IPA, 2003, Chicago by Turan Ertan: Psychogeriatrics in Turkey.

Figure 15.2 also shows the capacity distribution of elderly homes in Turkey by 2003. Not surprisingly, we observe that government institutions dominate with a big difference today. More than half of the total capacity is directed by government by 2003. Although expected to be more in the near future, private capacity is only 10%.

Ten per cent of the beds in some old people's homes run by the goverment and municipalities are designated for demented patients. These patients are separated from the rest of the building. However, people with mild dementia should not necessarily be segregated (Eker, 1995). We need the assessment wards and day-care centres to be more specialized in care at home and long-term care, with well-trained staff for these patients. There are no good segregated services for severe dementia which can pay special attention to the particular needs of sufferers and can develop special activities and programmes of care.

Social care developments, i.e. domestic and personal care, respite care, day care, overnight care, residential and nursing home care and support systems for relatives, are not sufficient and remarkably varied, both in content and volume, from one geographical area to another in Turkey. However, the community services have started to be used, especially in the three big cities of Istanbul, Ankara and Izmir.

The Turkish Alzheimer Society & Foundation founded the first care centre for patients with AD in Istanbul in 2002. The capacity of this centre is limited to 20 patients. In the care centre, patients are included in social activities such as sports, painting and music. There are full-time nurses, hospital attendants and a psychologist, while a neurologist visits the patients once a week. Caregiver support groups are also being held by the psychologist for the relatives and caretakers of the patients. Yasamkent is the name of the other care centre in Istanbul. The Alzheimer Foundation has signed a protocol for its section with AD patients. In Turkey, special day hospital care has not been developed to make it possible for patients with dementia to remain in their own homes as long as they wish and the family situation allows. In Ankara, there is a day hospital that provides medical treatment, social interaction training and care to the demented patients and relief and support to the carers.

There is no 24-hour crisis service for demented patients in Turkey. We need 24-hour responsive primary care teams with access to specialist advice quickly. General psychiatric services do not want to accept demented patients and general psychiatrists and neurologists do not want to take on the task of caring for these people. On the other hand, in Turkey, demented patients are seen by neurologists and psychiatrists at a late stage in outpatient clinics. Family members are more likely to report behavioural and psychological symptoms rather than memory problems in their patients. Caregivers in our community may underreport BPSD, because of fear of their relatives being mentally ill. They desire not to relinquish the caregiver role. As we mentioned earlier, relative caregivers of demented patients with behavioural and psychological symptoms do not want to place their patients in nursing homes. Recently, a taking care of the elderly having dementia at home project is under development in the big cities. Some educated voluntary groups are engaged in looking after these patients.

In Turkey, there are problems in identifying AD patients. There is lack of GP awareness and involvement. Some GPs have not yet realized how important it is that the diagnosis of dementia is made. Families complain that GPs, and even general psychiatrists and neurologists, do not listen to the actual practical problems they are coping with. There is urgent need for continuing the education of GPs and young psychiatrists and neurologists who are interested in dementia. The Turkish Society of Geriatric Psychiatry and the Alzheimer Foundation have started to organize some courses on AD.

There is poor coordination of specialist medical and psychiatric services for demented patients. Recently, there has been an improvement in professional training for primary and social care staff and education of the public. They exchange personal experience and emotions and receive understanding, support and confirmation. They receive advice from each other and from the trained members of the Turkish Alzheimer's Foundation on how to handle the problematic situations they encounter.

We have caregiver support groups in Istanbul, Ankara and Izmir. But voluntary organization for demented patients is insufficient. Caregivers receive information about dementia and about professional help they can call in. We need obligatory involvement of the independent sector in planning service development, training and quality assurance programmes. The private sector is not involved in specific service development for demented patients. We need specialist day centres to care for dementia sufferers. The private sector of care has grown to fill great gaps left by the public services; nursing services and live-in help has already begun in the big cities. The organizations which provide private help at home should be inspected in order to protect the vulnerable demented clients and their relatives.

In summary, the system in Turkey has not engaged voluntary groups, community organizations and other members of the local community in its activities. There are no district nurses who have special training and responsibility in carrying out nursing tasks in the patient's own home. There are no social workers who have specific roles in arranging admission to residential homes and who may be responsible for community care assessment and management. On the other hand, we have no health visitors who are planned to find cases of dementia, to assist in diagnosis by getting background information, to plan services and to support families. We have no social workers concerned with the care of the elderly.

We need trained community psychiatric nurses who can be involved in identifying the specific problems of demented patients and offer psychiatric nursing advice on management. There is a lack of practice nurses to be involved in specific nursing tasks such as dealing with incontinence, dressing, supervision of medicines or injections. There are not enough home helps who are being trained and given responsibilities for demented people and their problems. We have some volunteer helpers who are involved with the care of patients and with the support of relatives. The Alzheimer Foundation is trying to extend voluntary services for demented patients. We have a helpline that offers a 24-hour service organized by the Turkish Alzheimer Foundation. In particular, in the hospital of medical schools in the big cities, there are few geriatric services which look after demented patients if they have a major medical problem or need physical nursing care, but they cannot cope with patients who have some psychological and behavioural symptoms. They usually ask for a consultation from general psychiatrists. There is only one inpatient old age psychiatry department, which is run by our medical staff and ourselves in Istanbul. There is a good liaison between our old age psychiatry and geriatric service, which are sited in the same hospital. This good liaison eases transfer of patients between the two services and reduces misplacement.

References

Directorate of Population Registry. Data obtained from www.nvi.gov.tr, the website of the Directorate of Population Registry, Turkey, presented by Turan Ertan at the 11th Congress of the IPA, Chicago, USA; 2003.

Directorate of Social Services and Child Protection. Data obtained from www.shcek.gov.tr, the website of the Directorate of Social Services and Child Protection, Turkey, presented by Turan Ertan at the 11th Congress of the IPA, Chicago, USA; 2003.

Eker E. Services for elderly care in Turkey, oral presentation. 7th IPA Congress, Sydney, Australia; 1995.

chapter 16

The practice of dementia care: Belgium

Peter Paul De Deyn, Sebastiaan Engelborghs and Guy Nagels

Epidemiology of dementia in Belgium

Epidemiological studies on dementia in Belgium are rather scanty. Roelands et al (1994) studied a sample of 1736 community-dwelling individuals aged between 65 and 85 years old. Participants were screened with the Mini Mental State Examination (MMSE) and then subjected to a diagnostic process involving the CAMDEX and DSM III criteria. The prevalence of dementia in these populations was estimated at 9%. Age-specific prevalence was 0.6% for 65–69 year olds, 5.1% for 70–74 year olds, 7.6% for 75–79 year olds, 16.2% for 80–84 year olds and 33.6% in the elderly (over 85 years old). The ANCOG study is the only Belgian study evaluating prevalence as well as incidence of dementia in an elderly population (aged 75–80 years old) living in Antwerp (De Deyn et al, 2003). Prevalence of dementia in this community-dwelling population for the city of Antwerp was 9.6%, with a yearly incidence of 4%, as observed during a 4-year follow-up. The Belgian NADES study reported an estimated prevalence of 17.2% for the total population of individuals over 65 years old (Kurz et al, 1999; Scuvee-Moreau et al, 2002). Based on the available epidemiological data and on the demographic evolution as reported by the National Institute for Statistics, there will be approximately 175 000 individuals suffering from dementia in Belgium in 2010.

Facilities for patients with dementia in Belgium

Extramural facilities
Domestic care facilities aim to keep the patient as long as possible in the domiciliary environment by preserving or stimulating self-care and by providing (individualized) care facilities. Domestic care facilities include both structured (paid) supplies and volunteer aid.

Domestic care facilities for dementia are mainly provided by volunteers (spouse, children and other relatives), primary care physicians, medical specialists and home nurses. Among medical specialists, mainly neurologists, psychiatrists and geriatricians play a role in domestic care for dementia patients by making correct diagnosis, coaching multidisciplinary care and establishing optimal (pharmacological) treatment for dementia. Medical specialists can be consulted in private practices or in specialized care facilities such as memory clinics. The role of home nurses is not confined to nursing and caring tasks, but also involves counselling, monitoring of treatments and psychosocial coaching of the patient and family and volunteer carers. Occupational, physical and speech therapists also play a role in domestic caring.

Some of the home-care facilities are provided by services and networks for domestic caring, which are community-driven or private initiatives. Nurses, nurse aids, social workers and geriatric assistants provide domestic help, nursing and caring tasks as well as psychosocial coaching and counselling, thus preserving or stimulating self-care and providing (individualized) care facilities. These home-care facility networks often include a service for distribution of meals. Several organizations such as local service centres and health insurance companies provide a kind of elderly-minding service that aims to relieve the patient's family or volunteer aid and to help the patients in their activities of daily living.

Many districts have local service centres that are major constituents of the network for domestic caring. These local service centres provide a variety of services to local senior citizens that should allow them to preserve their autonomy and integration in society. They also organize recreational or educational events and meetings for both patients and caregivers.

In 1982, a new model for local healthcare was introduced in Belgium. All healthcare workers (primary care physicians, nurses and physical therapists) involved receive a fixed fee, based on the number of patients they are taking care off. This form of local health care is provided through regional centres and is free for patients, thus ensuring an easily accessible first-line healthcare system. Outpatients with psychological problems can seek help in regional centres for mental health where care is provided by a multidisciplinary team of psychiatrists, psychologists, occupational therapists and nurses.

Intramural facilities
Temporary intramural facilities

Some hospital wards are specifically intended for elderly and/or dementia patients. Geriatric inpatient wards (so-called G wards) are meant for elderly patients with severe disorders such as dementia that require specialized care. An active treatment is established in order to keep the duration of hospitalization as short as possible. The mean age of the hospitalized patients should be 75 years old and the maximal hospitalization term should not exceed 3 months. Medical care is provided under the supervision of a specialist in internal medicine/geriatrics. Furthermore, the multidisciplinary team consists of nurses and nurse aids, physical therapists, occupational therapists and sometimes psychologists.

Some psychogeriatric wards and specialized hospital wards offer specialized care for dementia patients (so-called SP wards). These wards are not confined to the elderly and patients with various disorders that affect all age categories can be hospitalized in this type of ward. In 1999, the number of beds in SP wards was 3150 (Flanders and Brussels). Furthermore, some specific geriatric institutions exist that consist of both G and SP wards.

Several day-care centres are provided by nursing homes and memory clinics and are confined to the elderly patient with and without dementia; they offer social/recreational and/or therapeutic activities (cognitive rehabilitation, psychotherapy, physical and occupational therapy). The number of patients that are able to benefit from day-care centres is limited by logistics (transport to and from the day-care centres) and by financial factors (reimbursement). Some nursing homes also provide night-care or short-stay facilities for the elderly with and without dementia; these facilities are provided for patients with acute needs or when volunteer aid is temporarily not sufficient or is unavailable.

Permanent intramural facilities

Nursing homes form the majority of institutions offering permanent inpatient facilities. Most nursing homes accept elderly patients with dementia and some even have specialized wards. Nursing homes are confined to patients with chronic disorders who need nursing or paramedical care as well as help with the activities of daily living. These institutions do not provide specialized medical care, and medical follow-up is offered by personal or institutional primary care physicians.

Psychiatric nursing homes are confined to patients with chronic but stabilized psychic disorders. Although dementia cannot be considered a stabilized psychic disorder, psychogeriatric patients form the majority of inpatients in such institutions.

Service flats offer individual residential facilities where the still-independent elderly can take benefit from a limited number of paid facilities such as meals, some nursing facilities and recreational activities. Only patients with a mild dementia or dementia patients and their spouses are eligible for service flats.

Memory clinics

The first Belgian memory clinic, the Memory Clinic of the OCMW Antwerp (MCA) was established in 1990, and has experienced a continual growth as a multidisciplinary functional unit ever since. Presently, more than 1000 new memory patients/year are examined, and supported regardless of age and aetiology. The objectives and functions, as well as the composition of the multidisciplinary MCA team, are representative of modern memory clinics. The objectives, tasks and functions of the MCA are shown in Table 16.1 (Pickut et al, 2000). Memory patients are referred by general practitioners, specialists, patient associations or by self-referral (patient and/or environment). The MCA has an ambulatory, polyclinical and intramural infrastructure as well as a day-care clinic and facilities for cognitive rehabilitation. It forms an interface between extra- and intramural care.

Medicinal treatment of dementia: Reimbursement in Belgium

In Belgium, cholinesterase inhibitors (donepezil, rivastigmine and galantamine) and the glutamatergic antagonist memantine are reimbursed under strict conditions. First, diagnosis of Alzheimer's disease (AD) should be established by a neurologist, psychiatrist or geriatrician according to the DSM IV criteria. Secondly, a cerebral infarction should have been excluded by computed tomography (CT) or magnetic resonance imaging (MRI). Thirdly, patients should have mild to moderate AD (MMSE 12–24 and, in case of a MMSE score >24, confirmation of diagnosis by ADAS-cog or CAMDEX), in case of reimbursement of cholinesterase inhibitors, or moderate to severe AD (MMSE <15 and >3), in case of reimbursement of memantine. Moreover, functional evaluation ((instrumental) activities of daily living) and behavioural assessment (NPI) should be performed and a multidisciplinary structure of care should be set up before a request for reimbursement can

Table 16.1 Objectives and activities of the Memory Clinic, Middelheim Antwerp

- Adjust service to memory patients, regardless of age and cause of the disease
- Multidisciplinary approach
- Intra- and extramural health care
- Hospitalization, polyclinic, day-room
- (Early) diagnosis of memory problems
- Treatment
- Medicinal and non-medicinal – rehabilitation, etc.
- Possibility for crisis intervention
- Short-term admission, 24-hour permanency
- Follow-up
- Social and psychological support
- Education of patients: familial and professional caregivers and physicians
- Sensibilization of general public and professionals
- Training of patients and family
- Scientific research
- Diagnostics (imaging, neuropsychological testing)
- Pathophysiological
- Epidemiological
- Therapeutical

eventually be granted. In Belgium, *Ginkgo Biloba* is reimbursed under the same conditions as the cholinesterase inhibitors.

Until today, cognitive rehabilitation is not reimbursed in Belgium and specific multidisciplinary teams have not yet been recognized or funded. We hope that the near future will bring changes in this situation.

Ethical and legal issues in dementia

In this short section, we refer to a couple of ethical and legal issues that may have been dealt with in Belgium in a manner slightly different from other European countries.

People suffering from dementia will of course at a certain time face difficulties in managing their assets. Under Belgian law, a patient who is still will-capable can bestow an *authorization*, granting someone else the right to take actions with his or her material goods. If this authorization covers property –

e.g. when the person holding the authorization has to be able to let the patient's house – the authorization should be formalized by a notary. When the patient becomes will-incompetent, use of the authorization becomes a violation.

Patients suffering from cognitive deterioration can be protected under the law of 18 July 1991. Under this law, the justice of the peace can appoint a *guardian* or 'voorlopig bewindvoerder', who is responsible for the financial affairs of the person put under protection. The request can be put to the justice of the peace by the district attorney, or by any concerned person. A medical statement, describing the health state of the person to be put under protection, has to be added to the request. This system has been in effect for a number of years. Since the law of 3 May 2003, people have the right to choose their guardian in advance. They can do this by deposing a statement with the justice of the peace of their place of residence, or with a notary. This deposition is added to a central register, which is kept by the Federation of Notaries. The justice of the peace can still appoint another guardian, but only if he has sound reasons to do this. Personnel of the institution in which the patient resides can never be appointed as guardian. The guardian has to take care that sufficient funds remain available to care for the protected person but does not make medical decisions for his ward.

The *spouse* of a demented patient can face specific legal problems. Under Belgian law, the consent of both partners is needed for actions such as selling property or signing a lease. The court (eerste aanleg) can grant the marriage partner of a demented patient the right to take these decisions without the consent of his or her spouse.

Dementia and driving

People suffering from a neurological disease which might influence driving ability are required to turn in their driver's licence until they receive positive advice from the Belgian Institute for Traffic Safety (CARA, law of 27 March 1998). The treating physician is required to inform the patient about this law, but is not required or even allowed to report the patient to CARA. CARA can grant unconditional permission to drive, or impose restrictions like the restriction to drive after dark or the restriction to drive within a certain distance from the patient's home. CARA's permissions are generally valid for 1–3 years.

Participation in clinical research

The Belgian Order of Physicians formulated an opinion (20 June 1998, tijd-schrift van de orde van geneesheren, p7) on informed consent in 'confused patients'. They were requested to do so by the secretary general of the Belgian Society for Gerontology and Geriatrics. The Order feels that the care-taker of a will-incapable patient usually does not have sufficient juridical qualifications to represent the patient, but that the caretaker's consent is a deontological requirement for inclusion into a trial. The Order also refers to the legal guardian which might have been appointed, although this guardian strictly speaking is not appointed to take medical decisions. Legal experts are clear on the fact that the guardian appointed by the justice of the peace is not empowered to take medical or other decisions about the patient but only about his material assets. Under current law, for instance, the guardian cannot decide to place the patient in an institution if he or she does not agree to be put there. The guardian is not a proxy-decider, and the justice of the peace cannot appoint him in that capacity.

The Order of Physicians feels that the legal or acting guardian should seek the advice of a physician who is not connected to the trial. It is interesting to note that the Order does not differentiate between clinical trials with and without possible therapeutic benefit.

The Belgian Advisory Committee for Bioethics formulated an opinion (No. 14, 10 December 2001) concerning 'ethical rules towards persons suffering from dementia'. The Committee pleads for an urgent legal con-struction, allowing for the appointment of legal representatives for people suffering from dementia: these representatives would be able to take medical decisions for the will-unable patient. The justice of the peace should be able to appoint the representative, providing that the patient chooses someone for this task when he or she is still able to do so. The representative might also decide whether the patient could take part in medical experiments with possible therapeutic benefit. The Committee remained divided on the question of medical experiments without possible therapeutic benefit.

Physical restraints

Patients suffering from dementia are sometimes restrained because of dis-ruptive or destructive behaviour. These restraining techniques pose a legal problem. Medical personnel sometimes resort to restraining techniques because this makes them feel safe concerning their responsibilities towards their patient. This does not appear to be the case in Belgium. The Court of Appeal in Ghent ruled that nurses were responsible for wounds a patient suffered while removing her restraints (Verrijcken, 2002).

End-of-life decisions

The Belgian Advisory Committee for Bioethics states in its Opinion No. 14 on ethical rules towards persons suffering from dementia that it would be absurd to employ important treatments to elongate the life of a severely demented person who has completely lost his or her autonomy.

Life-terminating interventions on incompetent patients remains a subject for debate in Belgium. An advice on the termination of life of incompetent patients was formulated by the Belgian Advisory Committee for Bioethics on 22 February 1999. This advice does not concern the withholding or with-drawing of futile treatment, but deals with active interventions to terminate life carried out by a physician on a patient who is incapable of making his or her wishes known. Several situations can arise. If the patient has made his or her wishes known by writing, an advance directive before the onset of incompetence, legal recognition of life termination should be possible. The physician can assess the opportunity for this together with a representative of the patient, or with the advance directive (Strubbe, 2000).

The first advice of the Belgian Advisory Committee for Bioethics was 'on the desirability of a legal framework for euthanasia'. It was published on 12 May 1997. Years of debate followed. Research showed that in spite of the strict Belgian law, medical intervention with the explicit intention of ending the patient's life were already taking place (Deliens et al, 2000).

On 28 May 2002, a law on euthanasia was approved by the Belgian par-liament, with 86 votes for 51 against, with 10 abstentions. An English trans-lation of the law has been published ('The Belgian act on euthanasia of May, 28th 2002'. *Eur J Health Law* 2003; 10(3): 329–35). The law was voted after years of debate (Deliens and van der Wal, 2003; Weber, 2001). It contains a procedure for non-terminally ill patients and for unconscious patients from whom a written advance directive is available, but not for conscious demented patients: the patient should suffer unbearably, and the clinical course should be hopeless. The law was contested by political and other groups. The 'pro vita' movement appealed to a high administrative court (the arbitragehof) to annul the law. One of the arguments for this appeal was directed towards Article 4 of the law, which gives capable people the right to formulate a written advance directive, which makes it possible for the treating physician, under a number of conditions, to practise euthanasia should they become unconscious, affected by a serious, irreversible and incurable illness. The appellants referred to Article 2 of the European Convention on Human Rights. On 14 January 2004, the court decided to reject the appeal. The court felt that 'pro vita' assumed that people asking for life-terminating actions are, per definition, mentally incapable, and that the law offers sufficient guarantees that patients should ask for euthanasia out of their own free will.

This law does not apply to patients suffering from dementia. Few patients suffering from a mild dementia will request euthanasia in a phase in which they are mentally competent. If they would ask for euthanasia in this stage, the criterion of unbearable suffering, stipulated in the law, is probably not met. The second scenario described in the law, where a patient can draw up an advance directive, is also not applicable, because the physician can only perform legal euthanasia based on an advance directive if the patient is in an irreversible unconscious state.

Because an important number of people want the right to take their own decisions concerning the end of their life, even or especially in case they become mentally incompetent, society needs to continue the debate on assisted suicide and euthanasia in dementia. This debate is presently ongoing in Belgium.

References

De Deyn PP, Goeman J, Dourcy-Belle-Rose B, Steppe A. De Antwerpse congnitie studie (ANCOG): prevalentie en incidentie van dementie bij een oudere bevolkingspopulatie. *Intern OCMW Rapport* 2003.

Deliens L, Mortier F, Bilsen J, et al. End-of-life decisions in medical practice in Flanders, Belgium: A nationwide survey. *Lancet* 2000; 356:1806–11.

Deliens L, van der Wal G. The euthanasia law in Belgium and the Netherlands. *Lancet* 2003; 362: 1239–40.

Kurz X, Broers M, Scuvée-Moreau J, et al. Methodological issues in a cost-of-dementia study in Belgium: The National Dementia Economic Study (NADES). *Acta Neurolog Belg* 1999; 99: 167–75.

Pickut BA, Verstraeten S, De Deyn PP. De geheugenkliniek: veelvuldige opdrachten waaronder een correcte diagnostiek van dementie. *Antene* 2000; 18: 5–8.

Roelands M, Wostyn P, Dom H, Baro F. The prevalence of dementia in Belgium: A population-based door-to-door survey in a rural community. *Neuroepidemiology* 1994; 13: 155–61.

Scuvee-Moreau J, Kurz X, Dresse A. National Dementia Economic Study Group. The economic impact of dementia in Belgium: Results of the National Dementia Economic Study (NADES). *Acta Neurol Belg* 2002; 102: 104–13.

Strubbe E. Toward legal recognition for termination of life without request? Remarks on Advice No. 9 of the Belgian Advisory Committee on Bioethics concerning termination of life of incompetent patients. *Eur J Health Law* 2000; 7(1): 57–71.

Weber W. Belgian euthanasia proposal meets resistance. *Lancet* 2001; 358:1168.

Verrychen M. (2002) De juridische bescherming van de feitelik onbekwamen. In: Scheiris J, Thiery E, De Deyn PP. Van Hove H (Eds.) *Gehengenstoornissen: revalidatie en psychosociale zorg.* 2003; Leuven: Acco.

chapter 17

The practice of dementia care: Sweden

Sture Eriksson

Dementia care in Sweden has been in the public focus for several years. There are a large number of media reports of how elderly people with dementia are treated less well, especially in various forms of nursing homes and group-living environments. Often the focus is on patients where a fracture has not been detected early enough, or patients staying in their beds during the whole day, locked in and not permitted to see sunshine, or how the food is too sparse and not well prepared, or how terrible it is that patients have chronic ulcers, and so on. The media are looking for simple solutions: common explanations are lack of staff or uneducated staff, and often managers are blamed for deficiencies in care. In some instances, local politicians are held responsible by the media, but often they blame the staff and are actively looking for scapegoats. On the other hand, there are also some happier stories, often presenting a fairly healthy elderly person living alone in a nice apartment, often after having been 'saved' from an institution or being treated with some new anti-dementia drug.

Is this a true picture? The answer is, as expected, both yes and no. Naturally, there are patients who are in bad conditions, in bad care situations where staff numbers and education may be insufficient, but from my point of view, seeing a large number of patients in various settings, most of the patients with dementia are taken care of in care settings that meet high standards.

But in a wider sense, what is the standard of dementia care in Sweden? There is no simple answer, but in this chapter I will present some aspects of dementia care in Sweden that can serve as indicators of the standard of care.

First, I will give some examples of general and national trends. Dementia care today and in the future is on the public agenda in Sweden. Media, central governmental organizations and a number of local organizations are active in this field. Examples of this are a recent work task force within

Ministry of Health and Social Affairs, who published a comprehensive review of present and future dementia care in Sweden (Ministry of Health and Social Affairs, 2003). Furthermore, SBU (The Swedish Council of Technology Assessment in Health Care) has a large project running that is intended to establish Swedish guidelines for evidence-based dementia care. Another indicator of standards of dementia care is the comprehensive Swedish research on very different aspects of dementia, from genetics to epidemiology, which also includes nursing sciences and a large number of intervention trials in dementia. It is not possible to review the research in this context, but it is of general interest to note that, recently, an official funding initiative (the Swedish brain power project) was launched providing research funds of 20 million SEK yearly for 5 years that is intended to develop early diagnosis and intervention in dementia. This project also seeks to increase the cooperation both between different research fields and between research groups and other parts of dementia care such as local authorities and the pharmaceutical industry.

Most basic dementia care is locally based and includes care in the family and by local authorities. When family support is insufficient, the local authorities have the responsibility of providing basic care. This can include social support in the home, day care, relief care and various forms of sheltered living such as group living, home-for-the aged and general nursing homes and homes for patients with severe BPSD (behavioural and psychological symptoms of dementia). The legal base for this service is the general social service support This also includes medical care, but only medical care *not* provided by physicians. The forms of care are also, to a various extent, supported by primary care and psychogeriatric specialist care. In some areas, for example Umeå, there are also specialist teams that support the BPSD care in both the home and local authorities settings.

Does this system of support provide enough support for those suffering from dementia? There is no national survey addressing this question exactly, but a recent national survey (National Board of Health and Social Welfare, 2003) on the correspondence between authorities' estimation and decision on need of support and provided support indicated that 4200 persons did not receive this form of social support even if they had the need and a formal decision to provide support. In 200 other cases, there was a decision not to give support even if the local authorities had found that a need was present. This number may seem high, but it is small in relation to all decisions taken (about 360 000 yearly) and thus may indicate that the vast majority of people are provided with sufficient support.

Another question is: if all these decisions are of good quality, do they meet a good standard? There a no known systematic follow-up of all these decisions, but some remarks can be made. An elected board (Sw 'Socialnämnden') of local politicians is responsible for each individual decision concerning the provided social support, including the setting for care (e.g. between home care, sheltered living or a nursing home). However, as a rule, these decisions are delegated to one person, who can take the decision on behalf of the political board. There are no formal regulations for qualifications of this person and, thus, knowledge of dementia care is not requested. Furthermore, these people are requested to do an investigation of the need of care as a basis for the decision. Naturally, this system gives some concerns about the quality of the service provided. Are the investigations done professionally? Are medical treatments provided in an appropriate way? Are the services provided, the most cost-efficient? Are they open to irrelevant argumentation, such as demands from angry family members? Are the services provided to those in most need of the service?

Other aspects of dementia care concern the diagnostic and treatment processes. What are the standards of early diagnostics, early intervention and follow-up during the progress of the diseases? There is a general, but not formalized, policy that every patient with cognitive decline should be investigated and, if appropriate, also treated. One estimate (Ministry of Health and Social Affairs, 2003) is that about one-third of people with Alzheimer's disease (AD) are treated with acetylcholinesterase inhibitors. This estimate is based on prescription data in relation to the estimated prevalence of AD in Sweden and, even if there is a large geographic variation in treatment policy, it is a fairly high proportion as regards both investigation and treatment. There is also a great variation in investigation policy between the different settings, such as university clinics and primary care, but the basic standard is fairly similar. It includes medical history, physical investigation, laboratory screening, a simple cognitive assessment such as mini mental state examination (MMSE) and the clock test and brain imaging such as computed tomography (CT), single-proton emission computed tomography (SPECT) or magnetic resonance imaging (MRI). Some centres use analysis of spinal fluid as a routine investigation. Specialized centres normally use a more comprehensive programme that includes neuropsychological, nursing, social and occupational assessments.

Support for the clinical management of dementia education is often regarded as a cornerstone of treatment. One interesting example of the Swedish educational approach is a CD-ROM-based educational package

(Eriksson, 2003), which has been used to train more than 10 000 persons, mainly primary care professionals, during the last years.

The policy for diagnosis and intervention in BPSD is not so well thought out. Only a few hospitals have a profiled organization for specialist management of BPSD and, thus, most BPSD is handled in the various dementia care settings. Thére are examples of well-functioning long-term care settings for severe BPSD, but they are few. A policy document on BPSD with a Scandinavian emphasis has been published and may have had some impact on Swedish BPSD care (Eriksson, 2000).

To conclude, my view is that, in general, Swedish dementia care is of a high standard. The comprehensive Swedish research in this field is also an important factor for the clinical praxis. Even if there are some obvious flaws, the intentions for improvement of Swedish dementia care are good and will in the future lead to further improvement of the situation.

References

Eriksson S. *Behavioural and psychological symptoms in dementia: a state-of-the-art document*. Göteborg: Janssen-Cilag AB; 2000.

Eriksson S. *Novartis Interaktiva forbildning demens*. Stockholm: Novartis AB; 2003.

Ministry of Health and Social Affairs. På väg mot en god demensvård. (*Report No. Ds 2003: 47*). Stockholm: Ministry of Health and Social Affairs; 2003.

National Board of Health and Social Welfare. *Ej verkställda domar och beslut enligt LSS and SoL 2003*. Stockholm: The National Board of Health and Social Welfare; 2004.

chapter 18

The practice of dementia care: Ukraine

Pinchuk Irina

'Do not leave me in old age,
Do not leave me weakened . . .'

Demography of Ukraine

Ukraine today may be referred to as a demographically old nation. The principle of three fives operates in Ukraine at present:

- every fifth inhabitant of Ukraine is a person of advanced age
- every fifth person of advanced age lives alone
- every fifth person of advanced age living alone has lost the ability to look after themselves and requires help and care.

Ukraine ranks 11th in the world in terms of population, but according to official statistics it is among the world's leaders in the number of elderly people, due to a substantial fall in the natural increase of the population.

Table 18.1 reflects the demographic tendencies in Ukraine as regards birth rate, mortality rate and natural increase/decrease of population per 1000 of population.

Table 18.1 Demography of Ukraine.

	Demographic data			
	1985	1990	1995	2000
Birth rate	15.0	12.7	9.6	7.8
Mortality rate	12.1	12.1	15.4	15.3
Natural increase/decrease of population	2.9	0.6	−5.8	−7.5

As can be seen from the table, annual birth rates have fallen since mid 1985. The birth rate declined from 15 live births per 1000 population in 1985 to 7.8 in 2000. The main reason for the sharp drop in the birth rate is associated with the social and economic conditions in the country. As a result of the drop of the birth rate, there was a substantial fall in the natural increase of population, since the mortality rate remained more or less stable at about 12–15 per 1000 population. Thus, the country has a high percentage of an ageing population.

The number of people of advanced age has already exceeded the number of children. Moreover, by 2050 the number of people over 60 years old is predicted to be three times the number of children under 15.

The growth of the ageing population inevitably results in the growth of age-related diseases such as dementia. As the frequency and prevalence of mental disorders is higher with age, the elderly require more psychiatric help. The changes taking place in Ukraine since its sovereignty was proclaimed in 1991 adversely negatively affected the mental state of the elderly. In addition, the dramatic changes in both social and economic life of Ukraine have greatly changed the role of the older generation. In general, moral values have also undergone considerable changes in society, particularly those of their offspring.

Many requirements of a medical, social and psychological nature require the development and introduction of complex nation-wide systems of medical aid and social services to elderly people through structural reorganization of public health services.

Until recently, there has been no uniform coordinated system of medical aid and social services for elderly people in Ukraine. The problems facing Ukraine in the field of organization of such a system differ greatly from those facing other European countries not in their character but in establishing priorities, considering the material means and financial resources needed to tackle the problems.

Owing to a critical shortage of the means for public health services and social protection under new economic conditions, the problem of creating a state system of geriatric help has become extremely difficult. On the one hand, it is the elderly who are least protected, both socially and financially; on the other hand, there is neither operative information support nor systematic work in geriatric services development.

According to statistics, 29% of the urban and 54% of the rural population over the age of 70 living alone do not require outside help. By contrast, 43.1% of the urban and 36.6% of the rural population need the public services to be provided as close to their home as possible; they also want social workers to help them fulfil domestic chores.

It should be noted that only 68.6% of the people over 70 years old, requiring social assistance, are provided with state-maintained medical aid and services; the others are taken care of by their nearest relatives – spouses, children or other people. Ten per cent of those under guardianship of the state social services are taken care of on condition of inheritance of their houses and flats.

The number of people requiring social help on the part of the state structures varies from 14.8 to 37.9% depending on their place of residence.

As they advance in years, the number of elderly people enjoying medical aid, chiefly at home, is growing. Home medical help is provided for the very old, those living in bad conditions, and those who are lonely. The rural population is much less served with medical aid at home compared with the urban population and doctors visit rural patients less often as in towns and cities.

According to official statistical data, mental disorders occupy 7th place among the causes leading to disability of the elderly: 11% of elderly people over 60 years old and 20% of those over 80 can't do without qualified psychiatric help. Half of the patients receiving long-term psychiatric treatment are over 65 years old; they constitute approximately one-fifth of all the patients taken into psychiatric hospital for the first time.

The number of patients suffering from chronic diseases such as dementia is growing, while the resources (both family and state) necessary to fight the most serious cases of it remain extremely limited.

In Ukraine early forms of dementia are not regarded as negatively affecting a patient's and his family's life. Cognitive deficiency characteristic of old age is regarded as typical for the elderly. On the contrary, more serious cases cause much graver problems, due to a limited choice of services available for the relatives of dementia patients. As a rule, they cannot afford to employ a person to take care of the chronic patient; specialized institutions such as old people's homes are rather scarce in the country.

Case study

Mrs M was widowed when she was still young. She didn't try getting married again. She devoted all her life to her only daughter. Later she got an economics education, got married and gave birth to a son. All of them, Mrs M and her daughter's family, lived in Mrs M's two-room apartment, Mrs M constantly giving a helping hand in running the house and bringing up her grandson. Her daughter thought her mother's help valuable. One day, Mrs M went shopping to the market and had much difficulty in finding her house on the way back. That incident made her daughter excited and watchful. That evening, Mrs M's mental state underwent a radical change. It was for the first time in her life that she was disturbed, restless; she saw some strangers in her room and asked her daughter to make them go away. The following day her daughter called for the local doctor, who recommended her to go to a neurologist. Mrs M's state gradually changed after a year's treatment. Among the most evident symptoms were helplessness, weakening memory and infantility. She could no longer run the house and bring up her grandson. All of these symptoms cautioned the family against the threatening danger: Mrs M would turn gas or water taps on and forget to turn them off. In addition, the boy refused to stay with his grandmother, saying that he was scared. He cried and got nervous. Mrs M's daughter was recommended to refer to a psychiatrist for help. The latter offered to take Mrs M to a psychiatric hospital. Later, after being discharged from hospital, she returned home, having spent 1 month there. She was silent, quiet and even more helpless than before. It took her much effort to find her bearing in the flat. She could no longer attend to her household duties. She spent all her time sitting quietly in her room. She was in this state for 6 months. Her daughter and son-in-law could do nothing but leave her alone in her room. Her grandson took care of her after coming back from school, his mother calling several times during the day to enquire how things were.

Soon, Mrs M's condition changed sharply for the worse. She became irritable, aggressive and capricious. Her daughter referred to the psychiatrist again. As a result, Mrs M found herself in the psychiatric clinic again.

The treatment lasted for 2 months and caused Mrs M indigestion and insomnia. She lost much weight and her rehabilitation potential decreased sharply. She could not do more without help and required an outside help. Sometimes, she did not even recognize her relatives. Her case was diagnosed as Alzheimer's disease, and she was recommended to be taken care of at home as she did not need active psychiatric treatment. Back home from hospital, she became a great burden for her family. They could not leave her at home alone. Her daughter applied for help to social services, but she was refused. They could not give her a nurse, as according to the law in force, only lonely elderly patients were given social help. Moreover, the law forbids taking patients with mental disorders under the trusteeship of social services. Mrs M's daughter applied for help for private care. The price of their services exceeded her salary three times. She took a month's holiday to take care of her mother. But when the holiday was over, the problem remained unsolved. Mrs M's state grew even worse: she did not recognize her daughter, stayed in bed all the time, was restless and did not have a good night's sleep. The daughter tried to have her mother taken to hospital again, but the mother was refused hospitalization; instead, she was offered consultancy at home in case of emergency.

In the face of these irreparable problems, the daughter's mental state also changed a lot: she was gloomy and depressed and often cried. Now she sometimes got angry with her mother; then she was repentant, and regretted her behaviour. Family life also underwent much change: they constantly quarreled and evidently she suffered a nervous breakdown. The husband complained of being neglected. Their 9-year-old son witnessing these conflicts made the situation still worse. The daughter had to find a more highly paid job to pay for a sitter — an elderly woman, living next door, who asked a reasonable price for her services.

Caring for the elderly

It is the problem of children's health that Ukraine focuses its efforts and money on. The health of adolescents is also paid due attention. But neither effort nor money is left for the elderly whose problems have coincided with a general reduction in public health services. Being old in Ukraine today attracts stigma, and having mental diseases is a double stigma: 40% of the people over 70 years old living in the Donetsk region, one of the largest and industrially developed areas in Ukraine, commit suicide.

According to the law, children are obliged to take care of their elderly parents. The problem of dementia is not regarded as serious, both on the part of the state and/or of society. Families consider it to be a characteristic of old age. There are no specialists in gerontopsychiatry in Ukraine. Elderly people with mental troubles have to apply for help to psychiatrists who have no special training in geriatrics. Moreover, there are no training programmes in this specialty. Medical treatment is clinically oriented, the main task being to recognize the symptoms and diagnose the illness. In fact, diagnosing the illness is almost all the help the patient can hope for.

Other characteristics of the situation in Ukraine today are:

- attention is focused on heavier forms of the pathology (heavy dementia, acute and chronic psychoses)

- treatment is based on biological methods
- priority is given to in-hospital forms of treatment
- multidisciplinary forms of help and the system of professional training in this sphere are both absent
- the increase of the number of beds for gerontopsychiatry patients in psychiatric hospitals coincides with the lack of specially trained staff.

To complete the picture, there is long-term treatment of elderly dementia patients in hospitals and insufficient contact with the patient's relatives.

Elderly people suffering from mental disorders cannot be expected to be registered by the organs of social trusteeship, their illness being a counter-indication according to the law. However, they have tried to overcome this obstacle in Kiev. It was here where the first department of social in-home help to elderly patients with mental troubles was created in 1998. A total of 102 social workers render services to more than 3000 patients who are under home nursing. Unfortunately, it is the only department of its kind in Ukraine.

Non-state systems play the leading role in rendering assistance to the elderly, their children carrying the main burden of care and expenses. However, the significance of the problems undermining the families' ability to maintain their elderly parents is growing. First, a sharp drop in birth rates means that one or two children will have to carry the burden of keeping their parents and taking care of them. Secondly, the number of working women in Ukraine is constantly growing, leaving the family less opportunities of rendering informal help to the elderly with psychiatry disorders (for it is women who carry the main burden of care). Thirdly, the migration of the young people of villages to towns and cities in search of jobs/employment results in a growing number of lonely elderly people in the rural regions with nobody to take care of them. All these factors mean that the creation of a public system of help is a real must.

The official system in Ukraine does not meet the necessary requirements, both in the scope of the appropriate contingency and the quality of services given. There is a network of public old people's homes in Ukraine for dementia patients but the need for them far exceeds their number. On the one hand, private institutions are extremely scarce and their services are sky-high expensive; on the other hand, there are a lot of families in Ukraine living from hand to mouth who cannot afford to maintain their elderly relatives, the old men's meagre pensions being the main source of keeping their body and soul together.

Ukraine today can boast of a powerful voluntary movement but has no experience in dealing with patients with psychiatry disorders. There was an interesting initiative by the Gerontology Institute of the Ukrainian Academy of Medical Sciences. They proposed, and even tried themselves, to select and train military servicemen to take care of the elderly (both in hospitals and at home). This initiative hasn't been supported by state structures, however.

The main emphasis in Ukraine today is put on a complex approach to provide the elderly with services and caring which is less expensive and more effective than creating specialized gerontological services for the elderly with mental disorders. A complex service infers uniting all the efforts aimed at satisfying fully the needs of the elderly as regards both their mental and physical health. Patients of this age group are known to have a combination of different kinds of pathology. Almost every elderly patient applying for help to the psychiatrist suffers from some physical disease or diseases. Since elderly patients tend to complain of their physical state rather than their psychological one, measures aimed at treating mental diseases will prove to be more effective provided they are part and parcel of the existing system of general medical service.

Conclusions

1. The present state of provision of both medical and social services in Ukraine does not meet the real needs of the elderly population in general and of those with mental disorders in particular. This has a high social demographic cost – the increase in sickness and death rates and a sharp drop of life expectancy.
2. A critical reduction of financing public health services in general, giving priority to maternity and child protection, as well as to men and women of younger age, characterize the state policy of the Ukraine public health services today.
3. Gerontopsychiatry as a specialty does not exist in Ukraine. The medical curriculum places little emphasis on psychiatric pathology of the elderly and trainee doctors in psychiatry do not study the fundamentals of gerontology.
4. Elderly people with mental disorders are deprived of opportunities to enjoy benefit from social services.
5. There are no official statistical data on the prevalence of mental disorders in the elderly.

6. Certain constructive changes to help the elderly with mental disorders have been outlined lately, including:
   - programmes of training for family doctors specializing in the mental pathology of the elderly are being developed
   - scientific research in gerontopsychiatry is being carried out in medical higher educational establishments
   - gerontopsychiatric consulting rooms have been opened in medical establishments
   - drafts of documents on measures of rehabilitation of the above-mentioned category of patients have been prepared for the approval of the Ministry of Health
   - more information is being given on the mental pathology of old age.
7. The problem of creating psychiatric services in local social community centres is being considered to provide lonely patients suffering from mental disorders with appropriate help.

chapter 19

The practice of dementia care: Norway

Knut Engedal

The elderly population

Norway is a large country with a small population of 4.5 million inhabitants. Except for the major cities, the population tends to be sparse. The retirement age is 67 years old. In the year 2000, about 700 000 people were aged 65 years old and above, and 200 000 were 80 years old and above. Mean life expectancy is 75.5 years for men and 81.1 years for women (Central Bureau of Statistics, 2001).

The health and social care system

The public sector plays the major role in providing health and social care to the inhabitants of Norway, and has its foundations in the social democratic welfare state. Until recently, the public healthcare system had been the only option offering healthcare services in Norway, ideally according to the need and independent of economic status and place of residence. The private market for health and social care services is growing, but still plays a modest role. Norway has a three-tier system for the provision of public health and social care, based on

- The Municipal Health Care Act, The Social Care Act
- The Hospital Act
- The National Insurance Act.

The responsibility for the Norwegian specialist healthcare service is devolved in five regions, and the state is responsible. The municipalities, 435 in all, are responsible for the social and primary healthcare services that include the care for the elderly at home (home help and home nursing) and in institutions for the elderly (care homes, group-living arrangements and nursing homes). In 2004, about 45 000 people live in institutions for the elderly, provided by the municipalities. About 150 000 people receive some kind of home care, provided by the local authorities.

National Insurance covers most of social care and primary healthcare expenses. For services in the municipalities, the customer has to pay a rather little part (pocket money) of the costs connected to medical examination and treatment. The same principles are used for provision of social services. The home nursing services are entirely covered by the municipality. The cost connected to long-term care in nursing homes and other residential homes is on a sliding scale, depending of the patient's annual income, and will in no case exceed the income. In all Norwegian hospitals, the accommodation and treatment, including medicines, are free.

Care for persons with dementia

It is calculated that about 60 000 to 70 000 Norwegians suffer from dementia, and that the incidence rate/year is 10 000 (Engedal and Haugen, 1993). About 40% are cared for in various institutions for the elderly, which is a rather high proportion compared to other European countries (Engedal and Haugen, 1993).

The care for persons suffering from dementia includes diagnostic assessment, support and advice to the patients and their family caregivers, day-care programmes, respite care and residential care.

Diagnostic assessment
The diagnosis and treatment of dementia should ideally be done in the primary healthcare sector. It is the general view that the family physician and a primary care district nurse should cooperate in the assessment of patients with *moderate or severe degree* of dementia, corresponding to a mini mental state examination (MMSE) score of 23 or below. A substantial number of family doctors have the expertise to carry out a dementia assessment. The Norwegian Centre for Dementia Research, Service Development and Education has produced a standard diagnostic assessment programme, and offer educational courses to health personnel in primary care services (Engedal, 1997). However, there is still a long way to go before all GPs are experienced in this field (Braekhus and Engedal, 2002). In many municipalities nurses have special competence in the field of dementia and organize assessment of demented patients together with occupational therapists.

Specialist healthcare teams should ideally assess patients with suspected dementia or dementia of *mild degree*, corresponding to an MMSE score of 24 and above. This is done in memory clinics or specialist outpatient clinics organized in geriatric medicine or old age psychiatry. There are such specialist outpatient clinics in most of the 19 counties in Norway, and the service seems to work well all over the country, except for some districts with very sparse populations. Specialists in old age psychiatry assess patients with severe behavioural disturbances or severe psychiatric symptoms co-morbid with dementia. Departments of old age psychiatry or sections of old age psychiatry exist in 17 of the 19 counties, and accomplish this task. Specialists in neurology seldom take part in assessment of demented patients. Only the very young patients with suspected dementia or patients with symptoms indicating a subcortical dementia are referred to a neurologist.

It is difficult to know whether the provision of diagnostic services meets the needs. Some people with suspected dementia will not come to examination; some will come in a moderate or severe stage of dementia. In general, it can be said that both primary and specialist healthcare services offer diagnostic assessment to a larger group of patients today, than 10 years ago.

Support and advice to patients and caregivers

Some memory clinics run support groups for patients and family caregivers. However, support and advice to caregivers is in most cases a matter of the Norwegian Alzheimer Society, called 'Demensforeningen'. The Norwegian Health Organization, a charitable organization, organizes the Alzheimer Society of the country. The organization disseminates information about dementia to family carers through more than 120 local dementia clubs, and a nationwide information telephone service. They also publish a journal *Agenda*, with 4–6 issues a year, and run educational programmes for family caregivers (caregiver school) with support from professional healthcare personnel in some major cities.

Individuals with dementia, regardless of whether they live with a spouse or child, are offered home-care service according to their needs. This is a truth with modifications. Many of the social and healthcare workers in the home-care service system are without formal education and have sparse knowledge of dementia and the special needs of individuals who are cognitively impaired. The provision of service is, therefore, not optimal. New quality assurance systems that could possibly identify persons with dementia and their needs are being implemented.

Day care and respite care

Day-care programmes for demented patients exist in the major cities but not in the countryside, except for some development activities called 'green care'. Green care is a new way of activating demented people who used to live on farms. The centres are organized affiliated to a farm, and the farmer is involved in the activity programme. Normally, a day-care centre is affiliated to a nursing home, and there are two kinds of programmes. One programme is dedicated to the elderly in general, including people with a mild degree of dementia. These programmes have usually more than 20 attendees a day. The other programme is dedicated to demented people only, and in these day-care centres the number of attendees is small, about 6–8 a day. The day-care centres offer social activities, transportation and three meals (breakfast, warm lunch and a coffee break in the afternoon) a day. The elderly patient normally attends the centre twice a week, but some, especially severely demented patients, may visit the centre on a daily basis. The normal opening hours are from 9 a.m. to 4 p.m. from Monday to Friday (Engedal, 1989).

Respite-care service is provided in nursing homes. Every municipality in the country has one or more nursing homes, which means that all demented patients and their family caregivers have access to respite care.

Institutional care

The institutional care for people with dementia is provided in nursing homes in either regular or special care units, in group-living accommodation or in care homes dedicated to demented patients. As already stated, about 40% of all patients with dementia are cared for in such institutions. Normally, demented patients are admitted to institutional care in a severe stage of the condition, and the length of stay is 2–3 years (the time from admittance to death). The prevalence of dementia in nursing homes is about 75% (Engedal and Haugen, 1993). On average, 18% of the beds are organized as special care units for demented people (Eek and Nygaard, 1999). Thus, most demented patients live in a regular unit where the prevalence of dementia is still above 65%.

The target group for special care units (SCUs) comprises demented patients with disturbed behaviour, severe communication problems and patients with psychiatric symptoms or delirium. An SCU is a small home-like unit for about 6–10 patients, ideally 8. Every patient has his own room with a toilet, and shares a sitting room and a combined kitchen/dining room. Normally, the sitting room and kitchen are located in the middle of the ward (Figures 19.1

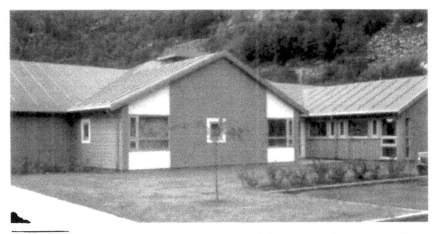

Figure 19.1 *The outside of a special care unit (SCU) for a person with dementia. This SCU is built in a small municipality on the west coast of Norway, and has been the model for other municipalities.*

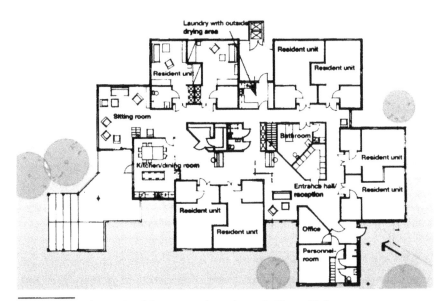

Figure 19.2 *The inside of the same unit as shown in Figure 19.1.*

and 19.2). The patients are offered social activities, and can work part in the kitchen. The SCUs are staffed a bit better than regular units in the nursing home, and normally staff are educated in dementia care.

Many municipalities have organized group-living accommodation for people with dementia. These are located outside the nursing home, often in a rebuilt villa. The group-living accommodations are in most cases organized as an SCU and offer the same services as an SCU in the nursing home.

In the last 5 years, a new kind of 'institution' for the elderly and elderly demented persons, called a care home, has been established. Actually, it is not an institution, but an organized way of giving home care to frail elderly people. When elderly people move to a care home, they have to pay a normal rent. The municipality offers all kinds of health and social services in the home. Some care homes are dedicated to people with dementia, and they are tailored to the disabled demented patients.

Measures that can improve the care for people with dementia

To support and educate social and health care personnel, the Norwegian Ministry of Social and Health Affairs decided in 1996 to give funding to a centre of excellence (knowledge) in the field of dementia. The Norwegian Centre for Dementia Research, Service Development and Education began to operate in 1997. In agreement with the Ministry, the Centre should develop new services to people suffering from dementia and their caregivers through research and experimental activities. This should be attained by an interaction between the development of new expertise and instruction and advice and guidance to the health sector. The Centre has four priority areas:

1. research and experimental activities towards a better health and social care service, including treatment for people suffering from dementia and their caregivers
2. advice and guidance to primary and specialist healthcare authorities regarding the development and evaluation of new care programmes
3. development and distribution of teaching materials
4. offering educational programmes in the field of dementia.

In 2004 the Centre is responsible for and runs 11 research projects with the aims of improving diagnostic assessment of dementia in primary care and treatment and support to family caregivers, developing new measures of home care and trying out technological assistive devices in the care of demented patients living at home. Advice and guidance are offered to local healthcare administrators in the municipalities, e.g. by building new institutions for demented patients or rebuilding of institutions, or by running educational programmes for health and social care personnel in the municipality. The Centre offers library services to health and social care personnel and caregivers from all over Norway. The home page (www.nordemens.no) is frequently used by the public, and for the time being, the Centre is developing distance learning programmes about dementia on the internet. The Centre publishes the periodical *DEMENTIA* with 4 issues a year, and 6–8 new publications a year, such as textbooks, reports and brochures. Some of the textbooks are for medical students and doctors, some are for nursing students and others for nurses' aids and social and health personnel with no formal education. In 2004, the Centre organized 23 conferences and courses about dementia for doctors, nurses, therapists, social workers and personnel without formal education. In addition, about 500 lectures were given to students at universities and colleges at graduate and postgraduate level.

Conclusions

Norway, as a welfare state, has established a variety of social and healthcare services to persons with dementia and their caregivers at specialist and primary healthcare level. A research, service development and education centre offers guidance and educational programmes to social and health personnel throughout the country. A charitable organization has organized the Alzheimer Society and runs more than 120 local clubs and a nationwide information telephone service. Healthcare professionals cooperate with the charitable organization in the education of family caregivers.

References

Brækhus A, Engedal K. Diagnostic work-up of dementia – a survey among Norwegian general practitioners. *Brain Aging* 2002; 4: 63–7.

Central Bureau of Statistics. *Statistical Yearbook 2001*. Oslo; 2001.

Eek A, Nygaard AM. Innsyn og utsyn. Tilbud til personer med demens i norske kommuner. *Sem: Nasjonalt kompetansesenter for aldersdemens* 1999.

Engedal K. Day-care for demented patients in general nursing homes: effects on admissions to institutions and mental capacity. *Scand J Prim Health Care* 1989; 7: 161–6.

Engedal K. Er det demens?. *Sem: Info-Banken* 1997 [In Norwegian].

Engedal K, Haugen PK. The prevalence of dementia in a sample of elderly Norwegians. *Int J Geriatr Psychiatry* 1993; 8: 565–70.

Multidisciplinary Working

chapter 20

Standard of care for dementia in nursing homes: The Dutch experience and views

Raymond TCM Koopmans

Introduction

The Dutch nursing home is a healthcare institution for most chronically ill people needing permanent medical and paramedical attention and complex nursing care, which is comparable to skilled nursing facilities in the United States (Hoek et al, 2000). It differs from nursing homes in other countries in that the staff includes specially trained nursing home physicians (1 full-time doctor per 100 patients), physical therapists, occupational therapists, speech therapists, pastoral workers, dietarians, psychologists, social workers and sometimes music therapists and psychomotor therapists, all of whom are employed by the nursing home (Hoek et al, 2000, 2001).

Dutch nursing home medicine consists of specific elements from various medical specialities, which are transformed and integrated to form an approach that best serves the characteristics of the patients in nursing homes (Hoek et al, 2001). The concepts of cure and care are uniquely balanced. Dutch nursing home medicine entails continuous, often long-term, systematic and multidisciplinary, problem-oriented medical care. An individual multidisciplinary care plan is made for every patient, usually based on the following domains: physical functioning, activities of daily living (ADL) and mobility, social functioning, psychological functioning and communication.

Treatment and care are mostly aimed at alleviating impairments and disabilities of diseases (e.g. dementia), in order to enhance or stabilize well-being and quality of life. In the multidisciplinary care plan problems, goals and treatment and care actions are formulated. Specific disciplines are involved in the care plan at the request of the nursing home physician. Care plans are evaluated in multidisciplinary team meetings at least twice a year, and more often if necessary. Patients and, in the case of dementia, family members have to give their consent to the care plan.

In my view, a specially trained nursing home physician is essential for good care for dementia patients in a nursing home. The nursing home physician should be skilled and competent in assessments, diagnostics, prognostics and interventions in dementia and has to be able to deal with complex medical–ethical dilemmas and moral problems.

Diagnostics and assessments

On admission to a nursing home, a full medical and neuropsychological investigation has to be carried out. A physical examination and laboratory testing should rule out treatable causes of dementia. The medication list should be screened for inappropriate medication (such as anticholinergics) and drugs with no indication should be discontinued. An attempt to discontinue psychotropics should always be made, because the nursing home environment is mostly more tolerant to behavioural problems and often specially designed (see below). Polypharmacy should be avoided, because of the adverse effects and interactions.

If the patient is admitted without a proper diagnosis of the type of dementia, the nursing home physician should establish the diagnosis based on all the information gathered, including neuropsychological testing and history-taking from relatives. The nursing home physician can use national consensus statements for diagnosing and should classify dementia according to international standards (e.g. National Institute of Neurological Disorders and Stroke/Alzheimer's Disease and Related Disorders Association (NINCDS-ARDRA) criteria for probable and possible Alzheimer's disease). One should be aware of the absence of diagnostic equipment such as computed tomography (CT) scanning in nursing homes. Therefore, one should be satisfied with the level of 'possible' diagnoses instead of 'probable' diagnoses.

I would advise the use of assessment scales on cognition, behaviour, functional status and quality of life. Assessments should take place at least when important treatment decisions have to be made. While dementia is progressing, one should shift from testing the patient to observational scales. Mini mental state examination (MMSE), cognitive screening test (CST) or, in the case of advanced dementia, the severe impairment battery (SIB) are reliable and international standardized instruments for assessing cognition. There is some discussion about whether all these scales are able to measure changes in time. Furthermore, MMSE, CST and even the SIB face bottom effects in patients with severe dementia. An alternative in these phases could be the Bedford Alzheimer Nursing Scale-Severity Subscale (BANS-S) or any other scale which can measure slight changes of the disease such as changes in emotional expression or response to stimulation (Magai et al, 1996). More research on the final stages of dementia is needed (Koopmans et al, 2003).

Behavioural problems can be assessed by the Neuropsychiatric Inventory Nursing Home version (NPI-NH) and the Cohen-Mansfield Agitation Inventory (CMAI). In my experience, these two scales cover the whole range of behavioural and psychological symptoms in dementia in nursing home patients. The advantages of the scales are that they offer clear terms and operational definitions of behavioural problems. This is especially important because nurses and even doctors mostly use words like 'confusion', or 'restlessness' without specifying the behaviour. Another advantage is that they assess behaviours that otherwise would not be mentioned spontaneously, such as sexually abusive behaviours.

Functional status assessment scales for nursing home patients should have a minimum of instrumental-ADL (I-ADL) items because most of the dementia patients in nursing homes have progressed to stage 5 of the Reisberg global deterioration scale (GDS) and therefore are no longer able to do these complex tasks. I would advise the modified 19-item Alzheimer Disease Cooperative Study-ADL-inventory (ADCS-ADL$_{19}$) or the Care Dependency Scale (Dijkstra et al, 1999). The latter scale is especially validated in nursing home patients with advanced dementia and has no I-ADL items.

Assessment of quality of life (QOL) is important for future treatment decisions and monitoring outcome of any intervention. An ideal instrument should measure QOL throughout the whole process of dementia and should have a part in which patients can assess themselves and a part for proxy assessment. In the Netherlands a research group from Amsterdam is now designing a new QOL instrument for demented nursing home patients. Measuring discomfort by means of the Discomfort Scale in Dementia of the Alzheimer Type (DS-DAT) is another approach to get an indication of well-being (Hurley et al, 1992).

Perhaps the minimum data set of resident assessment instrument (MDS-RAI) could replace all aforementioned assessments (Hawes et al, 1997). MDS-RAI is obligatory in US nursing homes and is widely used in other countries around the world. However, the MDS-RAI is not specifically designed for dementia patients and therefore less sensitive and complete, for instance, to assess behavioural problems or cognitive functions. However, the MDS-RAI ADL scale is very suitable to measure basic ADLs in advanced dementia patients.

Treatment and prevention of intercurrent health problems and co-morbidity

Most demented nursing home patients are over 80 years old and have several co-morbid diseases. Although it is presumed that Alzheimer patients are healthier than for instance patients with vascular dementia, there is a tendency for patients with no co-morbidity and hardly any behavioural problems to stay in their own homes or residential homes. This means that nursing homes are places for patients with multiple, complex problems, with much co-morbidity and many behavioural problems.

The nursing home physician should visit the wards at least twice a week. Once a week physical and psychological functioning should be evaluated, and once a month the medication list should be checked for medications that are no longer needed. Nurses should be trained in observation of the demented patients and should be aware of the non-specific symptoms these patients present, such as incontinence as a sign of urinary tract infection, acute confusion as a sign of delirium and of course pain assessment.

First of all, the nursing home physician has to treat chronic diseases such as diabetes, heart failure, atrial fibrillation and so on. It is very important to create a stable condition, because any problems in these diseases, for instance hyperglycaemia, could cause further deterioration and confusion. The nursing home physician should always look at the medication list to see whether the problem could be explained by any of the drugs prescribed. It is known that there is a relationship between the prevalence and incidence of intercurrent health problems and progression and mortality (Koopmans et al, 1994; Van Dijk et al, 1996). The five most frequently occurring health problems are urinary tract infection, adverse effects from medication, constipation, pneumonia and pressure ulcers.

One should try to prevent these problems as much as possible by means of good hygiene; prevent epidemic outbursts of influenza by vaccinating all nursing home patients; prevent polypharmacy as stated before; prevent pressure sores by using special mattresses and by frequent turning and lifting of immobile patients; prevent falls; and optimize nutrition.

Much attention has to be paid to good nutrition of demented patients. They should at least take 1.5 L of fluids and should have a balanced food intake, with enough calories, proteins, vitamins and fibres. One should know the personal preferences of the patients, to adjust their daily meals. There should be sufficient staffing and time to assist patients who can no longer eat independently. Music has a positive impact on food intake of demented patients. Weight has to be monitored every 3 months in order to signal weight loss. When problems with eating arise, a thorough analysis has to be made by the nursing home physician. Speech therapists can analyse swallowing problems and occupational therapists can look at posture and can give advice on adjusting spoons and cups and so on. Good mouth care is essential when eating problems arise. In my view, there should be a dentist in every nursing home and the nursing home physician should look for treatable causes such as oral candidiasis. When problems with chewing or swallowing arise, consistency of the food can be changed.

While dementia is progressing, most patients lose their ability to walk independently and the risk of falls increases. Everything should be done to preserve mobility and transfers. Physiotherapists have an important role in treating problems with mobility and therefore prevention of falls. However, the nursing home physician should always look at physical causes such as hypotension, adverse effects from benzodiazepines, antipsychotics, or pain caused by arthritis. Patients should use all kinds of walking aids and, if patients have lost mobility, specially adjusted and comfortable wheelchairs have to be prescribed. In the final phase of dementia, patients can become bedridden. Much can be done to enhance comfort for bedridden patients. Everything has to be done to prevent physical restraints, and one should always search for alternatives that do not limit the freedom of movement of the patients, such as electronic warning systems.

Paratonia, or 'gegenhalten' is a special problem that can arise in dementia patients (Kurlan et al, 2000). In the end, paratonia can result in a total flexure posture and muscle contractures, with the risk of skin problems and even pressure ulcers. Physiotherapists and occupational therapists can design special ortheses to prevent such problems. In the end, surgery by cutting the tendons is an option.

Improving well-being and prevention and treatment of behavioural problems

It is known from the literature that more than 90% of demented nursing home patients have some type of behavioural problem (Wagner et al, 1995). Behavioural problems are the main reason for admission to nursing homes. A

thorough analysis of the behavioural problems should take place before starting any intervention. The Dutch Association of Nursing Home Physicians has
developed a guideline and analysis should take place according to this guideline. The following issues should be addressed: description of the behaviour,
duration and frequency, place and circumstances, determinants (including
escalating factors, environmental factors and factors or interventions that
cause the behaviour to decrease or even disappear), consequences (including
the question: 'For whom is the behaviour problematic?') and possible explanations for the behaviour. The nursing home physician should always look for
a somatic cause (including medication), psychological, personal and environmental factors that could explain the behaviour. Neuropsychological testing is
an essential part of the analysis. A history should be taken from the relatives
to get information about the premorbid personality of the patient and to
know important life events, former habits and preferences. Knowing and
understanding patients as they were in the past is one of the main points for
treatment and should be a standard procedure at admission to a nursing
home. Every patient needs an individual analysis and treatment plan.
However, there are some general recommendations concerning environmental factors and communicating with dementia patients.

Psychogeriatric nursing homes should be specially designed for these
patients. One should create a home-like environment, ideally with small
units or houses where 6–8 patients live under supervision of trained nurses.
Every patient has to have his own (bed)room, with a separate shower unit.
Patients have to be allowed to bring their own furniture and other familiar
items. There should be a separate dining and living room on every ward,
where patients can meet and eat together. There also has to be a kitchen
where patients can prepare their own meals when appropriate. In larger
institutions there should be a walking circuit, so patients can pace. Lighting
should receive special attention, by using large windows and light colours on
the walls. Distressing noises such as loud television sets, radios or shouting
by the personnel should be prevented as much as possible. There should be
clearly visible orientation signs to guide the patients, e.g. to the lavatory or
their own rooms. Ideally, the patients should have enough room to walk
around, without being able to wander outside the institution. In smaller
units, doors have to be closed. However, the doors should be concealed so
that patients do not recognize them as exits.

Ideally, all units should be located on the ground floor and surrounded by
patios and gardens, which can be easily accessed by the patients. Whenever

possible, patients should be allowed to bring their own pets and keep animals like chickens and goats in the gardens.

I would recommend placing patients with similar stages of dementia together. In my experience, patients with mild to moderate dementia do not mix well with patients who have severe dementia and need other approaches and environments. Patients with young-onset dementia should not live together with elderly patients. A drawback of this policy is that patients have to move to another ward when the dementia is progressing. Another approach is to create groups of patients based on their cultural backgrounds.

All staff at the nursing home, especially nurses, should be trained in communication with dementia patients. Depending on the needs of the patients, they should use techniques such as reality orientation, validation therapy, reminiscence, sensory stimulation ('snoezelen'), music therapy and so on. In the Netherlands we speak of an 'emotion-oriented approach', which means that we always try to understand the emotions, beliefs and thoughts of the patients (de Lange, 2004). If they cannot enter our world, we must enter and affirm theirs.

I am convinced that the use of these forms of communication improves well-being and helps prevent behaviour problems. Dementia patients should always be treated with respect. It is important not to use rigid schedules, e.g. for waking up in the morning, having breakfast, or toileting. Patients who are used to sleeping until 11 a.m. should continue this habit in the nursing home. It is better to tolerate bizarre behaviour such as going to bed with the trousers on or eating mashed potatoes with one's fingers than arguing about it and provoking aggression.

Activity plans should be drawn up for every patient, based on former habits and actual needs. Individual activities and group activities should take place in and outside the wards. In some nursing homes 'clubs' of patients are formed, e.g. a bridge club or a club where people listen to classical music. Keeping patients active prevents loneliness and apathy and improves well-being. Spirituality is very important, especially for the elderly. Pastoral workers have to be intensively involved in the care of dementia patients. Every nursing home should have a chapel or at least a quiet room to pray. The smell of incense and burning candles are signs of recognition and sometimes patients with aphasia appear to be able to sing religious lyrics from the past. Of course, younger patients have different needs and, for these physically healthy patients, sports such as volleyball or jogging could be appropriate activities.

Music is essential in the nursing home and should be used actively and passively. Whenever possible, patients should be stimulated to play their own instruments and to bring them to the nursing home. Group singing often gives one a feeling of contentment.

In the case of severe behavioural problems, psychosocial intervention is the mainstay of treatment. After the thorough analysis as described above, an individual tailor-made psychosocial treatment plan has to be designed by the multidisciplinary team, in which the psychologist plays an important role. When determinants of specific behaviour are identified, the nurses have to be advised concerning communication with patients to alleviate agitation and possible intervention. Theoretically, all disciplines can have a role in the treatment plan. Finding the right solution requires some trial and error. Psychotropics should be reserved for those behaviours that cannot be influenced by psychosocial interventions. For the nursing home physician, it is essential to identify core symptoms such as psychosis, or agitation-aggression, or mood symptoms for choosing the right drug. Atypical antipsychotic drugs are preferred above typical antipsychotic drugs. However, recent evidence shows an increase in cerebrovascular problems and mortality with these agents. The adage is always 'start low and go slow'. The nursing home physician should always look at co-morbidity when making his choices. Psychotropic drugs with anticholinergic properties, antidepressants, such as tricyclics, should be avoided and one should be aware of side effects. One should always seek the lowest effective dose, with a minimum of adverse effects. After a stable phase of at least 2 months, the nursing home physician should try to discontinue the medication by gradually lowering the dosage and by intensively monitoring the behaviour, e.g. with NPI-NH and CMAI assessments.

In spite of this policy, the literature shows that about 60–80% of the Dutch nursing home patients with dementia have and receive at least one prescription of a psychotropic (Koopmans et al, 1996; van Dijk et al, 2000). Nursing home physicians should consider cholinesterase inhibitors or memantine too, although there is some reservation because of the high costs and the lack of evidence. To date, only 1 or 2% of Dutch nursing home patients with dementia have prescriptions for one of these drugs.

Advance care planning, living wills, shared care and end-of-life decisions

Within 2 weeks of admission, the nursing home physician should start with advance care planning concerning treatment policies in case the patient gets seriously ill. The nursing home physician should ask for a written living will and if there is one, he should speak with the patient or his relatives about whether the text is up to date. Agreements about whether or not to provide heart massage and/or artificial ventilation in case of cardiac arrest should be made. However, in my view cardiopulmonary resuscitation in dementia is a disproportionate treatment measure and should be avoided whenever possible. In the Netherlands, skin, organ and cornea donation is contraindicated in dementia patients; otherwise, these issues should be discussed.

Advance care planning can compromise three treatment options: curative treatment, which means treatment of all health problems including hospital admission; palliative treatment, which means treatment of health problems with certain restrictions, e.g. no admission to a hospital or no causal treatment such as surgery; and, finally, symptomatic treatment, which means merely relieving symptoms such as pain or dyspnoea, without causal treatment such as antibiotics for pneumonia or artificial nutrition and hydration (ANH) in the case of serious problems with drinking and food intake. In symptomatic treatment, extending life expectancy is contraindicated. These options should be discussed with the patient whenever possible and with the relatives, who are asked to reconstruct the will of their family member. This 'shared care' with respect to the wishes of the family is essential for good care in dementia patients. Right from the start of admission to the nursing home, it should be clear to the family that we will share the path of gradual deterioration together and that there is a strong need to keep in contact. On every occasion, the nursing home physician should inform relatives about prognosis and the course and complications that can be expected. In this way, relatives are prepared for future events, and decision-making gets easier when a life-threatening illness occurs or important end-of-life decisions have to be made. Of course, one cannot anticipate every possible complication; therefore, final treatment decisions have to be taken at the moment the event occurs.

Treatment policies should be evaluated at least twice a year and, in case of rapid progression, more often. While dementia is progressing, the treatment policy shifts from curative to finally symptomatic treatment. It is known from the literature that in Dutch nursing homes ANH by tube feeding is rarely started in patients with severe dementia (The et al, 2002). ANH is given mainly when there is an acute illness or a condition that needs medical treatment and which requires hydration to be effective. The medical condition of the patient, the wishes of the family and the interpretations of the patients' quality of life by their care providers are considered more than living wills and policy agreements.

It is also known from the literature that care for Dutch nursing home residents with lower respiratory tract infection (LRI) and dementia is less aggressive than care for US residents, particularly in residents with severe dementia (van der Steen et al, 2004). Treatment of LRI in US residents involves a larger number of antibiotics, more frequent hospitalization and greater use of intravenous antibiotics and rehydration therapy than in Dutch residents of equal dementia severity.

Euthanasia in dementia is prohibited. However, there are a few cases in the Netherlands where euthanasia in dementia patients has taken place and the doctor has not been prosecuted. There is an ongoing debate on this issue, since people tend to request euthanasia in their living wills.

Conclusions

In the Netherlands there is comprehensive experience with specialized dementia care. The cornerstone of this care is the multidisciplinary team under the direction of a specially trained nursing home physician. The living environment should be specially designed for the needs of these patients. Creating a safe, home-like environment, where patients are treated with respect, is one of the most important aspects of standard care of dementia in nursing homes.

References

Dijkstra A, Sipsma D, Dassen T. Predictors of care dependency in Alzheimer's disease after a two-year period. *Int J Nurs Stud* 1999; 36: 487–95.

Hawes C, Morris JN, Phillips CD, et al. Development of the nursing home Resident Assessment Instrument in the USA. *Age Ageing* 1997; 26: 19–25.

Hoek JF, Pennix BWJH, Ligthart GJ, Ribbe MW. Health care for older persons. A country profile: The Netherlands. *J Am Geriatr Soc* 2000; 48: 214–17.

Hoek JF, Ribbe MW, Hertogh CMPM, Vleuten van der CPM. The specialist training program for nursing home physicians: A new professional challenge. *JAMDA* 2001; 2: 326–30.

Hurley AC, Volicer BJ, Hanrahan PA, Houde S, Volicer L. Assessment of discomfort in advanced Alzheimer patients. *Res Nurs Health* 1992; 15: 369–77.

Koopmans RTCM, Ekkerink JLP, Hoogen HJM, van den Froeling PGAM, Weel C van. Indicators for progression of dementia in nursing home patients *Ned Tijdschr Geneeskd* 1994; 138: 1164–8. [in Dutch]

Koopmans RTCM, Ekkerink JLP, Weel van C. Survival to late dementia in Dutch nursing home patients. *J Am Geriatr Soc* 2003; 51:184–7.

Koopmans RTCM, Rossum JM van, Hoogen HJM van den, et al. Psychotropic drug use in a group of Dutch nursing home patients with dementia: Many users, long-term use, but low doses. *Pharm World Sci* 1996; 18: 42–7.

Kurlan R, Richard IH, Papka M, Marshall F. Movement disorders in Alzheimer's disease: more rigidity of definitions is needed. *Mov Disord* 2000; 15: 24–9.

Lange de J. Dealing with dementia. Effects of integrated emotion-oriented care on adaptation and coping of people with dementia in nursing homes; a qualitative study as part of a randomised clinical trial. Thesis, Rotterdam; 2004.

Magai C, Cohen C, Gomberg D, et al. Emotional expression during mid- to late stage dementia. *Int Psychogeriatr* 1996; 8: 383–95.

Steen van der JT, Kruse RL, Ooms ME, et al. Treatment of nursing home residents with dementia and lower respiratory tract infection in the United States and the Netherlands: An ocean apart. *J Am Geriatr Soc* 2004; 52: 691–9.

The AM, Pasman R, Onwuteaka-Philpsen B, Ribbe MW, Wal van der G. Withholding the artificial administration of fluids and food from elderly patients with dementia: Ethnographic study. *BMJ* 2002; 325: 1326.

van Dijk PT, Dippel DW, Van Der Meulen JH, Habbema JD. Co-morbidity and its effect on mortality in nursing home patients with dementia. *J Nerv Ment Dis* 1996; 184:180–7.

van Dijk KN, Vries de CS, Berg van den PB, Brouwers JRBJ, Jong de-Berg van den LTW. Drug utilisation in Dutch nursing homes. *Eur J Clin Pharmacol* 2000; 55: 765–71.

Wagner AW, Teri L, Orr-Rainey N. Behavior problems of residents with dementia in special care units. *Alzheimer Dis Assoc Disord* 1995; 9:121–7.

chapter 21

Recognizing and delivering quality nursing care for people with dementia

Anne-Françoise Dufey and Kevin Hope

Introduction

In considering the relationship between nursing and contemporary dementia care, images and metaphors that spring to mind are characterized by energy, growth, development and a realization of potential. Nurses working in dementia care exist in exciting times, enmeshed in a maelstrom of research and practice developments associated with the articulation of broad-based biopsychosocial discourses. The introduction of acetylcholinesterase inhibitors, the growth in the centrality of the subjective and lived experience of the person with dementia and the impact of psychosocial interventions for people with dementia and their carers are but a few of the many examples that can be identified. Work of this nature has facilitated a challenge to therapeutic nihilism previously characteristic of dementia care and energized the development of exciting initiatives for and by nurses working in the field.

Advanced nursing practice under the auspices of memory clinics, extended roles that include working in outreach settings, educating and modelling quality care and working with families and carers in a focused, evidence-based manner are but a few of the many examples on offer. Within this context, the provision of high-quality care is ascribed central importance. This tenet would appear to be a 'given' when analysed in relation to the history of dementia care. What has changed over time though is the operational definition of quality. Kitwood and Benson (1995) outlined 10 differences between what they describe as 'old' and 'new' cultures of care, the latter reflecting and encompassing person-centred approaches to care. Within the 'new' culture, caring is consequently intertwined with the maintenance and enhancement of personhood and reflects the broad discourse of the bio-psychosocial approaches cited above.

Recognizing and delivering such care though creates challenges, and problems in defining quality become manifest. Almarez (1994) highlights the multifaceted nature of the quality construct. On the one hand, cognitive approaches that recognize the abstract nature of the concept can be identified with the emergent theme that one will recognize good care when one sees it being evident. On the other hand, the case is made that the meaning of quality needs to be operationalized in some way. This debate is well represented in the dementia care field, with some commentators expressing frustration at the abstract nature of person-centred care while others have sought to address this.

Brooker (2004) has identified four basic tenets of person-centred care.

1. a value base which values people with dementia and those who care for them
2. individualized care which recognizes the uniqueness of the individual within a biopsychosocial framework
3. the perspective of the person with dementia directs intervention
4. supportive social environments which promote positive person work in the context of relationships

These tenets are welcome and provide some clarity and guidance although work is ongoing in relation to identifying relevant indicators for each component.

An alternative approach which has been widely used in evaluating healthcare quality was developed by Donabedian (1988a). This perspective promulgates the view that nurses can benefit from referring to outcomes and process standards in assessing the quality of their work. As Donabedian argues:

'This three-part approach to quality assessment is possible only because good structure increases the likelihood of good process, and good process increases the likelihood of a good outcome. It is necessary therefore, to have established such a relationship before any particular component of structure, process, or outcome can be used to assess quality. The activity of quality assessment is not itself designed to establish the presence of these relationships. There must be preexisting knowledge of the linkage between structure and process, and between process and outcome, before quality assessment can be undertaken.'

(Donabedian, 1988b: 1745)

Arguably, this is the case for all nursing functions, including practice, management, education, research and political activities. The following list explores these five functions, utilizing the process and outcomes model. It is not intended to be exhaustive or prescriptive but is offered as a framework to provide points of reference for nurses working across all care environments in which people with dementia are present and who wish to assess both their activities and results in the field of dementia nursing

The process standards (PS) and outcome

Clinical practice

PS – At all times, work in partnership with the client and their relatives/carers, promote their comfort, security, dignity and self-esteem.
Outcome – Mutual negotiation with all parties contributing to the decision-making process.

PS – Promote an environment that conveys a sense of belonging and of feeling valued to relatives/carers, one in which they are able to express emotions, acquire information and share experiences. Promote regular exchanges between staff and relatives/carers and with the client.
Outcome – Perception of support and control by carers/relatives, reduction of the perception of powerlessness, culpability, anxiety and sadness.

PS – Meaningfully collaborate with the client, his carers and other professionals for the process of assessment.
Outcome – Assessment located in the person's biography. Collaboration in identification of strengths and needs evident.

PS – Care plans are collaboratively generated, taking into account the strengths and needs of the client with clear objectives, plan of intervention and dates for review.
Outcome – Care based on negotiated understanding which reinforces the strengths and addresses the needs of the client.

PS – In association with other relevant professional groups and carers, identify the client's ability to support and maintain their activities of daily living and provide appropriate compensatory intervention commensurate with the client's wishes, physical and cognitive resources.

Outcome – Comfort and security while autonomy and dignity of the person with dementia are preserved and maintained.

PS – In association with other relevant professional groups and carers, maintain the efficiency and effectiveness of any prosthetic devices such as spectacles and hearing aids.

Outcome – Orientation and social integration of the client facilitated.

PS – Administer medication in the prescribed manner and assess and evaluate the intended and side effects.

Outcome – Safe and therapeutic use of medication, notably the effective monitoring of psychotropic drugs.

PS – In association with other relevant professional groups and carers, assist clients to engage in meaningful activity, occupation and therapy, which aligns with their strengths and needs.

Outcome – Enhanced indicators of wellness and promotion of his/her social integration.

PS – Manage the physical and human environment in such a way as to promote personhood by taking into consideration any sensory deficits of the client, their cognitive, physical and emotional status and the wishes of relatives and carers regarding their participation in the caring process. In some circumstances, for example with newly commissioned buildings or on discharge home, proactively involve professionals such as architects, occupational therapist, etc., in this process.

Outcome – Environment is appropriately adapted to meet the needs of the client and the relatives notably in terms of the layout of physical spaces, the choice of colours and lighting.

PS – In association with other disciplines, manage transitions in care provision in a manner that takes into account and is responsive to the wishes and desires of clients and carers, their resources and their coping mechanisms.

Outcome – Maintenance of feelings of security and control in clients and carers.

PS – In association with other relevant professional groups and carers, consider the utility of technological aids and devices in the context of promoting and maintaining personhood.

Outcome – Increased perception of physical and psychological security. Maintenance and development of autonomy in movement. Reduction of agitation due to a limiting environment.

Management

PS – Identify and publicize a shared philosophy of care for quality provision that takes account of the needs of people with dementia and which reflects evidence-based practice and available resources.
Outcome – Promotion of quality and continuity of care appropriate to the needs of the person with dementia.

PS – Promote models of caring based on meaningful partnership (with relatives and associated professionals) and networking (with all involved professionals and community services).
Outcome – Increased sense of ownership and belonging for all parties so that the human resources involved feel that their input is worthwhile and appreciated. Better perception and integration of people with dementia in the community.

PS – Promote an environment in which staff utilize their talents and capacities to the full and in which they feel supported to explore and develop new models of caring.
Outcome – Emergence of creative, innovative specific and efficient models in dementia care.

PS – Manage the skill mix of staff so that resources match demands in a manner commensurate with the philosophy of care.
Outcome – Staff feeling secure and turnover of staff minimized.

PS – Facilitate provision now and in the future for a practitioner in advanced practice (e.g. consultant nurse, clinical nurse specialist) with a remit for education, practice development and research.
Outcome – Evidence-based care, reflexive and reflective practice, innovation and creativity and synergy between theory and practice. Enhanced value of dementia care in the nursing profession, in the social environment and the population.

PS – Utilize benchmarking tools to guide staff provision.

Outcome – Objectivity in resource allocation.

PS – Utilize quality processes as frameworks to act as a catalyst to challenge the status quo in care provision and to acquire accreditation.
Outcome – Promotion of quality care provision within an external reference framework. Enhanced value of institutions providing dementia nursing.

PS – Provide an environment, establish and maintain links with education providers and act as a learning resource in theory and in practice.
Outcome – Learners identify and develop the knowledge attitude and skills commensurate with high-quality dementia care.

PS – Establish and maintain links with research centres.
Outcome – Raising awareness and contribution to the evidence base and development of new perspectives in models of care in this field of nursing.

Education

PS – Promote the development of education in mental health of the elderly at all levels of the educational system (non-professionally qualified, under-graduate, postgraduate) and service providers and across the spectrum of care provision.
Outcome – Raising awareness and understanding of the nature and impact of dementia so that appropriate attitudes and responses are widespread.

PS – Promote masters and doctoral programmes in dementia care.
Outcome – Enhanced value of dementia care and development of advanced practitioner pool.

PS – Promote interdisciplinary education.
Outcome – Improving awareness and skills using complementary approach in addressing the complexity of client situations.

PS – Promote education in empowerment models of dementia care.
Outcome – Development of a workforce inclined towards and able to recognize and facilitate partnership working with clients and carers which takes into account competencies already developed by clients and carers.

Research

PS – Motivate and develop nurses as future researchers in dementia care able to augment the knowledge base regarding the promotion of health, social integration and quality of life for people with dementia within an ethically sound framework.
Outcome – Further development of a workforce capable of contributing to a culture of inquiry in dementia care.

PS – Promote and educate staff in the systematic recording of nursing interventions in dementia care.
Outcome – Production of valid indicators for research.

PS – Develop research proposals which are cognizant of the perceptions of all parties collaborating in the care process and their resources.
Outcome – Prioritization of research endeavour and identification of resources.

PS – Develop research proposals related to the care of people with learning disability who also have a dementing illness.
Outcome – Proactive responses in this domain.

PS – Contribute to interdisciplinary research.
Outcome – Inclusion of a nursing perspective in the process.

PS – Dissemination of research findings and contribution to data collection.
Outcome – Increased knowledge about the impacts and appropriate responses in dementia care.

Political activities

PS – Educate clients and their relatives/carers on their rights. Identify sources for self-help, advocacy and welfare provision and promote an environment in which clients and their relatives/carers feel able and free to express their needs and wants.
Outcome – Promotion of an empowered clientele ready to assume increased responsibility and control of their situation to make proposals at a political level.

PS – Engage with the information and activities of professional, governmental and learned bodies.
Outcome – Contribution to policy and decision-making.

Conclusion

Dementia represents an important challenge for the future of nursing. Good quality care can substantially contribute to the improvement of quality of life of people with dementia and their relatives. In this respect, exciting developments are evident but many models of care show room for improvement and others need to emerge which truly reflect user-centred principles. Systematic assessment of quality in this area is needed to generate new ideas and pointers in overcoming the challenge.

Even though this chapter was specifically concerned with describing processes and outcomes, we are conscious that these can only be adequately attained if the structures, in terms of services and politics, are present and supportive of such goals. As the World Health Organization argues:

> 'New structures may well be required to enable new treatments to be used successfully . . . It is urgent that people responsible for health care policy development and implementation take note of the requirements and act accordingly. Responsive action should lead to the development, appropriate to local conditions, of the components of services which will adequately address these needs. Such components should be integrated and co-ordinated to serve older people with mental health problems and their carers and should be supported by adequate resources
>
> WHO, 1999

Such concerns though should not detract from the impact that nurses, both as individuals and within groups, can have on the genesis, provision and subsequent development of quality initiatives in dementia care and it is in this spirit that these indicators have been developed.

References

Almaraz J. Quality management and the process of change. J Organizat Change Manage 1994; 7: 6–14.

Brooker D. 'What is person-centered care in dementia?' *Rev Clin Gerontol* 2004; 13: 215–22.

Donabedian A. Quality assessment and assurance: unity of purpose, diversity of means. *Inquiry* 1988; 25: 173–92.

Donabedian A. The quality of care. How can it be assessed? *JAMA* 1988b; **260**: 1743–8.

Kitwood T, Benson S. *The new culture of dementia care*. London: Hawker Publications; 1995.

WHO, Department of Mental Health. *Lausanne Technical Statements on Psychiatry of the Elderly*. Geneva: WHO; 1999.

Further reading

Association Suisse des Infirmiers et infirmières, Secrétariat central. *Normes de qualité pour les soins et l'accompagnement des personnes âgées*. Berne: Association Suisse des Infirmiers et infirmières; 1994.

ICN. *International principles and framework for standards development in nursing*. Geneva: ICN; 2004.

Lévesque L, Roux C, Lauzon S. *Alzheimer. Comprendre pour mieux aider*. Montreal: Ed. du Renouveau pédagogique. 1990.

Nolan M, Gordon G, Keady J. The carers act: realising the potential. *Br J Community Health Nurs* 1996; **6**: 317–22.

Ordre des infirmières et infirmiers du Québec. *L'exercice infirmier en soins de longue durée. Au carrefour du milieu de soins et du milieu de vie*. Montréal: OIIQ; 2000.

Tang WK, Chiu H, Woo J, Hjelm M, Hui E. Telepsychiatry in psychogeriatric service: a pilot study. *Int J Geriatr Psychiatry* 2001; **16**: 88–93.

The Canadian Caregiver Coalition. http://www.ccc-ccan.ca/en/frame.html

Challenges for the treatment of demented patients from a geriatrician's point of view

Cornel C Sieber

Demographics

A steadily increasing life expectancy, paralleled by a low birth rate in the developed countries, is rapidly and profoundly changing the age pyramid. As most different forms of dementia show a clear age dependency, the number of demented patients will increase exponentially in the years and decades to come. With some time lapse, this will also be seen in many countries with rapid growing economies such as Mexico, India and China. All diagnostic and therapeutic new avenues in the field of dementia have therefore also to be seen in this context.

A specificity of geriatric medicine is the multimorbidity of the people it concerns. For a long time, classical geriatric syndromes such as the four to six 'I' – immobility, instability, incontinence, and intellectual problems and more recently isolation and iatrogenic problems – were handled mainly by geriatricians, whereas the problem of dementia was preferentially dealt with by gerontopsychiatrics. These two parallel avenues were and are often not interconnected enough, leading to deficient services on both sides. This situation is often topped by not close enough established services with neurologists. As a geriatrician, I see the need to establish interconnected services in order to help the patients with dementia and the families involved. In addition to the clear advantages of linked services on a quality assurance level, such services also help in that the patients and their caregivers do not have to move from one specialist to another, but that the specialties come to the patient. We recently established a 'Centre for Medicine for the Aged' in Nuremberg, a concept I would like to present in some more detail.

Centre for Medicine for the Aged

In order to overcome the above-mentioned network problems, we established a Centre for Medicine for the Aged in 2003, concentrating the specialties of geriatrics, neurology and psychogeriatrics in a single building with a coordinating desk person. The memory clinic is also incorporated in this building as well as conference rooms. The main referrals directly to the centre are patients with the possible diagnosis of dementia: the split now is about two-thirds of patients coming for a first diagnostic programme, and one-third on follow-up visits. The three core specialties mentioned above meet on a regular basis to coordinate the services and to discuss complex patient and family situations. In addition, the centre aims to be the platform for demented patients and their caregivers for both 'inside' and 'outside' diagnostic and therapeutic programmes.

'Inside' means the coordinating place for consults for elderly patients within the hospital (a 2500-bed hospital with all specialties at hand). It is evident that due to the demographic shift and the impact of always shorter hospitalization times within the acute care hospitals, longer-stay hospitalized patients are mainly elderly multimorbid patients. The centre therefore aims to help in the care of these elderly (demented) patients, especially also in the surgical departments. By 'outside', we see the centre as a platform for services outside the hospital, in the region. This mainly involves a close contact with general practitioners in town, with long-term care facilities and rehabilitation clinics and with institutions such as the town offices for the needs of the old.

In times when 'organ clinics' (e.g. hip replacement clinics, cardiology intervention units) become more and more fashionable, it is evident that a close collaboration with a core interdisciplinary team (geriatrics, psychogeriatrics) is important as often elderly people with dementia are in these patient groups. This not only holds true for an expert handling of these diseases but also as patients and families affected by dementia are in a special need also, from a psychological point of view, for a stringent and effective specialist team.

'Meeting point' of the different dementia syndromes

Years ago, when therapeutic drug therapies were scarce or even nearly missing for Alzheimer's disease, a clear and strict separation of the different dementia syndromes was reasonable, especially the differentiation from vascular dementias. Step by step, these more or less closed borders between 'dementia schools' have became permeable: cholinesterase inhibitors for mixed and even 'strict' vascular dementias (Erkinjuntti et al, 2002, 2004; Black et al, 2003), statins eventually for Alzheimer's disease (Rockwood et al, 2002; Li et al, 2004) and, more recently, even moderate alcohol intake (especially red wine with a high level of antioxidants such as reveratrol) not just for vascular dementia (Ruitenberg et al, 2002; Letemeur, 2004), underscore this tendency from a pharmacological point of view.

These new emerging pathophysiological and therapeutic understandings lead directly to a more interconnected need for collaboration between different specialties. Once again, the geriatrician and psychogeriatrician have to move closer together; as in the differential diagnosis as well as consecutive therapeutic strategies, the know-how of both expert groups are crucial.

It is to be hoped that this amalgamation may also help to bundle therapeutic strategies besides the mere pharmacological interventions. For an example, t'ai chi may prove a good method for both movement handicapped and fall-prone demented patients (Kressig et al, 2003). A closer collaboration between the two 'groups' may also prove helpful as a platform between ambulatory services and caregivers.

Rehabilitation of the demented patient

The demented patient has usually other (chronic) diseases besides the dementia itself, as mainly elderly people are affected. This especially holds true for vascular or mixed dementia, where the brain is just one of the target organs of vascular insults. Thus, ischaemic or haemorrhagic strokes are often seen with the need for rehabilitation. Another frequent problem is Parkinson's syndrome as a consequence of dementia or the inverse, dementia problems in the advanced stages of Parkinson's disease. Finally, Alzheimer's disease is itself often accompanied by specific geriatric problems such as repetitive falls. It is therefore not surprising that osteoporotic fractures are also seen more often in demented patients.

As 80% of demented patients in Germany are cared for within their families, rehabilitation successes are mandatory in order that these people may stay in their usual surroundings. Inadequate rehabilitation often results in institutionalization. Especially in the demented patient, removal from a well-known environment usually leads to a rapid deterioration of the situation.

By contrast, it is often said that demented patients are not well adapted for rehabilitation programmes. It is evident that in times of restriction in the resources allocated for rehabilitation programmes, demented patients are especially prone to become victims of 'ageist' behaviour. The literature with regard to rehabilitation successes in demented patients, e.g. after fall-induced fractures, is quite sparse. We therefore used the 'Bavarian geriatric database', which covers about 90% of all rehabilitation beds within Bavaria, to study this question retrospectively. We chose surgically treated proximal femur fractures in 110 patients with dementia compared with mentally healthy age-matched controls with the same fracture type. We were able to show that the severity of dementia measured by the mini-mental state examination (Folstein et al, 1975) was indeed an independent factor for the rehabilitation results in geriatric-specific rehabilitation units. Nevertheless, significant lower success rates (e.g. for Barthel index) were only seen for mini-mental state levels less than 18 points. For a wide range of dementia, the rehabilitation results were therefore not different to non-demented patients (Baier, 2004), showing that dementia in itself cannot be a reason to restrict rehabilitation programmes.

For all those working with demented patients, it is important to fight for the rights of our patients so that they get into rehabilitation programmes as already small amelioration (e.g. transfer from the bed to the toilet chair, eating without any help from another person) may separate those staying at home from those living in institutions, as the caregivers are also often old and frail.

Mobile geriatric rehabilitation for demented persons

Besides geriatric day clinics and ambulatory geriatric rehabilitation in specialized units, some frail elderly people cannot be rehabilitated outside their home. These are patients living too far away from a unit to be transported in any reasonable time frame, or patients and families being against therapies outside their homes. The most vulnerable patient group in this respect are mentally disturbed people, making rehabilitation programmes outside their known surroundings impossible. On top of that, rehabilitation programmes at home enable the specialist to see the patient in his known environment, where therapeutic programmes can be customized to the special needs of the patient. Often, the caregiver is also there and the health professional can also discuss care problems locally as an 'add-on' and is able to comfort the caregiver in times of signs of a 'burn-out'.

This construct is not only well-adapted for the patients and caregivers involved but it also helps to reduce resources going out of the health system budget, as inadequate referrals and hospitalization can be reduced. Such programmes are well established in countries such as the UK and France, but they are still missing in many countries, including Germany.

When (mentally) disabled persons get old

The demographic shift also covers – a huge success of modern medicine – more and more disabled people. This holds true for both innate disability as well as disabilities starting at a later stage of life. With regard to innate disabilities, Down syndrome may serve as a good example. The average life expectancy of mongoloid children was 7 years by 1920; it is now already more than 60 years. Down syndrome is also a good example in that these people have a significant increased risk of developing dementias of the Alzheimer type.

A special interest for us, as geriatricians, in these situations lies in the fact that multimorbidity in these people when they become old, demands special diagnostic and therapeutic skills.

From a more gerontological point of view, these patients have more and more been cared for by their families in the last decades. They are therefore not used to staying in specialized institutions for disabled people. When, now, the caregivers – mostly their parents – become old, the care system becomes vulnerable as a whole. More and more we face the situation of needing to look for a place for a mentally disabled person cared for by a family member suffering from an acute disease.

Concluding remarks

It is evident that, in this short chapter, only selected topics could be discussed. There is also a clear 'selection bias' in that I have considered factors especially important for my daily work with demented patients. Nevertheless, I hope to have shown that the field of dementia is still a challenge for all the professional groups involved. As dementia syndromes are probably the most prominent 'silent epidemic' in Western societies, with major impacts not just for the patients and families affected but also for the healthcare sector as a whole, I hope that I have described some relevant facets of the problem.

References

Baier F. *Der Einfluss von Demenzerkrankungen auf das Rehabilitationspotential von Patienten mit Oberschenkelfraktur.* Inaugural dissertation, Friedrich-Alexander-Universität Erlangen-Nürnberg; 2004.

Black S, Roman GC, Geldmacher DS, et al. Donezepil 307 Vascular Dementia Study Group. *Stroek* 2003; **34**: 2323–30.

Erkinjuntti T, Kurz A, Gauthier S, et al. Efficacy of galantamine in probable vascular dementia and Alzheimer's disease combined with cerebrovascular disease: A randomised trial. *Lancet* 2002; **359**: 1283–90.

Erkinjuntti T, Roman G, Gauthier S. Treatment of vascular dementia – evidence from clinical studies with cholinesterase inhibitors. *J Neurol Sci* 2004; **226**: 63–6.

Folstein MF, Folstein SE, McHugh PR. 'Mini-Mental State': a practical method for grading the cognitive state of patients for the clinician. *J Psychiatr Res* 1975; **12**: 189–98.

Kressig RW, Beauchet O, Tharicharu J. T'ai chi in the elderly: practical aspects. *Rev Med Suise Romande* 2003; **123**: 671–5.

Letenneur L. Risk of dementia and alcohol and wine consumption: A review of recent results. *Biol Res* 2004; **37**: 189–93.

Li G, Higdon R, Kukull WA, et al. Statin therapy and risk of dementia in the elderly: A community-based prospective cohort study. *Neurology* 2004; **63**: 1624–8.

Rockwood K, Kirkland S, Hogan DB, et al. Use of lipid-lowering agents, indication bias, and the risk of dementia in community-dwelling elderly people. *Arch Neurol* 2002; **59**: 223–7.

Ruitenberg A, van Swieten JC, et al. Alcohol consumption and risk of dementia: The Rotterdam Study. *Lancet* 2002; **359**: 281–6.

chapter 23

The role of the old age psychiatrist

Alistair Burns

Old age psychiatrists have a pivotal role in the diagnosis and management of people with dementia. In the UK this reflects the relative strength and coherence of old age psychiatry as a discipline stimulated, at least in part, by the seminal studies of Roth (1955) and Post in the 1960s and 1970s (Post, 1972), in addition to the pioneering work of practitioners such as David Jolley and Tom Arie (Jolley and Arie, 1978)

The role of old age psychiatry services in the UK has been described previously (Jolley and Arie, 1978), brought up to date (Dening, 1992, Jolley and Arie, 1992) and recently summarized internationally (Draper et al, 2005). The principle for all old age psychiatry services, in particular in relation to people with dementia, is that care in the community is most important and, while services throughout the UK differ in their style of organization, the common theme is community outreach, carried out by multidisciplinary teams, usually with a consultant old age psychiatrist as 'the nucleus of the service' (Jolley and Arie, 1992). The Royal College of Psychiatrists in the UK published norms some years ago for the approximate numbers of specialists and beds for a service, suggesting that one old age psychiatrist could serve a population of some 22 000 people over the age of 65 but more recently reflected an increase in the complexity of the service provided and in people's aspirations of care. A consultant might be expected to look after a population of between 10 000 and up to a maximum of 15 000 people over the age of 65. It is estimated that just over 20 acute beds with 45 continuing care beds and 45 day hospital places would be appropriate support for this (Royal College of Physicians and Royal College of Psychiatrists, 1989). However, the field changes on a regular basis and initiatives such as the NHS Plan and the National Service Framework for Older People have emphasized that services should be dynamic and should reflect the multidisciplinary nature of the work involved. This attests to the rising strength of other professions in the care for older people with mental health problems, in particular dementia.

Community mental health teams

The old age psychiatrist retains a pivotal role in leading the community mental health team which cares for older people with mental health problems in their own homes. A typical team is multidisciplinary, involving community nurses, social workers, physiotherapists, occupational therapists and chiropodists. The exact form of the team varies from centre to centre and depends often on the availability of local resources or how a team has grown over time. Old age psychiatry and old age psychiatrists are nothing if not adaptable, and inadequate resource provision over the years has led to the philosophy of services developing within the philosophy of 'the best service that could be offered within the constraints of existing facilities was the only meaningful aim possible' (Lennon and Jolley, 1991).

Challis et al (2002) found that 16% of old age psychiatrists felt that their services were not integrated with social services, with 11% saying that they were truly integrated with the rest in between. The aspiration is that integration, particularly with social care, offers advantages for individual patients referred to the service. A comparison with services available in Northern Ireland, where full integration is the norm (Reilly et al, 2003), showed that even when administrative integration is achieved, this does not always impact in terms of individual patient management. A survey has also shown the assessment instruments that old age psychiatrists use as a routine, with over 95% using a standard instrument for the assessment of cognitive function, 60% an instrument for assessing depression, 40% for assessing behaviour and 23% for assessing activities of daily living. Of those assessing for dementia, 95% used the mini mental state examination (MMSE), with 50% using the clock drawing test. In terms of assessing behaviour, 25% used the Clifton Assessment Procedures for the Elderly and nearly 20% used the Barthel Index (Mahoney and Barthel, 1965). The traditional vehicle for assessment at home is the domiciliary visit carried out by an old age psychiatrist. From a contractual point of view, this usually attracts an additional fee and therefore has become a target for rationalization in the health service. The outcomes of visits at home have been documented (Orrell et al, 1997).

Memory clinics

Memory clinics have become increasingly popular and they are now seen as a more or less integral part of old age psychiatry services and have been formally endorsed by the National Service Framework for Older People. Lindesay and colleagues (Wright and Lindesay, 1995; Lindesay et al, 2002) have carried out surveys of memory clinics, emphasizing the move away from a resource to attract people into taking part in clinical trials in dementia to services integrated with mainstream old age psychiatry provision and also involved in the initiation and monitoring of treatment with anti-dementia drugs.

Liaison psychiatry

An increasing number of older people with mental health problems are admitted to medical, surgical and geriatric wards in the general hospital. Old age psychiatrists are often asked to provide opinions as to the management and significance of behavioural problems. The usual model is one of consultation, i.e. the consultant in charge of the patient seeks advice about a specific problem but that consultant remains responsible for the patient's overall management and care. However, this provision is patchy throughout the UK and the infrastructure to support it does not reflect the volume of work. In some services, it can be upwards of a quarter to a third of all new referrals. A recent report (Holmes et al, 2002) underscored the huge need in this area and the requirement to have set time and resources within the old age psychiatry team to manage the workload. In some areas, nurses have begun to take on an enhanced role (Burgess and Page, 2003).

Nursing and residential homes

This is a sector of increasing importance in terms of old age psychiatry provision, largely reflecting the fact that more and more people in the residential and nursing home sector suffer from significant mental health problems. Our own studies have shown the success of old age psychiatry provision in terms of advice on the management of behavioural problems, largely related to dementia, in nursing and residential care (Proctor et al, 1999) and also in terms of the benefits of a pharmacy intervention in this sector (Furniss et al, 2000). Also, studies looking at the quality of life in nursing homes have emphasized that quality of care in this sector varies enormously (Mozely et al, 2004). This is obviously a sector where the role of psychiatric provision is increasing, as demonstrated by a recent national UK survey (Purandare et al, 2004) which found that the vast majority of home managers felt that there was a significant need for specialist advice and care for residents with mental health problems in their homes (Orrell et al, 1997). The philosophy is that assessing people in their own homes gives a better picture of their needs and therefore management can be targeted more specifically at their needs, with improved outcomes.

Services in the rest of Europe

It is difficult to find much information specifically about the role of the old age psychiatrist in the care of people with dementia; hence, the concentration in this chapter on the situation in the UK. However, some inferences can be drawn from descriptions of services in other countries. Bleeker and Diesfeldt (2000) describe the situation in Europe, describing four clusters or types of services that are characterized by a multidisciplinary approach, community orientation, coverage of the population and professional support of family carers. Denmark, Finland, Iceland and Sweden were found to score positive on all these factors. The profile of services in Holland is dominated by the profile described by Arie and Isaacs (1978) which emphasizes that the services should deal with the whole range of psychiatric morbidity in older people, may be confined to a geographic region, be responsible for the first contact, maintain the person at home wherever feasible, have multidisciplinary assessment in the person's own home, have hospital and community carers to complement the work of family doctors, have professionals to support families and operate an active day hospital. The Netherlands has a long-standing tradition of nursing home care for older people with mental health problems which has grown out of the medical model of care delivery. In Germany, it was noted that facilities for older people with mental health problems tended to be secondary to those available in general psychiatry (Weyerer et al, 2000). The vast majority of care for older people with mental health problems takes place in nursing homes, although there are old age psychiatry wards for short-term assessment and psychiatric hospitals where the length of stay is up to 3 weeks and a large number of admissions suffer from behavioural disturbances associated with dementia. In Italy, an Alzheimer plan was described in the Lombardy region up till 1996 with a view to the model spreading to the rest of the country (Paduoani and De Leo, 2000). The idea was to have five regional centres for the diagnosis of people with dementia, 40 Alzheimer units and 9 day hospitals and outpatient services linked to the regional Alzheimer centres.

Reifler and Cohen (1998) described the development of geriatric psychiatry, noting a number of stages of development of the specialty in the care of people with dementia. Ritchie et al (2005) has summarized some of the main services in France, Germany, Poland, Romania and Sweden as being representative of both Eastern and Western Europe. In France, old age psychiatry is not a specialty, and care is undertaken in general psychiatry or in specialist geriatric units or, in the presence of dementia, by neurologists. Long-term hospital care was the norm until recently. Most care takes place in people's own homes. In Germany, geriatric psychiatry is one part of psychiatry and neurological care is not a specific medical specialty. Informal care at home is the mainstay of the service with memory clinics recently becoming more important. Several multi-professional psychogeriatric centres are around, attached to psychiatric or general hospitals (Weyerer et al, 2000). In Poland, until the 1990s there was no statutory old age psychiatry service but since then things have developed and while there is no recognized specialization in psychogeriatrics, of 3100 psychiatrists in Poland, between 60 and 80 specialize in old age psychiatry. The usual range of inpatient facilities and outpatient clinics exist and there are aspirations to combine medical and social care. In Romania, old age psychiatry has been recognized as a specialty since 2001 and, of around 1000 psychiatrists, 27 are old age (or geronto-) psychiatrists. The first memory clinic has opened and a Romanian Association for Gerontopsychiatry was established in 1999. In Sweden, there is no specific specialty covering the field of old age psychiatry, treatments being undertaken in either geriatric medicine or general psychiatry with old age psychiatry incorporated into training.

Antidementia drugs

In the UK, old age psychiatrists are at the forefront of the prescription of antidementia drugs and for their monitoring and follow-up. The UK National Institute for Clinical Excellence (www.nice.org.uk) has recommended that regular monitoring of the effects of the drugs are put in place and, of the specialties cited as being able to do this, old age psychiatrists are mentioned along with geriatricians and neurologists. However, in practice in the NHS, the associated resources to allow for monitoring and follow-up of the effects of treatment are nested within old age psychiatry services. It attests to the interest and the relative power of old age psychiatry as a discipline that, in the UK, a major part of the prescribing and monitoring of antidementia drugs takes place in that specialty.

Conclusion

Old age psychiatry as a discipline has a great deal to offer in terms of the assessment and management of people with dementia. In the UK, it takes a key role in early diagnosis, organization of services, outreach of services and monitoring of treatment effects. The role has extended far beyond that which is often perceived by others as being the discipline's core contribution, i.e. the assessment and management of psychiatric symptoms and behavioural disturbances associated with dementia. An increased role in the treatment and management of people with a variety of antidementia drugs is likely, with the discipline having the most experience and having the administrative infrastructure to manage this regulated process.

References

Arie T, Isaacs A. A development of psychiatric services for the elderly in Britain. In: Isaacs A, Post F, eds. *Studies in geriatric psychiatry*. Chichester: John Wiley and Sons; 1978: 251–2.

Bleeker J, Diesfeldt H. Services for dementia in continental Europe: a Dutch view. In: O'Brien J, Ames D, Burns A, eds. *Dementia*, 2nd edn. London: Arnold; 2000: 300–2.

Burgess L, Page S. Educating nursing staff involved in the provision of dementia care. *Nurs Times* 2003; 99: 34–7.

Challis D, Reilly S, Hughes J, et al. Policy, organisation and practice of specialist old age psychiatry in England. *Int J Geriatr Psychiatry* 2002; 17: 1018–26.

Dening T. Community Psychiatry of Old Age: a UK perspective. *International Journal of Geriatric Psychiatry* 1992; 7(10): 757–765.

Draper B, Melding P, Brodaty H, eds. *Psychogeriatric service delivery*. Oxford: Oxford University Press; 2005.

Furniss L, Burns A, Cooke J, et al. The effect of a pharmacist's medication review in nursing homes. *Br J Psychiatry* 2000; 176: 563–67.

Holmes J, Bentley K, Cameron I. *Between two stools: Psychiatric services for older people in general hospitals*. Report of a UK Survey. University of Leeds; 2002.

Jolley D, Arie T. Organisation of psychogeriatric services. *Br J Psychiatry* 1978; 32: 1–11.

Jolley D, Arie T. Developments in psychogeriatric services. In: Arie T, ed. *Recent advances in psychogeriatrics 2*. Edinburgh: Churchill Livingstone; 1992: 117–35.

Lennon S, Jolley D. An urban service in South Manchester. In: Levy R, Oppenheimer C, eds. *Psychiatry in the elderly*. Oxford: Oxford University Press; 1991: 322–38.

Lindesay J, Marudkar M, Diepen E, Wilcock G. The second Leicester survey of memory clinics in the British Isles. *Int J Geriatr Psychiatry* 2002; 17: 41–7.

Mahoney FI, Barthel DW. Functional evaluation: The BARTHEL index. *Maryland State Med J* 1965; 14: 61–5.

Mozeley C, Sutcliffe C, Bagley H, et al. *Towards quality care: outcomes for older people in care homes*. Ashgate, Aldershot: PSSRU; 2004.

Orrell MW, Hardy-Thompson C, Bergmann K. Comparison between general practitioners with high or low use of a psychogeriatric domiciliary visit service. *Int J Geriatr Psychiatry* 1997; 12: 885–9.

Paduoani W, De Leo D, Bleeker J, Diesfeldt H. Services for dementia in continental Europe: an Italian view: In: O'Brien J, Ames D, Burns A. eds. *Dementia*, 2nd edn. London: Arnold; 2000: 306–7.

Post F. The management and nature of depressive illness in late life: A follow-through study. *Br J Psychiatry* 1972; 121: 292–404.

Proctor R, Burns A, Stratton-Powell H, et al. Behavioural management in nursing and residential homes. A randomised controlled trial. *Lancet* 1999; 354: 26–9.

Purandare N, Burns A, Challis D, Morris J. Perceived mental health needs and adequacy of service provision to older people in care homes in the UK: A national survey. *Int J Geriatr Psychiatry* 2004; 19: 549–53.

Reifler B, Cohen GD. Practice of geriatric psychiatry in mental health services for the elderly: Results of an international survey. *Int Psychogeriatr* 1998; 10: 351–7.

Reilly S, Challis D, Burns A. Does integration really make a difference? A comparison of old age psychiatry services in England and Northern Ireland. *Int J Geriatr Psychiatry* 2003; 18: 887–93.

Ritchie K, Norton J, Kurz A, et al. *Psychogeriatric services: Current trends in Europe*. Oxford: Oxford University Press; 2005: 161–75.

Roth M. The natural history of mental disorder in old age. *J Mental Sci* 1955; **April**: 281–301.

Royal College of Physicians and Royal College of Psychiatrists. *Care of elderly people with mental Illness: Specialist services and medical training*. London: Royal College of Physicians and Royal College of Psychiatrists; 1989.

Weyerer S, Schaufeler M, Bleeker J, Diesfeldt H. Services for dementia in continental Europe: a German view: In: O'Brien J, Ames D, Burns A. *Dementia*, 2nd edn. London: Arnold; 2000: 303–5.

Wright N, Lindesay J. A survey of memory clinics in the British Isles. *Int J Geriatr Psychiatry* 1995; 10: 379–85.

chapter 24

Neurology

Gunhild Waldemar

Introduction

The early identification, diagnosis, treatment and long-term management of dementia requires a multidisciplinary approach, which includes the skills of physicians as well as many other professionals, including, among others, specialist nurses, district nurses, neuropsychologists, therapists, social counsellors, legal advisors and district nurses. In recognition of the need for specialization and of the complexity of the task, many multidisciplinary memory clinics or dementia services have been developed throughout Europe during the past two decades. They typically offer a comprehensive service from early diagnosis to long-term management and caregiver training.

The role of neurologists in Europe

The particular contributions of the neurologist comprise the early identification and differential diagnosis of rare and common brain disorders causing cognitive and behavioural symptoms, the referral for and interpretation of certain ancillary investigations and the management of concomitant neurological complications.

For some patients, the neurologist provides the specialist advice for the primary care physician, geriatrician or psychiatrist caring for the patient; for others, the neurologist is the primary physician responsible for diagnosis and treatment. In general, neurologists see patients of younger age or those with a rapid progression, unusual clinical presentation, additional neurological symptoms or abnormal brain imaging. Some neurologists, however, may see a broader spectrum of patients of all ages.

The role of neurologists varies considerably across Europe, both in general and specifically in relation to dementia (Waldemar et al, 2000). The relative involvement of psychiatrists, geriatricians and neurologists in dementia research and patient care vary to a great extent. Also, the emphasis on primary care or direct self-referral to specialists has a major influence. Most neurologists are involved to some extent in the diagnosis of dementia, usually in the ongoing care but only a minority in long-term and residential care. Clearly, the number of patients per year seen by neurologists varies with the specific interests of the individual, with the setting and with the number of neurologists in the country. The latter varies considerably in European countries from 1 in 15 000 to 1 in 200 000 (Waldemar et al, 2000).

The contribution of the neurologist in the multidisciplinary setting

A wide array of neurological diseases may present with cognitive impairment or dementia. The large majority of dementias are caused by vascular dementia and degenerative brain diseases, of which Alzheimer's disease, frontotemporal degeneration and dementia with Lewy bodies are the most prevalent. The identification of more rare symptomatic causes of dementia, e.g. neuroinflammatory and neuroinfectious diseases, intracranial tumour or normal pressure hydrocephalus, also relies on the neurologist.

The diagnostic evaluation of patients with mild to moderate cognitive symptoms and possible dementia is an integrated multidisciplinary task. It should focus on the identification of non-progressive and potentially reversible aetiologies, co-morbidity, selective cognitive deficits and rare or atypical neurological conditions, as well as on the early identification of common progressive dementia disorders.

Thus, in the diagnostic work-up of dementia the role of the neurologist should be an active one, but what could the specific role of the neurologist be in the diagnosis and management of dementia? In general, the specific roles of neurologists may involve (Waldemar et al, 2000):

- general history-taking, with special reference to previous neurological events, of the patient and a close informant
- the neurological examination, with emphasis on focal signs, disturbances of eye movements, extrapyramidal signs and gait disturbances
- referral for and interpretation of specific ancillary investigations, such as neuropsychological tests, neuroimaging, lumbar puncture, electroencephalography (EEG), electromyography (EMG) and brain biopsy
- the identification and treatment of vascular factors in dementia

- diagnosis and treatment of seizures and extrapyramidal disturbances
- advice to referring physician, patient and caregivers on neurological aspects of diagnosis and treatment.

For some patients the neurologist is the primary physician in charge of the treatment and care. In these circumstances the neurologist should take part in the general management and in specific psychosocial treatments and assure the organization of psychosocial interventions for patients as well as for caregivers in collaboration with the community facilities. For most patients the neurologist acts as a consultant, but the neurologist should be aware of available psychosocial treatment principles and caregiver intervention programmes and refer the patients to appropriate programmes.

The neurologist in multidisciplinary versus monodisciplinary teams

Many multidisciplinary services have been developed as multidisciplinary teams in the monodisciplinary setting of either old age psychiatry, geriatrics, neurology or of a primary care centre. These services then rely on referral to specialists in other relevant medical fields, when necessary. There are concerns, however, that if referral between specialists, particularly neurologists and old age psychiatrists, is incomplete, patients may be underinvestigated or inappropriately followed up.

A recent British survey (Cordery et al, 2002) on the management of young patients concluded that, currently, the ideal of full collaboration between old age psychiatrists and neurologists is not achieved. Young patients may be underinvestigated if managed solely by an old age psychiatrist and may not receive adequate follow-up services if managed solely by a neurologist. (Cordery et al, 2002).

That the diagnosis and management of young patients with cognitive symptoms, in particular, call for an integrated multidisciplinary setting was also suggested in a study by Elberling et al (2002). With the objective of characterizing the cognitive profiles and underlying conditions in younger patients with cognitive symptoms, 314 consecutive patients (aged <60 years old) referred to a multidisciplinary memory clinic were studied: 15% of the patients fulfilled international criteria for dementia, 17% had selective cognitive deficits and 55% had no cognitive deficits. Thus, cognitive symptoms in younger patients rarely reflect dementia but more often other medical and psychiatric conditions (Elberling et al, 2002).

Likewise, in elderly patients, there is also evidence that an integrated multidisciplinary approach may improve diagnosis and follow-up. Verhey et al (1993) investigated referrals from different specialists to a memory clinic service. In patients referred by psychiatrists, sensitivity rates for dementia and Alzheimer's disease were low; in patients referred by neurologists, depression often went unreported. The results underscored the need for more frequent use of integrated multidisciplinary services for cognitively disturbed patients (Verhey et al, 1993).

Hejl et al (2003) investigated the effect of systematic psychiatric evaluation in patients referred to a memory clinic in a neurological setting. Psychiatric conditions and symptoms are frequent in elderly patients with cognitive symptoms, including those referred to a neurological memory clinic. The data provided evidence that a systematic multispecialty and multidisciplinary approach to the diagnosis and management of patients with possible dementia enhanced the identification of cognitive and psychiatric symptoms (Hejl et al, 2003).

Thus, there is a general consensus that the management of dementia should be handled by multidisciplinary teams.

Neurological guidelines for the diagnosis and management of dementia

With continuous advances in neuroscience, new methods and techniques for diagnosis and treatment of neurodegenerative brain disorders will frequently come into clinical practice. Hence, the development of evidence-based guidelines for the diagnosis and management of dementia will be crucial for summarizing and updating evidence for the clinicians who are involved in the management of dementia (Qizilbash et al, 2002). Guidelines may also serve to identify aspects of care where there is a lack of evidence. National or international guidelines are useful in order to develop uniform management practices, to set the standard for quality health care and for the evaluation of quality of care. Regional guidelines may serve to define the role of different professionals and specialists. Evidence-based guidelines for neurologists have been developed in several countries, and some of them have been published in international journals. The American Academy of Neurology recently published their revised guideline in three parts (Petersen et al, 2001; Knopman et al, 2001; Doody et al, 2001): mild cognitive impairment, diagnosis of dementia and management of dementia. The

Italian Neurological Society recently published their revised guideline (Musicco et al, 2004). An international group under the auspices of the European Federation of Neurological Societies (EFNS) published the first European guideline for neurologists (Waldemar et al, 2000), a guideline which is now being revised by the EFNS with the involvement of other specialists.

Training of neurologists

With the significant advances in neuroscience research, particularly in the field of behavioural neurology, and with the increasing prevalence of dementia, the need for appropriate and timely neurological involvement will increase. Hence, it is essential that diagnostic evaluation and management of dementia should be included in the training of all neurologists. The training should include individual patient-based training under competent mentoring, as well as the teaching of updated information on basic science issues relevant to dementia, and on diagnostic evaluation and treatment of Alzheimer's disease and other dementia disorders (Waldemar et al, 2000).

Concluding remarks

Ideally, a dementia service should be multidisciplinary not only across professions but also across medical specialties. Specialists from geriatrics, neurology and old age psychiatry should all be members of the team. Further progress in understanding brain diseases and behaviour will demand even fuller collaboration and integration of these fields, as the tools they use, the questions they ask and the theoretical frameworks they employ come closer.

References

Cordery R, Harvey R, Frost C, Rossor M. National survey to assess current practices in the diagnosis and management of young people with dementia. *Int J Geriatr Psychiatry* 2002; 17: 124–7.

Doody RC, Stevens JC, Beck RN, et al. Practice parameter: Management of dementia (an evidence-based review). Report of the quality standards subcommittee of the Amerian Academy of Neurology. *Neurology* 2001; 56: 1154–66.

Elberling TV, Stokholm J, Høgh P, Waldemar G. Diagnostic profile of young and middle-aged memory clinic patients. *Neurology* 2002; 59:1259–62.

Hejl AM, Hørding M, Hasselbalch E, et al. Psychiatric morbidity in a neurology-based memory clinic: the impact of systematic psychiatric evaluations. *J Am Geriatr Soc* 2003; 51: 1773–8.

Knopman DS, DeKosky ST, Cummings JL, et al. Practice parameter: Diagnosis of dementia (an evidence-based review). Report of the Quality Standards Subcommittee of the Amerian Academy of Neurology. *Neurology* 2001; 56: 1143–53.

Musicco M, Caltagirone C, Sorbi S, Bonavita V. Dementia Study Group of the Italian Neurological Society. Italian Neurological Society guidelines for the diagnosis of dementia: Revision I. *Neurol Sci* 2004; 25: 154–82.

Petersen RC, Stevens JC, Ganguli M, et al. Practice parameter: Early detection of dementia: Mild cognitive impairment (an evidence-based review). Report of the Quality Standards Subcommittee of the Amerian Academy of Neurology. *Neurology* 2001; 56: 1133–42.

Qizilbash N, Schneider L, Chui H, et al. *Evidence-based dementia practice.* Oxford: Blackwell Science; 2002.

Verhey FRJ, Jolles J, Ponds RWHM, et al. Diagnosing dementia: Comparison between monodisciplinary and a multidisciplinary approach. *J Neuropsychiatr Neurosc* 1993; 5: 78–85.

Waldemar G, Dubois B, Emre M, et al. Diagnosis and management of Alzheimer's disease and related disorders: The role of neurologists in Europe. *Eur J Neurol* 2000; 7: 133–4.

chapter 25

Primary care: Fit for the dementia challenge?

Gabriela Stoppe

Family physicians are in the key position

There is no doubt that family physicians (FPs) are in the key position for early recognition and management of dementia (Table 25.1). This holds especially true for health systems with gatekeepers, such as in the Netherlands, Finland or Denmark. In contrast to many of the specialists' services, primary care is available in urban and rural areas and provides home visits and continuity of care (e.g. Consensus Statement, 1997; Audit Commission, 2000). The elderly often suffer from one or more somatic disorders, for the treatment of which they visit their FP on a regular basis. Just to give an example, even in the urban area of Berlin, according to the Berlin Ageing Study, 85% of the over 70-year-old elderly visit the FP more than 20 times a year on average. Of the 60% who also visit a specialist, only 4% visit a neuropsychiatrist (Mayer and Baltes, 1996).

However, while patients contact a memory clinic to get a check for memory complaints, they do not explicitly 'bring' this symptom to the FP. Typically, the FP and the practice personnel should be 'searching' for (early) signs of dementia. This means a more active approach (Löppönen et al, 2003). Searching means that, when 'finding' is the consequence, diagnostics should be applied and a disclosure of a diagnosis might arise as the consequence. This seems to be a problem not only for many FPs, because they regard the diagnosis as not very relevant against a background of abundant nihilism and doubts of the efficacy of available treatments (Riedel-Heller et al, 1999; Turner et al, 2004; van Hout et al, 2000). In Germany (and other countries), budgetary restrictions also play a role. In our own investigation, we asked primary care physicians for their opinion on cholinesterase

Table 25.1 Tasks of a family physician and the necessary knowledge

Task	Knowledge/skill
Recognize early symptoms of dementia	Epidemiology, early signs, role of informant's information
(Opportunistic) screening and further diagnostic assessment	Reversible causes leading to memory complaints (depression, drugs, thyroid dysfunction, vitamin deficiency, etc.)
Disclosure of diagnosis	How to disclose, provide hope and help
Start of treatment, counselling	Which drugs (choice, side effects, dosage), impact of day structuring, light exposure, nutrition, etc.
Organize support for patients and caregivers	Information about people and institutions available in the region
Check the caregivers' health	Knowledge about caregiver strain
Check the patient's health	Awareness of changed/different way or absence of complaining
Legal consequences	Knowledge on legal conditions

inhibitors (ChEIs). When comparing real practice data to the answers in the interview of the same physicians, 69% would treat a relative suffering from Alzheimer's disease, 35% a patient, but – according to prescribing data and chart review – only 13% prescribed a ChEI to a demented patient in reality (Stoppe and Pirk, 2002).

Competence of primary care physicians

Recently, empirical studies have qualified the conventional wisdom that knowledge about dementia (epidemiology, diagnosis, therapy, etc.) is associated with more confidence and communication on the diagnosis (Turner et al, 2004; Cody et al, 2002). Many studies, using varying methods, consistently showed that early diagnosis is far from being reached in primary care. According to German, Swedish, Finnish and US studies, less than one-third of dementia cases is recognized, with increasing rates from about 20–33% in mild and up to 80% in moderate to severe stages (Stoppe et al, 1994; Olafsdottir et al, 2001; Löppönen et al, 2003; Boise et al, 2004). Referral to a specialist was considered in more advanced cases and in younger patients (Löppönen et al, 2003; Stoppe et al, 1998). Confidence, especially in the management of behavioural problems, and knowledge on the availability and organization of (local) support systems are even much lower than diagnostic confidence in the FPs studied (Turner et al, 2004; Riedel-Heller et al, 1999; Olafsdottir et al, 2001). That diagnosis and/or screening alone is useless, when there is not enough knowledge on the management thereafter, is also highlighted by the fact that the prescription rate of ChEI is much lower than recognition rate (Iliffe et al, 2003; Boise et al, 2004).

When considering the competence of FPs, the competence of primary care specialists should also not be neglected. In our own representative investigations comparing neuropsychiatric and FP competence, we could not find large differences with regards to awareness; however, there were many discrepancies considering diagnostic assessment (unpublished work). One US study compared 17 FP and 14 neurologists and – validated to neuropathological diagnosis – found a clinical diagnostic accuracy of 84% in FPs and only 77.5% in the specialists (Mok et al, 2004). This could explain the increasing relevance of memory clinics as the population learns more about dementia!

What is to be done for a better management of dementia in primary care?

Some researchers believe that existing guidelines could help. Evidence-based guidelines are also said to increase adherence (Grol et al, 1998). However, recently, one large implementation trial that included 727 FPs in Denmark could not detect an increase of practice adherence, at least in the short run, although the guideline was developed by general practice and 89% of the participating physicians regarded it as 'applicable' (Waldorff et al, 2003).

In a situation where available evidence points to a bad management of memory disorders in primary care and to a low adherence to guidelines, it is important to find clues on how to change the situation. The capacity and availability of specialist services are limited in all health systems, and underlines the major role for primary care. If however, like in Denmark, ChEI may be prescribed by specialists only, this means limited access to helpful treatments, especially to the rural and immobile demented population. There is a

Table 25.2 Some criteria for referral to a specialist as recommended by the German healthcare system

- Patients younger than 70 years old
- Suspicion of non-Alzheimer origin of dementia (acute onset, rapid progression, stroke or abrupt deterioration, focal neurological signs)
- Indication for (expensive) instrumental diagnostics: neuroimaging, genetics, cerebrospinal fluid, etc.
- Antidementia treatment shows no clear benefit
- Newly occurring behavioural symptoms
- Planned or upcoming nursing home admission, especially when symptoms such as nocturnal confusion, aggression or incontinence occur

Source: Stoppe et al, 2004.

need to define the interface in the cooperation between FP and specialists for each healthcare system. We did so in Germany by leaving diagnosis and treatment of a typical dementia patient to the FP and defining operational criteria for involvement of a specialist (Stoppe et al, 2004). Some criteria for referral are given in Table 25.2.

Although most FPs regard the management of dementia as their task and also agree that early diagnosis is important and much can be done for the patients and carers, there seem to be obstacles hindering FPs to do what seems to be necessary (Turner et al, 2004; Iliffe et al, 2003; Waldorff et al, 2003).

As pointed out, knowledge and skills contribute to confidence in the diagnostic and therapeutic skills and also correlate to nihilism and pessimism! Knowledge and skills are key domains of (postgraduate) education and point to the relevance of the medical teaching and training system. However, there is not much training available. In many countries, FPs do not have an obligatory training in geriatric medicine, psychiatry or neurology. In Europe, only in the UK is old age psychiatry established as a discipline: neither geriatric medicine nor old age psychiatry are present at the majority of German medical faculties. Thus, at best, the obligation to teach knowledge on dementia is spread over many disciplines and one might rely on the other. Teachers and trainers are heavily needed not only for the education of physicians but also for teaching other health professionals. In addition, the skill to talk to a patient about the diagnosis of a debilitating disease needs psychosocial training and is not only relevant for the dementias. To talk about taboos and to tackle persisting ageism are relevant topics for the education of physicians in a changing and ageing society.

References

Audit Commission. *Forget me not.* London: Audit Commission; 2000. Available at www.audit-commission.gov.uk

Boise L, Neal MB, Kaye J. Dementia assessment in primary care: Results from a study in managed care systems. *J Gerontol A Biol Sci Med Sci* 2004; 59: M621–6.

Cody M, Beck C, Shue VM, Pope S. Reported practices of primary care physicians in the diagnosis and management of dementia. *Aging Ment Health* 2002; 6: 72–6.

Consensus Statement of the American Association for Geriatric Psychiatry, the Alzheimer's Association, and the American Geriatrics Society. Diagnosis and treatment of Alzheimer disease and related disorders. *JAMA* 1997; 278: 1363–71.

Grol R, Dalhuijsen J, Thomas S, et al. Attributes of clinical guidelines in general practice: Observational study. *Br Med J* 1998; 317: 802–8.

Iliffe S, Manthorpe J, Eden A. Sooner or later? Issues in the early diagnosis of dementia in general practice: A qualitative study. *Family Pract* 2003; 20: 376–81.

Löppönen M, Raiha I, Isoaho R, Vahlberg T, Kivela SL. Diagnosing cognitive impairment and dementia in primary health care – a more active approach is needed. *Age Ageing* 2003; 32: 606–12.

Mayer KU, Baltes PB. *Die Berliner Altersstudie.* Berlin: Akademie Verlag; 1996.

Mok W, Chow TW, Zheng L, Mack WJ, Miller C. Clinicopathological concordance of dementia diagnoses by community versus tertiary care clinicians. *Am J Alzheimers Dis Other Demen* 2004; 19: 161–5.

Olafsdottir M, Foldevi M, Marcusson J. Dementia in primary care: Why the low detection rate? *Scand J Prim Health Care* 2001; 19: 194–8.

Riedel-Heller SG, Schork A, Matschinger H, Angermeyer MC. The role of referrals in diagnosing dementia at the primary care level. *Int Psychogeriatr* 1999; 11: 251–62.

Stoppe G, Bergmann F, Bohlken J, et al. Ambulante Versorgung von Demenzkranken. Ein Vorschlag zur Gestaltung der Schnittstelle zwischen HausärztInnen und ÄrztInnen für Psychiatrie und Neurologie in Deutschland. *Psychoneuro* 2004; 30: 489–96 [abstract in English].

Stoppe G, Pirk O. Praxisstudie: Therapie von Alzheimer Patienten. *Der Allgemeinarzt* 2002; 12: 884–6.

Stoppe G, Sandholzer H, Staedt J, et al. Diagnosis of dementia in primary care: Results of a representative survey in lower Saxony, Germany. *Eur Arch Psychiatry Clin Neurosci* 1994; 244: 278–83.

Stoppe G, Sandholzer H, Winter S, Kiefer J, Staedt J. Treatment of the memory disturbed elderly in primary care. *Primary Care Psychiatry* 1998; 4: 205–9.

Turner S, Iliffe S, Downs M, et al. General practitioners' knowledge, confidence and attitudes in diagnosis and management of dementia. *Age Ageing* 2004; 33: 461–7.

Van Hout H, Vernooij-Dassen M, Bakker K, Blom M, Grol R. General practitioners on dementia: Tasks, practices, and obstacles. *Patient Educ Couns* 2000; 39: 219–25.

Waldorff FB, Almind G, Makela M, Moller S. Waldemar G. Implementation of a clinical dementia guideline. A controlled effect of a multifaceted strategy. *Scand J Prim Health Care* 2003; 21: 142–7.

chapter 26

The occupational therapy contribution to interventions for people with dementias

Sylvie Meyer

Occupational therapy

Occupational therapists are health professionals interested in everyday life. Their patients are essentially those who, consequent to a disease, accident or developmental disorder experience difficulties in performing their occupations at home, at their workplace or in the community. Treatments are intended to help people to choose and engage in occupations they find satisfying. In practice, the occupational therapists propose to their patients activities that allow them to train their skills, give advice on how to act in different circumstances, suggest and realize change of environment and support adaptative strategies to new health conditions. Treatment is always a cooperative process between the occupational therapist and the patient (Canadian Association of Occupational Therapists, 1999). From an outside point of view, treatment often comprises ordinary everyday occupations such as using a lift or getting up from a chair, or exercises that are a little bit sophisticated such as moving special pieces on different targets, or games, or creative activities such as painting, or conversations (not always serious), or environment modifications such as reorganizing the contents of a cupboard (Meyer, 1996).

Old people, made frail by age or by disorders that alter their physical or mental functions, are an important population in occupational therapy. Occupational therapists meet them in hospitals, usually in rehabilitation facilities but also in psychiatric facilities or in special care units for Alzheimer patients; at home; in day-care service; and in residential long-term care (Glogoski-Williams et al, 1998; Meyer, 1996). People suffering from difficulties resulting from Alzheimer's disease or another dementia are traditionally part of an occupational therapist's clients, but not all of them need such an intervention and they do not always have access to it.

How occupational therapists understand dementia

Professionals who offer services to demented people share, in some measure, the same knowledge and the same competencies, but they also have, and simultaneously, specific ways of conceiving patients' problems and of solving them (Rufini and Gaillard, 1997). Some therapists are interested in cognitive aspects, others in medical diagnostics and medications and yet others in affective or emotional aspects of treatment. Occupational therapists are concerned in promoting the independence and autonomy of demented people in the context of their everyday occupations and daily life, according to their interests and to the impact of their cognitive deficiencies upon their actions and upon their relationship to others or to the physical environment. They are also involved in supporting the heavy work accomplished by the caregivers, either at home or in nursing homes (Dassié et al, 1999; American Occupational Therapy Association, 1996).

The beginning: to manage the occupations and prevention

During the first stage of the disease, the patient seldom has access to occupational therapy services, either because the diagnosis has not been given or because the case has not been referred to this kind of specialist. Nevertheless, when there are only light episodic memory troubles and executive functions troubles, the person has learning capacities, solving problems capacities and verbal and written communication skills that open a number of doors to managing in advance part of the problems that are to come (Mulligan et al, 2003). To be precise, the first subjective strategy used to adjust to the disease is to manage the patient's everyday occupations so that they do not become unbearable. The occupational therapist can help patients to list the stressful situations, to reflect upon them, to decide what to change, and then to modify their habits accordingly. The patient can then learn new routines that could be very precious later; e.g. to use public transport. In these cases, the occupational therapist's role is to sustain the preparation and the accomplishment of such learning (Nygard and Ohman, 2002; American Occupational Therapy Association, 1994).

An early intervention also offers people an opportunity to think of their needs and interests and to communicate them to their relatives. We know that most demented patients like to engage in meaningful and satisfying activities (Nygard and Ohman, 2002; Zgola, 1999). But the meaning that people give to their occupations varies a lot from one person to another and, furthermore, is taken for granted, so without reasoning and discussion, it stays inaccessible. It will be particularly hard to find the meaning of an activity for people who have not known the patient before he entered hospital and was no more able to reason and to communicate. For instance, when a person says, 'my favourite activity is playing violin', nothing indicates what he finds in this activity, but one knows that his performance will decrease, probably until its abandonment. The caregivers, professional or otherwise, will probably ask themselves what is the best choice to substitute for it: to play a simpler music instrument; to go to concerts; to participate in a choral society; to listen to the violin; or to clean the dishes? The better the work done to understand and to explore the meaning of the activity, the better will be the proposal of the caregivers.

Development of the disease: simplifying everyday activities and designing the environment

As the disease develops, the patient cannot manage everyday life alone. He is disorientated in the spatial environment, and faces the risk of being lost in his own surroundings. He experiences lots of difficulties: e.g. to learn to find his way in a nursing home. Patients are confused about their own history and they no longer know the temporal organization of the day. They inadequately plan activities, are lost in their actions and frequently fail, all of which generates frustration, withdrawal and sometimes violence against caregivers. The patient needs to be supervised or directed in his everyday routines such as shopping or cooking. The most common methods and familiar activities of the occupational therapist with these patients concerns these specific aspects of treatment (Santo Pietro and Ostuni, 2003; American Occupational Therapy Association, 1996; Zgola, 1999).

These methods have been widely disseminated, in particular by the Alzheimer associations. To tackle spatial disorientation, i.e. the person loses his way or cannot find the things he needs, the occupational therapist works on the learning process and on the environment. The environment must become more meaningful and indicators must be learned or relearned. One can clear the environment by removing useless objects, underline the function of the different spaces as explicitly as possible, e.g. by refusing to serve meals in the rooms of a nursing home, and increase the visibility and the access to desirable places, e.g. by leaving the toilet door open (American Occupational Therapy Association, 1996; Zgola, 1999). Temporal disorientation is harder to manage because this kind of orientation needs quite elaborate mental representation; nevertheless, it is possible to use an agenda or other forms of memory prosthesis (Holmes, 2000).

When programming an activity becomes problematic, the complexity of the activity must be decreased: e.g. when two things such as speaking about the weather and cooking rice cannot be executed together. It is often necessary to break tasks into pieces and do them step by step. Each part must stay understandable in itself and in relation to the entire activity so that it must have interest for the person; otherwise, it is nonsense. Very concrete and ordinary occupations such as ironing, gardening, wandering or painting a tin soldier (if the patient used to do it) have to be selected. Unusual tasks, especially those offered in some kind of treatment such as classifying images, must be avoided because they have no impact on everyday life (Josephsson, et al, 1995). To go from one part of an activity to another, one must give verbal indications that are simple, short, without ambiguity and include nonverbal cues (Santo Pietro and Ostuni, 2003).

Occupational therapists as educators more than therapists

The role of occupational therapists is not really to treat directly or to attend demented persons performing everyday occupations, but to delineate with them and their relatives those activities that must and can be accomplished, then to observe the performance to determine the supervision needed and the environment modifications required. Finally, the occupational therapist has to teach the most effective methods elicited to caregivers (American Occupational Therapy Association, 1996; Glogoski-Williams et al, 1998; Zgola, 1999). This behavioural observation must be sufficiently accurate and put in relation to the context and to cognitive deficiencies identified because a strictly functional analysis is not sufficient to determine the best means and ways to support performance of a specific patient. In this sense, the occupational therapist ought sometimes to reject old conceptions of Alzheimer's disease and what they have learned in their professional training to develop more evidence-based practice in their evaluations and treatment proposals.

In the end, and as dementia is a social problem that goes beyond both families and hospitals, we underline that acting to help those with dementia is not very difficult. One can even, for a while, make the mistake of regarding how a patient is understood without dramatic outcomes as it is usually possible to adjust an incorrect intervention, because treatment is more a continuing adaptation than a series of planned decisions to execute. For the therapist, the most difficult part of the process is to stay constant and consistent when always giving the same help so many times. Caregivers, at home or in nursing home, who stay so long with patients are not recognized enough for their heavy work. In the future, it is essential that the knowledge intended to remedy a demented person's difficulties should be further disseminated to people that meet these people in the community: policemen, shop assistants, public transport drivers, etc. In this manner, maintaining some autonomy and some quality of life for demented people and their caregivers will be achievable.

References

American Occupational Therapy Association. Statement: Occupational therapy services for persons with Alzheimer's disease and other dementia. *Am J Occup Ther* 1994; **48**: 1029–31.

American Occupational Therapy Association. *ROTE: The role of occupational therapy with the elderly*. Bethesda, MD: American Occupational Therapy Association; 1996.

Canadian Association of Occupational Therapists. *Enabling occupation: An occupational therapy perspective*, 3rd edn. Ottawa: Canadian Association of Occupational Therapists; 1999.

Glogoski-Williams, C, Foti D, Covault M. Dementia. In: Cara E, MacRae A, eds. *Psychosocial occupational therapy, a clinical practice*. Albany: Delmar; 1998.

Holmes T. Use of a memory notebook to help Alzheimer caregivers manage behavioral excesses. *Phys Occup Ther Geriatr* 2000; **17**: 67–80.

Josephsson S, Bäckman L, Borell L. Effectiveness of an intervention to improve occupational performance in dementia. *Occup Ther J Res* 1995; **15**: 36–49.

Meyer S. Etudes des conceptions de l'activité en ergothérapie auprès des personnes âgées. *J d'ergothérapie* 1996; **18**: 142–8.

Mulligan R, Van der Linden M, Juillerat A-C. *The clinical management of early Alzheimer's disease: A handbook*. Mahwah, NJ: L. Elbaum; 2003.

Nygard L, Ohman A. Managing changes in everyday occupations: The experience of persons with Alzheimer disease. *Occup Ther J Res* 2002; **22**: 70–81.

Rufini J, Gaillard M. *Pratiques psychogériatriques: La genèse d'une équipe interdisciplinaire*. Paris: L'harmattan; 1997.

Santo Pietro MJ, Ostuni E. *Successful communication with persons with Alzheimer disease*, 2nd edn. St Louis: Butterworth-Heinemann; 2003.

Zgola JM. *Care that works: a relationship approach to persons with dementia*. Baltimore: Johns Hopkins University Press; 1999.

chapter 27

Social work

Jane Hughes, Caroline Sutcliffe and David Challis

Introduction

The medical and social care of older people with dementia has become an international concern. As life expectancy continues to rise in European countries, the number of people with dementia is forecast to grow steadily over the next 25 years and this will require greater input from professional services and informal carers alike. Thus, it is important to promote international collaboration to exchange information and practice and to develop culturally appropriate dementia services (Alzheimer's Society, 2004). Specialist care management for older people with dementia is an area of practice in which there is much scope for innovation and development. However, a national survey of old age psychiatry services in England and Northern Ireland revealed that just 24% of old age services had specialist dementia services with designated members of staff and that links between health and social care provision were frequently poor (Challis et al, 2002a).

Prior to the introduction of care management, descriptions of social work in services for adults, including older people, tended to focus on profession-specific activities, to the neglect of outputs such as the function of linking the individual to networks of care, and these were typically short term in nature. The advent of care management has required a useful redefinition of social work in relation to long-term care of older people. It originated in North America in response to the shift in the balance of care away from institutional to community-based provision, and it can be most simply defined as a strategy for organizing and coordinating care services at the level of the individual client/patient. It has proven applicability to older people with dementia (Eggert et al, 1990; Challis et al, 2002b), and may be explained in terms of the six characteristics described in Table 27.1. Thus, care management is a model of long-term care, contrasting with short-term task-centred social work, as illustrated in Figure 27.1. This defining feature of case management renders it particularly relevant to the provision of community care

Table 27.1 Key characteristics of care management

Characteristics	Description
Functions	Coordination and linkage of care services
Goals	Providing continuity and integrated care; increased opportunity for home-based care; promote patient well-being; making better use of resources
Core tasks	Case-finding and screening; assessment; care planning; monitoring and review; case closure
Characteristics of recipients	Long-term care needs; multiple service need
Main features	Intensity of involvement; breadth of services spanned; lengthy duration of involvement
Multi-level response	Linking practice-level activities with broader resource and agency-level activities

Source: Challis et al, 1995: 20.

for older people with dementia whose need for long-term care is clearly demonstrated by their declining health status.

Donabedian (1980) described a model using the criteria of structure, process and outcome to address the quality agenda, which could also provide a useful framework to examine patterns of care for older people with dementia.

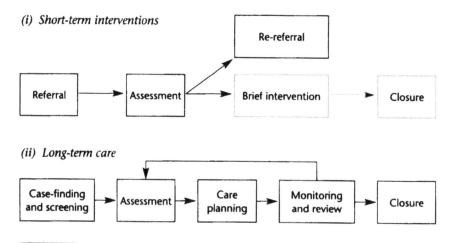

Figure 27.1 *A model of care. (Reproduced with permission from Challis et al. 1990.)*

Although primarily orientated to health care, this model can be applied to social care and, arguably, integrated health and social care, a concept of increasing importance. Indeed, in terms of the first two components of Donabedian's model, it is possible to describe elements of good practice for the care of older people with dementia using eight standards. Criteria of structure, which provide the first four standards, describe the framework in which care management for older people is undertaken. These include:

- the structure of teams
- arrangements for commissioning services, such as domiciliary care and respite care
- the financial arrangements which underpin these specialist services for older people with dementia, particularly the extent to which they facilitate integrated health and social care provision
- organizational arrangements which promote a differentiated response to individual need.

Process criteria describe the means by which core components of care management are delivered, namely:

- targeting
- assessment
- implementing the care plan
- monitoring and review.

These provide the remaining four standards, each of which is defined and described below.

Standards

Standard One
Care management should be provided by members of a multidisciplinary team specializing in the care of older people with mental health problems.

The provision of care management through specialist teams for older people rather than generic adult teams was found to be necessary for the development of intensive care management (Challis et al, 2001), a prerequisite for the provision of complex packages of care to enable older people with dementia to continue to live in their own homes as an alternative to residential and nursing home care. The benefits of locating a service within a multidisciplinary specialist mental health team have been clearly demonstrated (Challis et al, 2002b). In this context, care managers had small caseloads, access to a range of resources and provided care to older people on a long-term basis. Care management is not the exclusive preserve of social workers. It can be undertaken by nurses and, for older people with mental health problems, it is appropriate for them to have specialist training (Eggert et al, 1990; Weiner et al, 2003).

Standard Two

Services for older people with dementia require an integrated and informed approach to commissioning that embraces both their health and social care needs.

Clear goals are required in order to provide a framework for the commissioning of services for older people with dementia, such as day, outpatient, residential and hospital services. Moreover, adequate information must be available to inform the service-commissioning process in the locality incorporating the user/carer perspective. Whereas data on prevalence can be inferred from national sources, information on service use, particularly social care services such as respite and domiciliary care, may be difficult to obtain. Moreover, it is imperative that if health and social care for older people with dementia is not commissioned by a single agency, robust joint planning mechanisms must exist to ensure that the provision of appropriate services for this group of people is not neglected.

Standard Three

Financial arrangements are required which facilitate an integrated approach to the provision of health and social care for older people with dementia.

Financial arrangements which promote the provision of integrated care to older people with dementia are important. In the UK, recent legislative changes have created new opportunities to remove the financial barriers to joint working by promoting pooled budgets between health and social care, delegated commissioning and integration between services. Each brings potential benefits for older people with dementia by:

- the development of more flexible and idiosyncratic packages of care for individuals
- improved service commissioning at a local level
- greater continuity of care achieved by a single organization that provides both community nursing and domiciliary care.

This demonstrates the importance of establishing financial incentives which promote integrated service provision.

Standard Four

A differentiated approach to care management is necessary to ensure that older people with dementia receive a level of response appropriate to their health and social care needs.

In terms of degree of differentiation within care management arrangements, there are five defining features:

- provision by a specialist team
- variability in response to need in terms of level of staff and resource provided
- some staff with small caseloads
- the presence of intensive care management and, concurrently,
- the provision of care management to a wider group of patients (Challis et al, 1998).

A differentiated approach to the mode of assessment and care management is one in which a distinction is made between service users with complex needs often requiring a multi-service response and those with less complex needs which are often met by a single service response provided by one agency. Older people with dementia typically have complex health and social care needs and it is important that agencies have in place procedures and protocols within care management arrangements which facilitate an appropriate response.

Standard Five

Targeting within care management arrangements is required to ensure that vulnerable older people with complex needs, such as those with dementia, receive the care package they require to enable them to live at home.

The process of targeting resources occurs at two points in the care management process: on entry into the service and within initial assessment. It ensures that older people with dementia can receive services which differ both in content and intensity to those received by others with less complex needs. Care management services are intended for those people at risk of admission to long-term care, such as older people with dementia, reflecting the policy of 'downward substitution' by the provision of more cost-effective community-based alternatives. Therefore, the targeting of services on frail older people in greatest need, in particular older people with dementia, is a recurrent theme in the evolution of care management arrangements and is of paramount importance, both in terms of cost and, particularly, outcomes for patients.

Standard Six

Assessment as a precursor to a care plan must be multidisciplinary and appropriate in terms of content and timing to ensure that older people with dementia receive the requisite assistance to maintain their community tenure.

Assessment within care management has three elements:

- collection of information about a patient's situation and functioning
- the evaluation of this in the context of the patient's abilities, existing support and the need for additional assistance
- a care plan coordinating informal and formal services to maximize the patient's independence (Golden and Tropman, 2000).

It is important that assessment for care management is not regarded as a one-off process, that its elements are undertaken within a timescale appropriate to circumstances and that it is fit for purpose. This requires the clear identification of domains of assessment embracing patients' health status and their capacity to perform tasks associated with daily living; the support they receive from family, friends and formal services; and their quality of life in the context of their clinical condition. It thus requires a structured approach with the use of suitable standardized tools. Contributions to the assessment may be necessary from more than one source but should be appropriate to the nature of the problem and should facilitate the end product of the assessment, the care plan.

Standard Seven

Care plans are required to support, sustain and enhance the quality of life of older people with dementia in their own home, following an assessment of need and also to provide assistance to their carers.

Care planning is recognized as an important function of case management and incorporates two elements:

- negotiating the most appropriate means to achieve the goals identified in the assessment
- securing the necessary services or resources to meet them.

In an intensive case management service for older people with dementia the most frequently reported goals of intervention were supportive, therapeutic and practical. Supportive goals were mainly for the benefit of carers, to relieve their burden and provide respite. Therapeutic interventions were used to benefit both older people with dementia and their carers, including strategies to reduce the problem behaviours associated with the patient's deteriorating mental state. Practical goals were geared towards the individual patient, with assistance with personal care, health care and domestic care being the most frequently reported goals (Challis and Hughes, 2000).

Standard Eight
Monitoring and review in care management is required to ensure the timely and appropriate adjustment of the care plan in order to maintain older people with dementia at home in response to changing circumstances

Monitoring and review within case management are the means by which changes in circumstances and health status are noted and the components of the care plan are adjusted accordingly. They constitute one of the hallmarks of intensive care management: namely, the coordination of a variety of related functions over time (Challis et al, 1995). Regular systems of review are important for older people with dementia for three reasons. First, due to their vulnerability and their impaired ability to report any sudden changes in their circumstances, regular monitoring of services for older people with dementia is essential. Secondly, it provides a means of gaining enhanced knowledge of patients and their circumstances, thereby increasing the likelihood that the care plan will be closely tailored to patient need. Thirdly, it promotes maintenance of the care network by providing support to both informal and formal carers and is also a component of quality assurance in respect of services provided.

Conclusion

Overall, internationally, there is little documented evidence of progress towards a model of care management for vulnerable older people within a specialist multidisciplinary framework spanning health and social care. The challenge is to develop a model of care management based on the eight standards described above, in order to ensure that older people with dementia are enabled to remain in their own homes, thereby preventing inappropriate admission to long-stay facilities, and receive services appropriate to their complex health and social care needs.

References

Alzheimer's Society. Policy positions. 2004.
http://www.alzheimers.org.uk/News and Campaigns/Policy Watch/demography.htm

Challis D, Chessum R, Chesterman J, Luckett R, Traske K. *Case management in social and health care: The Gateshead Community Care Scheme.* Personal Social Services Research Unit, University of Kent at Canterbury; 1990.

Challis D, Darton R, Johnson L, Stone M, Traske K. *Care management and health care of older people: The Darlington Community Care Project.* Ashgate, Aldershot; 1995.

Challis D, Darton R, Hughes J, Huxley P, Stewart K. Emerging models of care management for older people and those with mental health problems in the United Kingdom. *J Case Manage* 1998; 7: 153–60.

Challis D, Hughes J. Multidisciplinary approaches in the management of dementia b) Social Work. In: O'Brien J, Ames D, Burns A. eds, *Dementia,* 2nd edn. London: Arnold; 2000.

Challis D, Darton R, Hughes J, Stewart K, Weiner K. Intensive care-management at home: An alternative to institutional care? *Age Ageing* 2001; 30: 409–13.

Challis D, Reilly, S, Hughes J, et al. Policy, organisation and practice of specialist old age psychiatry in England. *Int J Geriatr Psychiatry* 2002a; 17: 1018–26.

Challis D, von Abendorff R, Brown P, Chesterman J, Hughes J. Care management, dementia care and specialist mental health services: an evaluation. *Int J Geriatr Psychiatry* 2002b; 17: 315–25.

Donabedian A. (1980) *Explorations in quality assessment and monitoring Vol I: The definition of quality and approaches to its assessment.* Ann Arbor: Health Administration Press; 1980.

Eggert GM, Friedman B, Zimmer JG. Models of intensive case management. In: Reif L, Trager B, eds. *Health care of the aged: Needs, policies, and services.* New York: The Haworth Press; 1990.

Golden RL, Tropman P. The search for the perfect assessment. In: Applebaum R, White M, eds. *Case management around the globe.* California: American Society on Aging; 2000.

Weiner K, Hughes J, Challis D, Pederson I. Integrating health and social care at the micro level: Health care professionals as care managers for older people. *Social Policy and Administration* 2003; 37: 498–515.

chapter 28

Dementia – The view of social policy science

Frank Schulz-Nieswandt

Dementia in a no-care zone of public social law

Although the German government introduced a statutory social insurance system for nursing care – with a limited budget and a continuous complementary financial role of the public poverty transfer system – there is no satisfying solution in the case of care for dementia. The German nursing social insurance law has a very controversial definition of nursing need. The combination of activities of daily living and instrumental activities of daily living (ADLs and IADLs) do not cover the problems of dementia.

The social policy problems are broad:

- Dementia is a very strong risk factor for institutionalization in long-time nursing care. Long-term care institutions are not able to cope with dementia on a quality level that is acceptable.
- Private households and private informal social networks are overburdened to cope with dementia at home. The positive impact of the ambulatory system of nursing staff is limited.
- We think that wrong (or problematic) priorities have been developed by the goverment and by society as a whole. The national economic importance of dementia is well-known. The costs for dementia constitute more than 1% of the gross national product (GNP).

The dominant costs are the opportunity costs of the private households and networks. Society and the government do not like to cover the risk of dementia to such an extent that will be acceptable from the perspectives of nursing research and ethical reflections regarding the quality of life of persons with dementia and the living conditions of the overburdened social networks which have to cope with the problems. The problems are characterized by risk privatization and feminization of the care responsibilities.

Dementia from the perspective of broken transsectoral pathways

German social law clearly separates the health care sector and the nursing care sector. The path of many patients, especially geriatric patients, are characterized by broken transsectoral caring processes. It is not only a problem in Germany: it is a standard problem throughout Europe. But there are differences: in Germany, it is a huge problem.

Is the way to more competition a big step to unbroken transsectoral pathways? An ageing society must optimize the relationships in the socio-demographic structure of society, including the epidemiological implications on the one hand and the structure of the health care (and nursing) system on the other. The very high prevalance of dementia in the age group >80 years old has to be seen in combination with the fact that the numbers of the very old people will increase in the next decades. German healthcare reform policy is going along the path to a system of more competition, to optimize the economic efficiency of the allocation of scarce resources. To induce more competition into the system, the German healthcare policy is changing the institutional patterns of allocation. Now there is the possibility for individual and selective contract management of the health insurance enterprises. The government and central reformers hopes that they can induce a radical transformation of the care system according to the sociodemographic and epidemiological transitions of an ageing society.

Healthcare policy changes the economic incentives and offers the possibility of a new morphology of healthcare suppliers (integrated care systems, pathway management, disease management, etc.). I (F.S.-N.) have the opinion that this will be a very important precondition to realizing the optimization of the care system. But will it happen? I think that the big transformation of the healthcare system needs radical changes in medical culture: i.e. a more fundamental question than the question of the introduction of the new economic incentives and of new possibilities of contract management. Will the ageing society be able to realize an adequate medical anthropology? The societal answer can be generated during the next two decades and depends on the path taken following the new structural reform policy from the beginning of the new millenium.

Further reading

Schulz-Nieswandt F, Kurscheid C. Integrationsversorgung. Münster et al.: Lit Verlag 2004

Bundesministerium für Familie, Senioren, Frauen und Jugend (ed.) (2002). Vierter Bericht zur Lage der älteren Generation. Berlin

chapter 29

Training in care homes in the UK

Lynne Phair

The law which governs care homes in the UK changed in 2001. All care homes are now under the jurisdiction of the Commission for Social Care Inspection (CSCI), who work to the Care Standards Act 2000. This Act has a number of regulations and standards of care which are measured by the NCSC when they inspect the care home twice a year.

Homes have to be registered according to the client group they care for, and have to be able to demonstrate that staff are competent to care for that particular client group.

The legislation makes a requirement that all homes that offer registered nursing must have a registered nurse on duty 24 hours a day, and that the home must demonstrate a capability to meet the persons' assessed needs (NMS 2001).

For care staff, there is now a requirement that a minimum of 50% of care staff (on duty) must have National Vocational Training (NVQ) Level 2 or above, excluding the manager or registered nurses.

Care staff also have to complete induction and foundation standards training after 6 weeks and 6 months, respectively. These standards reflect basic training in human rights, abuse, health & safety and communication.

Training for care staff

National Vocational Qualifications
Launched in 1986 in order to create a coherent national system of qualifications, NVQs relate to specific occupational areas that can easily be understood, give credit for what people do as well as what they know and can be achieved independently from any formal programme of learning.

NVQs are competency-based which is described by the 'Unit for the development of Audit Continuing education' whereby 'competence is concerned with what people can do rather than what they know' (Flanagan, 2000). NVQs are based on skills, knowledge and understanding required, and are concerned with outcomes rather than the learning process.

The levels of National Vocational Qualifications
- Level 1 – the acquisition of a foundation of knowledge, etc., in a limited range of predictable and structure contexts.
- Level 2 – the acquisition of a broader range of knowledge, etc., which demonstrate the extension of previous abilities and are less predictable (GCSE).
- Level 3 – the acquisition of a more complex range of skills, etc., which develop autonomous, analytical and critical abilities (A Level).
- Level 4 – the acquisition of a broad range of complex technical or professional activities in a wide variety of contexts, with a substantial degree of personal responsibility (Diploma).
- Level 5 – the acquisition of knowledge, etc., involving substantial autonomous analytical and critical abilities (Degree). (There is no level 5 in care.)

Despite the system being in place for the past 16 years, recent research from the Centre for Policy on Ageing, which surveyed 418 homes employing 13 204 staff (older peoples services), identified that only 21% of care staff had an NVQ. Although managers felt that training the workforce did confer benefits, there was concern about the issue of funding and that the standards of training varied widely (Dalley and Deniss 2001).

There are 31 units that the candidate can select 6 from: not one of the units is dementia-specific, and there is no NVQ in the care of people with dementia at any level.

The learning environment

The contribution of NVQs to the learning milieu of the workplace and thus the impact of training on the quality of life of the resident has to be questioned. Stephenson et al (1999) examined the nature of a healthy learning milieu and the relationship between an NVQ and a healthy learning milieu. Although their work was not care-specific, the findings bear importance in relation to how to create a learning milieu and thus a better care experience for the client and their family.

Working with 2000 people from 10 organizations, the study identified eight features of healthy learning milieu (from a literature review) and the study placed evidence against them. The outcomes were that two features of a healthy learning milieu were commonly associated with NVQ activities:

- learning activities promote personal growth
- learning interacts with work.

However, the six remaining features discriminated between the cases showing different levels of overlap between NVQ activity:

- learning is prioritized
- learning is shared
- learning is for all
- learning is one's own responsibility
- learning pays
- learning is continuous.

The study also found that NVQs are more likely to be associated with organization-driven learning activities and less likely to be driven by learner-driven activities, recommending that organizations pay particular attention to the discriminators which are not in place. Thus, the culture of the organization will directly affect the success of the NVQ.

Dementia-specific training

A study by Lintern et al (2000a and b) examined whether training alone improves the quality of life of people with dementia, with an assumption that training alone would make a difference. The findings were that training alone did not lead to improved outcomes for residents and that improved attitudes and skills shown by staff were not enough to improve life for residents if organizational obstacles were in the way. There is very little evidence that just training staff in dementia care makes any difference to the quality of care for the residents. After 16 years of NVQ there are still initiatives being developed to improve basic care skills and quality issues:

- the NMS has a standard which states 'that people can wear their own clothes' (NMS, 2002, Standard 10)
- care workers in care homes continue to abuse – action on elder abuse (Jenkins et al, 2000)

- the Department of Health has written a document, *The essence of care*, benchmarking fundamental care issues for the NHS for quality assurance.

Training for registered nurses

Under their Professional Code of Conduct (Nursing and Midwifery Council, 2002), registered nurses must ensure they are competent to care for the patient. The pre-registration diploma or degree in nursing has four main branches: general nursing, community nursing, mental health and paediatric nursing. Despite many debates, there are still no plans to introduce a gerontology branch, which would include people with dementia.

Until April 2002, the Educational Boards of UK Nursing (National Boards) had a dementia care post-registration qualification. However, all of the National Board courses have been withdrawn and there are no plans to replace them. Thus, today, apart for doing an academic diploma, or degree, there are no dementia-specific qualifications for nurses to obtain. Equally, there are currently no long-term care of the older person specific qualifications either.

Support staff who work in a care home

There is very little evidence to identify specific training available for support (ancillary) staff in a care home. Lintern et al (2000a and b) identified the need for all staff to receive dementia care specific training, and one training programme has been validated for this purpose (AgeCare, 2002). However, the impact that support staff can have on the quality of life of the resident is often ignored.

It is essential that there is a national training and development programme for everyone that works with people in health and care settings. It is essential that care settings do no harm, and that a positive culture is embedded in the organization.

I have not yet found the evidence to convince me that any type of NVQ (yet alone a generalist one) is the best way of achieving this and, until the whole team (registered nurses and support staff) receive specialist training, the needs of people with dementia will continue to be unmet.

References

AgeCare. *AgeCare Awards Project*. London: AgeCare; contact 020-763-74577.

Dalley G, Deniss M. Trained to care. London: Centre for Policy on Ageing; 2001.

Flanagan J, Baldwin S, Clarke D. Work-based learning as a means of developing and assessing nursing competencies. *J Clin Nurs* 2000; 360–8.

Jenkins G, Asif Z, Bennett G. *Listening is not enough*. London: Action on Elder Abuse; 2000.

Lintern T, Woods B, Phair L. Training is not enough to change care practice (1). *J Dementia Care* 2000a; 8(2): 15–17.

Lintern T, Woods B, Phair L. Training is not enough to change care practice (2). J *Dementia Care* 2000b; 8(3): 15–17.

National Minimum Standards (NMS) Care homes for older people. London: Department of Health; 2001.

Nursing and Midwifery Council. *Code of Professional Conduct*. London: NMC; 2002.

Stephenson J, Williams R, Cairns L, Critten L. University of Middlesex. Contact address: J. Stephenson@mdx.ac.uk.

chapter 30

Implementation of standards in dementia care: Combating stigma attached to dementia

Myrra Vernooij-Dassen and AW Wind

Introduction

Standards or guidelines are developed to guide and support the professionals in daily practice. They are important to maintain and improve the quality of care (Burgers and Boluyt, 2004). Guidelines are especially important in dementia care, since both diagnosis and management of dementia are very complicated. Standards or guidelines are not self-implementing. Efforts to implement guidelines are often not successful. A general lesson from implementation studies was that no strategy was superior (Grol, 2001a). Crucial efforts to implement guidelines are the involvement of potential users in the development of the guideline, the study of current practice and studying and addressing facilitators and obstacles to its use (Grol, 2001b). The aim of this chapter is to describe the development of dementia guidelines, current practice and obstacles to the use of dementia guidelines. In addition, suggestions will be derived from these data for future improvement of dementia care.

Development of dementia guidelines

The development of dementia guidelines requires great efforts because they should comply with quality requirements. Guidelines should rely on evidence or on consensus when no evidence is available. Despite efforts to conscientiously examine available literature, guidelines are on average less than 40% evidence based (Grol, 2001b). A special instrument has been developed to assess the quality of guidelines, the AGREE instrument (Appraisal of Guidelines for Research and Evaluation). This instrument includes domains such as rigour of development, applicability, clarity and presentation and stakeholder involvement (Burgers and Boluyt, 2004; AGREE, 2003). No information is available on evaluation of dementia guidelines by the AGREE instrument.

Dementia guidelines have been developed for general practitioners (GPs) and medical specialists. In many EU countries GPs are gatekeepers in the healthcare system (Vernooij-Dassen et al 2005). GPs navigate patients to self-care, primary care and hospital or nursing home care. Therefore, special attention is needed for the development and implementation of guidelines for GPs. Without GPs recognizing dementia symptoms and taking action, in many EU countries the patient and the informal carer will struggle without professional support in dealing with this incomprehensible disease.

The content of dementia guidelines should provide information for professionals to deal with both diagnosis and management. The current focus in dementia guidelines is often on diagnosis rather than on management. The weakness of evidence on management of dementia care is mentioned as an argument for this focus. However, the evidence on care is growing and might not be substantially weaker than the evidence on diagnosis. Care research is maturing by acknowledging that complex problems need differentiated solutions. Recent results indicate that support programmes focusing on individual problems of patients and informal carers are most effective (Brodaty et al, 2003). A model that allows us to address the specific problems of patient and informal carer caused by the disease is the model of personal disease management (Vernooij-Dassen and Olde Rikkert, 2004). This person-focused care has the potential to make life with dementia bearable and even enjoyable here and now. Personal disease management often requires collaboration between several disciplines to provide transmural care that aims at providing the best care for the specific patient and carer.

Since dementia is characterized by deficits in memory, cognitive functioning including functional deficits and social functioning, experts in all these fields should be involved in guideline development and consider both diagnosis and treatment or management of dementia. Disciplines such as general practice, geriatric medicine, neurology, old age psychiatry, psychology, nursing, home help, occupational therapy, mental health services and nursing home medicine and medical sociology should be involved in the development of guidelines and in dementia care. Information on how to support the person with dementia and the informal carer should be part of future dementia guidelines.

Current practice

Guidelines for GPs are present in most EU countries, except for Portugal and Ireland (Vernooij-Dassen 2005). EU countries can benefit from knowledge and positive and negative experiences in other countries. Therefore, it is necessary that at least guidelines are available in the English language. This is not the case now.

The current practice of use of guidelines shows different faces in different countries. In France only one-third of GPs knew of the existence of the dementia guideline, which is a prerequisite for its application (Cantegreil et al, 2004). In the Netherlands with a long and rich tradition in development of guidelines, the average application rate of the dementia guideline was 86% (Van Hout et al, 2001). However, this application rate was considerably higher than that of other national guidelines (86% v 61%) (Grol et al, 1998) and did not reflect the average application by GPs, since the participating GPs were encouraged to work according to the guideline (Van Hout et al, 2001). In addition, the diagnostic criteria provided little guidance to GPs' decision-making (Van Hout et al, 2001). In the USA, dementia guidelines on diagnosis were followed by the majority of clinicians, and practices to support informal carers were implemented by half of the clinicians (Rosen et al, 2002). These figures seem to indicate a reasonable application rate of dementia guidelines. However, a major problem in dementia care is the late start of the diagnostic process, and thus delayed use of guidelines. It takes on average 30 months from the initial symptoms noticed by either patient or relative before a medical evaluation takes place (Haley et al, 1992).

Obstacles

Obstacles perceived by GPs to diagnosing dementia were the problems that patients did not mention symptoms, diagnostic uncertainty in early stages, constraints in 8-minute consultation and embarrassment at performing cognitive tests (Van Hout et al, 2000). Obstacles relating to the diagnosis to patients were stigma associated with dementia and embarrassment at discussing losses caused by the disease (Iliffe et al, 2004; Mendonca Lima et al, 2003). A prominent obstacle is professionals' feelings that they have nothing to offer (Van Hout et al, 2000; Iliffe et al, 2004). These obstacles perceived by GPs show a pessimistic and almost reluctant attitude towards dementia care.

Little is known about specific obstacles in actually managed dementia care, except that 39% of the GPs felt capable of managing and supporting the carers (Van Hout et al, 2000). Most GPs (94%) perceived it as their task to manage the problems of informal carers. However, in practice, 25% were proactive in paying attention to informal carers without medical complaints (Simon and Kendrich, 2001).

Until now there has been little evidence on the effects of systematic efforts to implement dementia guidelines and the available evidence does not show improvement in patient outcomes (Waldorff et al, 2003).

In order to implement dementia guidelines effectively, further analysis of the 'black box' of factors influencing the implementation of dementia guidelines is needed: focusing on the perspective of the culture of dementia care might provide more insight into these factors.

Culture of dementia care

The culture of dementia care is one of reactive care, meaning that reactive care is considered to be acceptable according to the opinions, norms and values of professionals. Reactive care is motivated by the fear of stigmatizing the patient. Yet, the fear of professionals to stigmatize the patients by considering them as persons not being sensitive for any treatment seriously threatens the quality of care and deprives patients and their carers of adequate care. Stigma reflects a process of disqualification whereby a normal person is reduced to a person with whom something is wrong (Goffman, 1963). Persons with dementia are often stigmatized by being perceived as having no quality of life or capacity for pleasure (Graham et al, 2003).

Stigma is a variably distributed phenomenon both within and among countries (Iliffe et al, 2004). In some countries, such as Portugal, the dementia label is avoided as this deprives people from nursing home admission, because nursing homes refuse to accept people with dementia (Iliffe et al, 2004). Stigma associated with dementia seems to be the overriding factor in delaying timely diagnosis in EU member states (Dassen et al 2005). In conclusion, the development of guidelines, current practice and the actual implementation of dementia guidelines are hampered by a negative stigma on dementia.

Future care

The implementation of guidelines can be obstructed by the prevalent culture in dementia care, but updated guidelines can also address these obstacles. Making a guideline is more than providing evidence or giving consensus-based instructions. Guidelines set norms. It is reconsidering old norms and setting new norms for the group of professionals on how to deal with a specific disease. Professionals are supposed to adhere to new culture norms in dementia care set in guidelines. In dementia care the cultural change to be made is the shift from reactive to proactive care. This might significantly improve the quality of care. This shift can be encouraged in guidelines both by explicitly setting this norm and giving information on how to carry out proactive care. A prerequisite for this proactive approach of dementia in general practice is that GPs are convinced of the utility of such a proactive approach. The growing evidence on the usefulness of personal disease management can motivate to make the shift to proactive care.

Changing a culture goes slowly and is complex. Providing the tools to set feasible goals and means to reach these goals in supporting the patient and informal carer might help to change the stigma of dementia as an untreatable disaster. An example on how to encourage a change from a pessimistic culture into a more optimistic proactive culture can be found in the recently updated Dutch dementia guideline for GPs (Wind et al, 2003) in which proactive dementia care is one of its explicit aims. This guideline addresses previously found obstacles (Van Hout et al, 2000) and provides means to encourage proactive care through:

- stimulating stepwise diagnosis by first confirming signals before further examination
- providing options to diagnose dementia in general practice or to refer the patient to a memory clinic
- providing advice for management of behavioural problems of patients and carer support
- stimulating collaboration with other professionals.

In addition, stigma can be combated by educational programmes that discuss personal beliefs and images of stigma in dementia such as the double-negative labelling of being old and having a psychiatric disorder (Sartorius, 2003; Iliffe et al, 2004), the association of dementia with its last phase (Iliffe et al, 2004) and the perception of people with dementia as people having no capacity for pleasure (Graham et al, 2003) and lacking awareness (Clare, 2003). Combatting stigma is important to improve dementia care and make life with dementia and living with a person with dementia bearable.

Efforts to implement new guidelines are an encounter and often a confrontation with local habits, facilitators and obstacles. These factors should be considered seriously, especially the local face of stigma as perceived by professionals. Doing so, the update and implementation of guidelines offer a major chance to set a culture of proactive dementia care.

Conclusions

- Implementation of dementia guidelines is hampered by a negative stigma on dementia.
- Guidelines set norms and can help to make the necessary shift in dementia care: from a reactive to a proactive approach.
- The growing evidence on the usefulness of personal dementia management can motivate to making this shift.
- Combating stigma is important to improve dementia care and make life with dementia and with a demented patient bearable.

References

AGREE collaboration, writing group, Cluzeau FA, Burgers JS, Brouwers M, Grol R et al, Development and validation of an international instrument for assessing the quality of clinical practice guidelines: the AGREE project. *Qual Saf Health Care* 2003; 12: 18–23.

Brodaty H, Green A, Koschera A. Meta-analysis of psychosocial interventions for caregivers of people with dementia. *J Am Geriatr Soc* 2003; 51: 657–64.

Burgers JS, Boluyt N. De kwaliteit van CBO-richtlijnen en NHG-standaarden beoordeeld met het AGREE instrument. *Huisarts Wet* 2004; 47: 394–9.

Cantegreil I, Lieberherr D, Garcia A, et al. La détection de la maladie d'Alzheimer par le médecin généraliste: résultats d'une enquête préliminaire auprès des médecins du réseau Sentinelles [Detection of Alzheimer's disease in general medicine: preliminary results of a Sentinelles general practitioner's network survey]. *Revue de Medecine Interne* 2004; 25: 548–55.

Clare L. Managing threats to self awareness in early stage Alzheimer's disease. *Soc Sci Med* 2003; 57: 1017–29.

Goffman GE. *Stigma: Notes on the management of spoiled identity.* New York: Prentice Hall; 1963.

Graham N, Lindesay J, Katona C, et al. Reducing stigma and discrimination against older people with mental disorders: A technical consensus statement. *Int J Geriatr Psychiatry* 2003; 18: 670–8.

Grol R. Effectieve organisatie van de implementatie. In: Grol R, Wensing M, eds. *Implementatie. Effectieve verandering in de patiëntenzorg.* Nijmegen: Elsevier; 2001b: 317.

Grol R. Improving the quality of medical care: building bridges among professional pride, payer profit, and patient satisfaction. *JAMA* 2001a; 286: 2578–85.

Grol R, Dalhuijsen J, Thomas S, et al. Attributes of clinical guidelines that influence use of guidelines in general practice: observational study. *BMJ* 1998; 317: 858–61.

Haley WE, Clair JM, Saulsberry K. Family caregiver satisfaction with medical care of their demented relatives. *Gerontologist* 1992; 32: 219–26.

Iliffe S, De Lepeleire J, Hout van H, et al. Understanding obstacles to the recognition of and response to dementia in different European countries: A modified focus group approach using multinational, multi-disciplinary expert groups. *Aging Ment Health* 2005; 9(1): 1–6.

Mendonca Lima CA, Levav I, Jacobsson L, Rutz W. Stigma and discrimination against older people with mental disorders in Europe. *Int J Geriatr Psychiatry* 2003; 18: 679–82.

Rosen CS, Chow HC, Greenbaum MA, et al. How well are clinicians following dementia practice guidelines? *Alzheimer Dis Assoc Disord* 2002; 16: 15–23.

Sartorious N. Introduction: Stigma and discrimination against older people with mental disorders. *Int J Geriatr Psychiatry* 2003; 18: 669.

Simon C, Kendrich T. Informal carers and the role of general practitioners and district nurses. *Br J Gen Pract* 2001; 52: 655–7.

van Hout H, Vernooij-Dassen M, Bakker K, Blom M, Grol R. General practitioners on dementia: tasks, practices and obstacles. *Pat Educ Couns* 2000; 39: 219–25.

van Hout H, Vernooij-Dassen M, Poels P, Hoefnagels W, Grol R. Applicability of diagnostic recommendations on dementia in family practice. *Int J Qual Health Care* 2001; 13: 127–33.

Vernooij-Dassen M, Olde Rikkert MG. Personal disease management in dementia care. *Int J Geriatr Psychiatry* 2004; 19: 715–17.

Vernooij-Dassen M, Moniz-Cook ED, Woods B, et al, and the Interdem Group. Factors affecting the timely recognition and diagnosis of dementia in primary care across eight European States: A modified focus group study. *Int J Geriatr Psychiatry* 2005 20(4): 377–86.

Waldorff FB, Almind G, Makela M, Moller S, Waldemar G. Implementation of a clinical dementia guideline. A controlled study on the effect of a multifaceted strategy. *Scand J Prim Health Care* 2003; 21: 142–7.

Wind AW, Gussekloo J, Vernooij-Dassen MJFJ, et al, NHG-Standaard dementie. *Huisarts en Wetenschap* 2003; 46: 754–66.

chapter 31

Psychological cornerstones for a standard of dementia caregiving[*]

Bère Miesen

Introduction

From the knowledge that behavioural changes in dementia patients have specific organic correlates in the brain, more understanding arose for people with dementia. Today the behavioural changes of dementia patients are also understood within the wholeness of the patient as a person. That means that at least a part of the patient's behaviour is seen in the light of (normal) coping with the (disease of) dementia. The patient's perception (and thus coping) with dementia is now understood as an interplay between the cause of the brain damage, the stage of the dementia process, the individual life-history (including amongst others, attachment history and eventual old psychic pain), personality and the way the patient has been dealt with by his (social) environment both before and after the assessment of the disease. Nowadays, dementia has been recognized as an individual trauma, drama and tragedy both for the people with dementia and for their family; and, along with that, the social status of the disease is increasing and the possibilities for intervention by amongst others psychoeducation and psychotherapy/counselling are overwhelming.

A brief psychology of caregiving in dementia[†]

The term 'dementia' is used when there are specific permanent (tissue) changes in the brain. It is only possible to determine whether phenomena

[*] Based on Chapter 19 of Jones GMM, Miesen BML, eds. *Care-giving in dementia. Research and applications. Vol. 3*. London: Brunner-Routledge; 2004.

[†] Based on Miesen B. *Dementia in close-up. Understanding and caring for people with dementia*. London: Routledge/Tavistock; 1999: 231

such as forgetfulness, restlessness, mistrust and confusion are due to dementia by extensively screening the person in question. If dementia is diagnosed, this means that an irreversible process has been triggered in the brain, for which there is currently no medical cure. This has far-reaching consequences for the person who has been diagnosed, as well as for his or her family. Care for dementia sufferers should mainly be aimed at making sure they are dealt with and managed as pleasantly and satisfactorily as possible. Insight and understanding are necessary, so that care can be given that is satisfactory for the patient as well as for his or her family.

Memory impairment forces people with dementia to seek structures to hold on to in their actual lives or in memories. They hold on to what they perceive for as long as they are able to perceive. Staying in contact with dementia sufferers means quite literally staying close to them. If you want to comprehend and understand them as an outsider, you must always make sure that you are in contact via the various senses. They must be able to perceive – to touch, smell, feel, see and hear, as it were – what you want to say.

People with dementia remain attached to what is actually happening to them for longer than has so far been assumed. We refer to this as their awareness, or 'awareness context'. Denial and avoidance do not mean there is no awareness. Because their memory is beginning to desert them, they often have feelings of upheaval and not belonging. And this makes them look for security, which can be expressed for instance through attachment and proximity-seeking behaviour. Parent fixation and parent orientation are examples of this. In cases where these phenomena are apparent, it is important to comfort the dementia sufferer and offer him or her security, helping to overcome the parent fixation and restlessness.

It is not just dementia sufferers who find it difficult – their families and in particular partners have a very difficult time. They have to tackle a whole host of practical as well as emotional problems. They have to slowly say goodbye to their nearest and dearest, whether they want to or not. It involves a process of dealing with their loss, a grieving process, with all the inherent behaviours and feelings. The thing that makes the dementia process all the more difficult for the family to bear is the lack of clarity. This situation is similar to what is felt if a loved one goes missing indefinitely: the person with dementia may well still be alive, but all emotional contact has now disappeared. It is only possible to say goodbye properly when the dementia sufferer has actually 'gone': in other words, when he or she has died.

Giving care to a person with dementia involves more than just offering help. Over the course of time, a closer and deeper relationship builds up between most caregivers – whether professional and volunteer carers or members of the family – and their patients. This bond can sometimes become so strong that it leads to a kind of adoption. In other words, the caregiver feels that he or she has become a member of the patient's family as it were. It is only possible to look after another person effectively if you look after yourself effectively. So it is important that caregivers accept their own skills and limitations. They should, therefore, whether in conjunction with each other or not, keep an eye on their own behaviour, be aware of their own motives for giving care and look into ways to put their skills into practice and develop them.

To ensure effective caregiving, in other words to give care that meets the needs of dementia sufferers, it is important that caregivers (professional and volunteer carers and members of the family) impartially take on board the various experiences of patients as well as their feelings and needs. In practice, professional and volunteer carers and members of the family usually all manage in their own way to take this on board without partiality. Both caregivers and dementia sufferers tend to project emotions and experiences from the past onto the present. This greatly affects the relationship between caregiver and dementia sufferer. We refer to this situation using terms such as transfer and countertransfer. It is important that caregivers are aware of possible transfer or countertransfer situations they may find themselves in, and that they have insight into the effect of these projections. In other words, they must be aware of how experiences and unresolved losses may affect their own behaviour and that of dementia sufferers.

When dealing with dementia sufferers on a daily basis, there are frequently occasions when certain forms of power (may) become apparent: e.g. when family or professional staff have to take decisions on behalf of the dementia sufferer, which they are forced to, given the dependence of the person with dementia. But power also resides in concern and a paternalistic attitude. Whatever decisions the family or staff have to take, they have to be taken to the best of their belief. All is well if decisions are made in an atmosphere of understanding, respect and acceptance of the limitations of the patient, as well as those of the family or member of staff. If decisions are not taken in this atmosphere, the patient will be excluded.

As their cognitive skills are declining, people with dementia increasingly use non-verbal means of communication to express what they are thinking, wanting or feeling. Touch then becomes the most important way of communicating, because dementia sufferers are starting to show more proximity-seeking behaviour. The relationship between the caregiver and patient increases in intimacy as the dependence grows. In such a situation, it is easy to misinterpret expressions of intimacy and sexuality as 'undesired intimacies'. It is important for caregivers to realize that these sorts of expression are not usually meant in that way, but more as a desire for warmth and tenderness on the part of the dementia sufferer. The extent to which caregivers accept 'awkward' situations like these depends on their own limitations, values and norms.

People with dementia may display aggressive behaviour. This causes difficulties in their dealings with family members and caregivers. If the family and caregivers are able to understand and identify the possible causes, they will be able to have a better idea of the patient's own perception of the world. This gives them a means of preventing aggression. The dementia sufferer does not degenerate into an unknown stranger. And a natural progression of this is that the aggressive behaviour is not felt to be directed at oneself. What is more, feelings of insecurity or one's own guilt tend to decrease and it is still possible to see the dementia sufferer as a nice, friendly, likeable or endearing person.

Dealing with people with dementia cannot be separated from dealing with the next of kin. It is important to note that the perspective from which the family experiences and perceives the situation is different to that of the caregiver. The main reason for this is that caregivers are busy dealing with the care aspect and do not have to free themselves from the emotional bond built up by the shared life history, whatever this may be. The family looking after a dementia sufferer has to do that out of necessity. And in my opinion, this affects their behaviour, both as regards the person with dementia and as regards the professional caregiver. It is therefore important that care staff take into account the process of dealing with loss on the part of the family when they decide what to do and what not to do, as well as what to say and what not to say.

The caregiving plan: From victim to survivor

If we view the dementia disease from a (psycho)trauma perspective, one can imagine the continuous battle against powerlessness, disruption and upheaval that only ends once the person with dementia is dead. From there it is clear that an individual disaster scenario – i.e. the caregiving plan – has to be drawn up for every person with dementia as well as for the family. The way in which this individual caregiving plan is handled requires expertise in the psychosocial field without any question. At the same time, it can be said that continuity in treatment, support and care is a prerequisite. From the beginning, if possible, the same multidisciplinary (treatment) team should stand by the family going through the dementia, regardless of (changes in) living situation, although continuity in the care team is not feasible for the entire course of the dementia. This continuity in caregiving is needed because the whole thing is about always giving treatment in the short term but from a long-term point of view. In the beginning, expertise is needed about everything that is going to happen. In the end, expertise is needed about everything that has happened. It is only with this support that people with dementia and their families can find the security and control they need to continue living their lives as normally as possible for as long as possible, despite the disease dementia: the victims have become survivors. No wonder that dementia has always a special impact on caregivers or care staff. And some can deal with it better than others.

The impact of (caregiving in) dementia makes everybody vulnerable: a practical model

The way in which patients cope with their suffering can be effectively identified after multidisciplinary examination: i.e. their vulnerability can be assessed by carefully identifying the factors which effect their coping. This examination leads to a main and/or an individual guideline or care plan.

Patients/residents

For the majority of patients, the main guidelines given on how to understand and manage their coping with the disease – provided that staff are properly prepared – are sufficient for the support of the patient and the caregiving. From time to time, these guidelines need to be adjusted. After all, dementia is a chronic disease of the brain. Sometimes, unexpected problems arise with patients or residents: then, a care staff meeting has to be called. The impact of an unexpected problem may be so great that care staff's own vulnerability requires support and guidance in so-called TimeOut Meetings.

For a small group of patients, it is possible to see that there are more than the usual amount of problems in their coping with the dementia or that such problems will sooner or later arise: e.g. patients with a specific personality or with old psychic pain. Then, the main guidelines are not sufficient to support the patients. These patients could be described as extra vulnerable. A care staff meeting has to be organized in advance to develop the guidelines into a special approach. And the impact to be expected and the corresponding behaviour of the patients are such that care staff's own vulnerability has to be supported on a regular basis (TimeOut Meetings).

For a few patients, it is possible to see that they are more than extra vulnerable, which may be for a variety of reasons: e.g. they may have a pathological personality or serious frontal lobe defects. In these instances, neither the main guidelines nor the care staff's meetings will be satisfactory. These patients will continue to be extra vulnerable and little or nothing can be done about their suffering. The vulnerability of the care staff themselves is at issue here from the start. TimeOut Meetings are needed right from the beginning.

Family

For most members of the family, a general package of information and support, followed by normal contact (empathetic and expert) with care staff, is sufficient to give them guidance. Sometimes, family members experience unexpected problems, in which case a care staff meeting is organized to tackle them. Sometimes, the impact of these unexpected problems are such that the care staff themselves need guidance and support (TimeOut Meetings).

For a small group of family members, it is possible to anticipate that they will have more than the usual difficulty in coping with the dementia or that problems will soon arise. For instance, if there is a situation in their own lives or if they have fragile health, a specific personality, a special attachment or an old trauma. They could be described as extra vulnerable. In these instances, the general package of information and support are not sufficient to support these families. A care staff meeting has to be organized in advance to develop a special approach. And the impact to be expected and the corresponding behaviour of the family are such that the care staff's own vulnerability has to be supported on a regular basis (TimeOut Meetings).

For a few family members, it is possible to anticipate their more than extra vulnerability, which may be for a variety of reasons: e.g. they may have a pathological personality or an insecure attachment with the patient. In these instances, neither a special approach nor holding a care staff meeting will be a satisfactory solution. They will continue to be extra vulnerable and little or nothing can be done about their suffering. The vulnerability of the carestaff themselves is at issue here from the start. TimeOut Meetings are needed right from the beginning.

Care staff

For most care staff, sufficient support is provided by the main and/or individual guidelines specifying how to deal with the patient and the family, and by care staff meetings. By adopting the guideliness, care staff find they will not encounter any problems in the provision of support and care, assuming they have sufficient knowledge and expertise. However, if for instance a patient is showing abrupt cognitive decline and the guidelines specifying how to deal with the patient are not adjusted quickly, then care staff find it frustrating to comply with them, although this frustration is manageable. Most care staff can handle these kind of frustrations when regular TimeOut Meetings have been held. Through this, most also can handle situations in which the impact of an unexpected (behavioural) problem on the part of the patient or family is particularly great.

For a small group of care staff, it is possible to foresee (on most occasions) that they will sooner or later encounter more than the usual amount of frustrations in dealing with the patient and family. For instance, if there are language difficulties, limited intelligence, inadequate knowledge and experience, a specific personality, an old trauma, too intense an 'adoption' or bond, etc. Straight away this makes them more vulnerable than their colleagues in carrying out their work. Regular, individual coaching and training are essential.

A few caregivers never learn or are never able to cope with the frustrations that are inherent in working with people with dementia and their families. They are simply 'unsuited' to this sort of work from the start. For a variety of factors – such as a disturbed personality, limited (practical) intelligence, previous frustrations that they have not yet worked out and countertransfer – they are too vulnerable for the (behavioural) problems and powerlessness they may encounter in their work. An effective personnel policy should save (both parties) a lot of misery.

Conclusion

Despite progress in the management of dementia disease, it is not easy for the patient to maintain control over his life and therefore maintain a feeling of safety or security. Therefore, it is important first of all that the patient receives a rapid and reliable diagnosis, so that he knows what he is up against. The second thing for him to do is to waste as little time as possible denying and avoiding what he is up against. It is here, in particular, that professionals and caregivers must focus. Because if denial persists – and there may be all kinds of reasons for this – many different forms of interventions (treatment, support and care) will either be impossible, barely possible or simply too late. It is therefore a matter of caregivers helping people with dementia and their families to take control of their fate (again).

As I have pointed out before, caregiving to people with dementia will sooner or later always have an (emotional) impact on the caregivers. They will have to constantly be aware of this impact and the way in which they deal with it, to ensure they prevent countertransfer (projections) which may end in burn-out. To help them in this, they need supervision, an encouragement of expertise and, above all, an open approach to the specific and complex (difficult and fascinating) aspects of this field of work (e.g. by regular TimeOut Meetings). And that makes caregiving in dementia a special field of its own that requires multidisciplinary cooperation beforehand.

Further reading

Jones GMM, Miesen BML, eds. *Care-giving in dementia. Research and applications, Vol. 1.* London: Routledge/Tavistock; 1992.

Jones GMM, Miesen BML, eds. *Care-giving in dementia. Research and applications, Vol. 3.* London: Brunner/Routledge; 2004.

Miesen BML, Jones GMM, eds. *Care-giving in dementia. Research and applications, Vol. 2.* London: Routledge/Tavistock; 1997.

Miesen BML, Jones GMM, eds. *Care-giving in dementia. Research and applications, Vol. 4.* London: Brunner/Routledge; 2006.

chapter 32

How to improve care for the elderly with cognitive decline and feeding difficulties

Sylvie Lauque

Introduction

Alzheimer's disease (AD) is a form of dementia characterized by a progressive loss of cognitive function (memory, reasoning and behaviour) caused by the degeneration of neurons in the brain. It affects 5% of the population after the age of 65 and 30% after 85. This already high percentage will certainly rise further because of an ageing population and through earlier diagnosis.

Recent studies have demonstrated that malnutrition, associated with low nutrient and calorie intake, is common among elderly people. Comparison of elderly people with younger age groups seems to indicate that age is a major risk factor for malnutrition. Furthermore, among the elderly with AD, inadequate energy and protein intake is frequent and is a predictive factor of morbidity and mortality (White et al, 1998). The final result is weight loss and undernourishment. This decline in the patient's nutritional status leads to further complications (increased fragility, decreased resistance to infections, greater dependence on others) and increases the burden experienced by caregivers.

Therefore, the nutritional status of the elderly patient with cognitive decline must be regularly monitored. Caregivers play an important role in providing well-chosen and specially adapted meals. They should be informed on the preparation of appropriate food and must be able to cope with behavioural problems associated with eating. They must also ensure that the patient has regular physical exercise.

The behavioural disturbances associated with Alzheimer's disease often have important implications for the intake of food. In general, these psychiatric symptoms vary according to the stages of the disease. First, patients may lose appetite, feeling depressed because they are aware of their own cognitive failures. Next, they find it difficult to cope with shopping, cooking, peeling vegetables and fruit, using cutlery or glasses, or even chewing and swallowing. In moderate or severe stages of dementia, patients sometimes refuse to remain seated during a meal, mix food together or refuse to eat at all. They are often distracted and slow, forgetting whether they have already eaten or had something to drink, thinking they had dinner when in fact they have not, or the contrary. In addition, they are less able to tell us when they are hungry or thirsty.

How to cope with these elderly people during meals

Whenever possible, patients should be involved in meal preparation for their own enjoyment, to stimulate their intellectual functions and also their memory. The help needed during meals varies from person to person and should be adapted to each individual patient. Their desire to feed themselves must be respected. It is better for nutrition and self-esteem that people should eat as independently as possible.

There are many reasons underlying the importance of good meal care in the daily life of patients suffering from dementia: meals are one of the basic pleasures in life and a time for social interaction with others are the most important ones. However, because of the loss of functional performance, there are several prerequisites for good meal care in dementia:

1. Food should be culturally appropriate.
2. Feeding should be appropriate to the patient's needs in relation to swallowing, eating and drinking problems, apraxia or weight loss.
3. It is useful to keep former rituals, such as washing hands before eating and saying grace before a meal.
4. It is better if the food offered is familiar.
5. It is also very important that food should be attractively presented. For instance, if food is served in the form of a purée, this can be made thicker and reshaped to look like the original food. If the consistency of food has changed, this should be explained.
6. If the family can help at mealtimes, encourage them to participate.
7. We have to watch for the cues that tell us when the patient wants to slow down or to have a rest.

8. There is no point in trying to encourage eating when a person is agitated; they may be consoled verbally or with small gestures.
9. Do not hesitate to let the patient eat standing up or even while walking, and if necessary postpone the mealtime.
10. In general, whatever happens, we must be available, stay calm and not show signs of impatience. It is also important to check that the patient has actually swallowed the food. Unnecessarily strict diets, such as no sugar or no salt diets, should be avoided. These simple rules may serve as the 10 Commandments at the table of the frail elderly.

Assistance during meals

Assisted feeding does not mean that a person has to have help in eating all the time. The assistance should be adapted according to the circumstances: during a crisis period, the patient may need to be fed, while at another time only supervision or a little help may be required. Independent eating should be encouraged and it avoids aspiration of food. Appropriate feeding aides can be of great help: stay-warm plates, non-slip mats, dysphagia cups, glasses with a heavy base, beakers, glasses with a handle or with a spout. When it is necessary to feed the patient, the person assisting needs to appear relaxed. He or she should sit in front of the patient, and not at the side. When possible, the actual dishes which are on offer should be shown to the patient. This helps people to make a real choice. Conversation should focus on meals and on the immediate environment. Verbal encouragement is helpful. Give step-by-step indications: 'keep your mouth closed, chew, swallow'. We have to demonstrate to the patient what we expect of them, leaning forward, and offering the food slowly and calmly. While feeding the patient, we can open our own mouths to show them what is expected. When a pause is necessary, we lean back to rest. Give the patient a smile and encourage them. Use touch to redirect the patient when they are distracted. The hand-over-hand technique is useful to help the patient to start feeding himself or herself. The spoon, fork or cup should be placed in the patient's hand, and appropriate utensils should be used.

If possible, the patient should sit in a proper chair (not a wheelchair). The feet should be on the floor and posture should be correct. The back of a wheelchair is a little concave, which is not as safe a position for swallowing and digestion. The table itself should be adapted to the physical disability of the patient: pleasant and functional with a tablecloth and place mats, and laid with crockery of a contrasting colour. Plates and glasses should be robust and cutlery appropriate. Anti-slip plastic mats to put under the crockery can be found in certain specialist shops. The place at the table should be considered to avoid further disorientation, and good lighting is recommended. It is preferable to serve each course separately rather than to put the whole meal on a tray. Indeed, some patients can become disorientated if there are several different types of food on the same plate. During the meal, it is necessary to check the temperature of the food and to name and describe each dish, with its taste, smell and consistency. If the patient has glasses, a hearing aid, or even more essential, dentures, make sure they are in place. For sight or hearing deficiencies, or mouth or dental problems, he or she should be referred to a specialist. Noise and distraction have a negative effect on food intake. Other people should not be allowed to pass through the dining room, and while meals are being served, no other activity should be going on in the same room. A structured environment and landmarks are necessary for disorientated elderly people, but it is sometimes necessary, and may even be useful, to change the patient's place at table, and even to change the carer (Amella, 2002).

Last but not least, mealtimes are not only for nutrition but also provide a routine and maintain relationships with friends and family (avoid excluding the patient). We must not be rigid in our way of thinking, we must always adapt and, after all, the best meal for all of us is a meal we enjoy (Altus et al, 2002).

Dietetic consultation

It is always useful to consult the dietitians (Keller et al, 2003), as they can provide helpful advice and ideas. Finger food is easy to eat, and can help better nutrition. Moreover, it preserves the patient's self-esteem if he or she can eat without assistance. Where there is a loss of appetite or weight loss, it is necessary to nutritionally enrich the meals and divide the portions (Lauque et al, 2004). Alzheimer's disease can also lead to taste and smell disorders (Murphy, 1999). If taste and smell are impaired, this is a potential cause of deterioration of appetite, food/nutrient intake and nutritional status. This sensory impairment must be taken seriously and it increases with age, particularly in men. One of the many possible ways of dealing with impaired taste and smell is by adding flavour to food (Koskinen et al, 2003). Dietitians can suggest flavours which make food more palatable and better accepted. This also yields greater release of digestive enzymes, by which micronutrients are better absorbed, and salivary flow and the secretion of salivary immuno-globulins are also increased (Schiffman and Miletic, 1999).

Beneficial effects of better nutrition

The effects of improvement in nutritional status can be found in a wide range of interacting domains. Some are frequently overlooked. For example, lymphocyte counts are improved, which makes a person less prone to infections. Next, energy intake increases muscle power. In turn, muscle power stimulates physical activity, and physical activity maintains appetite and muscle and bone strength. A walk a day keeps the doctor away, and is the most economical appetizer. So, a short walk every day is highly recommended, but a dance a day also fulfils this goal.

End of life

While providing comfort and dignity to the person with Alzheimer's disease is the priority at all stages of the disease, it becomes especially important during the late stage and end-of-life care. Difficult decisions often need to be made. Respect for the expressed wishes of the person with Alzheimer's disease should guide all end-of-life care decisions. A guiding principle should be to uphold the person's dignity, privacy and safety. When making decisions on behalf of someone else, it is important to follow their wishes, if these are known. If their desires have not been communicated, knowing the person's values and beliefs can assist in making a decision that most closely resembles the one the person would have made had he or she been capable of doing so. And even if a patient is incompetent to decide according to legal standards, he or she may take part in decision-making, especially if the professionals themselves realize that they do not know what would be the best decision to make (Olde-Rikkert, 2004).

In end stages of dementia, feeding tubes do have serious risks and can cause pneumonia, infection and discomfort, making no difference in a patient's survival. Moreover, patients who try to remove the tubes can injure themselves or have to be physically or chemically restrained (Monteleoni and Clark, 2004). Therefore, in general, artificial feeding is not indicated in end stages of the disease.

Sometimes, however, there is confusion about the nature of the feeding problems. In general, weight loss precedes dementia. Patients with advanced illnesses such as Alzheimer's disease feel less hunger or thirst and their appetites naturally diminish as death approaches. It is important to realize that it is not because the patient doesn't eat that they are going to die, but it is because they are going to die that they do not eat!

Conclusion

Much can be done to optimize care for the elderly person with cognitive decline and nutritional problems. Five cornerstones of nutritional support can be identified:

1. We can act directly towards the elderly person. Each person is unique, so there is not only one solution. Moreover, behavioural problems change as the disease progresses. It is up to us to adapt our care to the patient all the time during the illness, as the patient can no longer adapt himself or herself.
2. We can act on the quality, consistency and quantity of the food and drink provided.
3. Hospital workers and care assistants need to be trained in helping these trusting, vulnerable and touching patients. These staff have an important role to play during meals, to cope with the various behavioural problems associated with eating.
4. We can adapt the environment as necessary: the dining room, chairs, eating utensils and the time allowed to eat.
5. Finally, we have to care for the patient as a whole person. This means that all the professionals have to work together: doctors, nurses, speech and language therapists, social workers, dietitians, dentists, occupational therapists, physical therapists and podologists (Rypkema et al, 2004).

The joy that demented patients and their professional and informal carers perceive in meals may well serve as a quality indicator of care as a whole. The well-being of patients, the interaction with others, in sum the quality of life, is directly dependent on the quality of food. In this, patients with dementia are not at all different from us! Maybe we should have a new Michelin system, with stars for quality of care of meals and clients, not only for the happy few, but also for the unhappy many.

References

Amella EJ. Resistance at mealtimes for persons with dementia. *J Nutr Health Aging* 2002; 2: 117–22.

Altus DE, Engelman KK, Mathews RM. Using family-style meals to increase participation and communication in persons with dementia. *J Gerontol Nurs* 2002; 9:47–53.

Keller HH, Gibbs AJ, Boudreau LD, et al. Prevention of weight loss in dementia with comprehensive nutritional treatment. *J Am Geriatr Soc* 2003; 7: 945–52.

Koskinen S, Kalviainen N, Tuorila H. Flavor enhancement as a tool for increasing pleasantness and intake of a snack product among the elderly. *Appetite* 2003; 1: 87–96.

Lauque S, Arnaud-Battandier F, Gillette S. Improvement of weight and fat-free mass with oral nutritional supplementation in patients with Alzheimer's disease at risk of malnutrition: A prospective randomized study. *J Am Geriatr Soc* 2004; 10: 1702–8.

Monteleoni C, Clark E. Using rapid-cycle quality improvement methodology to reduce feeding tubes in patients with advanced dementia: Before and after study. *BMJ* 2004; 7464: 491–4.

Murphy C. Loss of olfactory function in dementing disease. *Physiol Behav* 1999; 2: 177–82.

Olde Rikkert MGM. Hospital based palliative care and dementia. In: ten Have HAAM, Portillo R, eds. *Ethic foundations of palliative care of Alzheimer diseases*. Baltimore: Johns Hopkins University Press; 2004: 80–96.

Rypkema G, Adang E, Dicke H, et al. Cost-effectiveness of an interdisciplinary intervention in geriatric inpatients to prevent malnutrition. *J Nutr Health Aging* 2004; 2: 122–7.

Schiffman SS, Miletic ID. Effect of taste and smell on secretion rate of salivary IgA in elderly and young persons. *J Nutr Health Aging* 1999; 3: 158–64.

White H, Pieper C, Schmader K. The association of weight change in Alzheimer's disease with severity of disease and mortality: A longitudinal analysis. *J Am Geriatr Soc* 1998; 10: 1223–7.

Carer Stress

chapter 33

Carer stress – overview

Rebekah Proctor and Ingelin Testad

It is widely recognized that caring for a family member with dementia can be both challenging and stressful. While caring can be rewarding, the strains and responsibilities of the role can have an impact on the carer's own psychological and physical health. There are consistent reports that caring for a family member with dementia is associated with high levels of strain, distress and depression (Donaldson et al, 1997). Developing a thorough understanding of the factors that determine carer stress is a major priority, as high levels of stress have been linked to increased use of primary care and respite services and earlier admittance to institutional care for the person with dementia (Brown et al, 1990).

Recognition of the importance of the role of carers has led to a surge of research studies and innovations in clinical practice to find the most effective ways of supporting carers and alleviating some of the distress associated with the role. In the last two decades, there have been a vast number of studies published in this area, with huge variation in methodology, design and research findings. Despite the cumbersome nature of the evidence base for interventions for carer stress, efforts have been made to consolidate what we know to develop much-needed care standards in this area (Department of Health, 1999a). This chapter is an opportunity to take stock of existing care standards, to examine the links between research and practice and to try to integrate this with our clinical experience of working with carers who are stressed. We know that carer stress is the product of an interaction of care-related stressors, the resources available to families and psychosocial variables. These factors interact to increase, maintain or reduce strain experienced by carers of patients with dementia and, as a result, carers in seemingly similar situations have vastly different experiences of the stress process. Consequently, the development of high-quality services for carers should involve taking the time to listen and learn from carers themselves, so that the basis of what we do is grounded in the experiences of those individuals who know most about what interventions work and for whom.

Detecting stress and health promotion

Early detection of signs of carer stress is a crucial first step in helping carers to access help and to learn how to cope with some of the demands of the role (Department of Health, 1999a). Many carers are socially isolated and there is great variation in what carers know about available services and support. There is often an important gap in the communication of information and the promotion of services that are available to help carers. Despite this, we know that carers are regularly in touch with the health service, and that primary care teams have the most frequent contact (Henwood, 1998). This means that primary care staff are not only in a key position to detect signs of stress in carers but also can take an important role in health promotion and education about service availability. In the UK, it has been proposed that primary care teams take steps to identify those patients who are carers and use a recommended checklist to ensure that the physical and emotional health of carers is screened and that information about available services is given (Department of Health, 1999b). In principle, this proposal should mean that more carers are aware of their rights to individual assessment and that problems with stress are detected and treated earlier.

However, in practice, primary care staff need to develop the skills to detect signs of stress in a patient group who may try to manage without acknowledging the need for help, or may, initially, be reluctant to engage with services. In view of this, there seems to be a clear role for training and support from specialist mental health and social services to help primary care staff to develop skills for screening assessments, encouraging service use and developing programmes of health promotion for carers of people with dementia. This is vitally important in ensuring that healthcare professionals not only have the necessary skills to detect and manage carer stress but also can promote well-being in carers through education about how to access help and manage stress effectively.

Individual needs assessments

Gathering information about the carer as part of an assessment is an important precursor to providing appropriate means of help and support. Carers are entitled to an individual needs assessment from social services to help them to maintain their own physical health and psychological well-being. Assessment requires a good awareness of the factors which increase carer stress and how these interact to make the situation of each carer unique. Using what we know from clinical practice and research evidence, it is possible to say that it is important that there is an understanding of:

- the person with dementia and their symptoms, particularly the non-cognitive features (Donaldson et al, 1997)
- the carer's demographic variables, their coping strategies, knowledge and psychological well-being
- the relationship between the carer and the person with dementia
- the support systems which are available to the carer, and the carer's perception of the quality of the relief that is offered (Coen et al, 1997).

Thorough assessment of carers' needs is important, but it is critical that the needs of both the carer and the person with dementia are considered together. It should not be assumed that what benefits one member of the dyad will be of benefit to the other member. The needs of the carer and the person with dementia are inevitably intertwined and can sometimes conflict. Furthermore, regular reviews are important, as the needs of carers and the person with dementia can change over time. Understanding the individual needs of carers and the person with dementia is important, as interventions which are tailored to meet the needs of specific populations are likely to be more productive than trying to provide a blanket approach to support all carers. At the very least, there should be an annual individual review of both the person with dementia and the carer's needs to ensure that changes are monitored and support is adapted appropriately over time.

Social and psychological support

Family caregivers are at risk of depression, which is often linked to lack of sufficient support and the behavioural symptoms of the person with dementia (Teri et al, 1988). In view of this, an effective, evidence-based intervention for family caregivers should be provided based on the following principles (Mittelman et al, 1996):

- each family has unique problems
- most caregivers should benefit from more understanding and support from their families

- most caregivers run the risk of isolation
- most caregivers are at risk of financial problems
- it is necessary to continue to provide support for caregivers throughout the duration of the disease rather than for only a short period of time.

Following assessment, health and social services have a responsibility towards carers in helping them to remain healthy. Part of this responsibility is manifest in the provision of practical help to relieve carers of some of the demands of their role. Various kinds of practical help are available, such as day centres, sitting services, respite care and domiciliary relief care, as well as community nursing and paramedical services. There is still some progress to be made in the development of a flexible and integrated network of support services which can be tailored to meet the individual needs of carers and family members with dementia. Within this network of services, it is crucially important that the staff who are employed to provide care for people with dementia are offered appropriate training and regular supervision to ensure that standards of care are not compromised. The provision of formal education and clinical supervision for care staff has been shown to improve the quality of care provided to people with dementia and to reduce the stress experienced by care staff in this role (Proctor et al, 1999). This is also supported by a study conducted in Norway where staff training led to a significant reduction in use of coercion towards patients with dementia and challenging behaviour (Testad et al, 2002). In view of this, a training programme for staff providing domiciliary care in patients' homes and for those working in residential and respite care settings should be a part of a care standard for dementia.

Many carers become socially isolated, and this has been linked to higher levels of reported stress (Thompson et al, 1993). Support groups for carers provide social contact and emotional support, which can help to alleviate feelings of isolation and promote well-being. Many carers value the guidance and help that this contact with other carers provides. However, social support is only part of the range of psychosocial interventions which can be used to help carers to cope with the demands of the caring role.

Psychological and social interventions incorporate a diverse set of approaches, including stress management, education about dementia, problem-solving and behaviour management. Counselling and support can reduce stress and help carers to manage their reactions to the behaviour of the person with dementia. Counselling and support lead to sustained benefits in reducing depressive symptoms in spouse–caregivers of patients with

Alzheimer's disease, and in delaying nursing home placement (Mittelman et al, 2004).

Despite the large body of research in this area, there is limited evidence that psychosocial interventions consistently produce a positive benefit for the psychological well-being of carers. This is because there is a huge variation in the assessment of the effects of interventions, how research studies are designed and the profile of the carers involved in studies. This inconsistency can impede insight into how to go about developing a standard for the provision of psychosocial interventions for carers. In view of this, it is important to consider what is already known, so that research and clinical questions are focused to help us to learn about the diverse psychological and social needs of carers. For example, carers face different tasks at different stages of the caregiving career, and psychosocial interventions should be offered to address these changing needs. For example, a post-diagnostic counselling group will be most helpful to those who face the task of adjusting to a diagnosis of dementia; behavioural management will be helpful for carers of family members who are exhibiting behavioural symptoms; and an intervention focusing on issues of loss and bereavement may be most effective at later stages in caregiving. A recent review of the literature on psychosocial interventions for carers suggested that a combination of social support and cognitive interventions such as problem-solving and stress management are relatively effective (Cooke et al, 2001). However, it is important that we develop an evidence base of more specific types of interventions which are focused on different needs of carers at different times. It is only with development in this area that we can establish clearly what psychosocial interventions work and for whom.

Education about dementia

Most psychosocial intervention packages for carers appear to include some educational component with the aim of increasing knowledge about dementia in some way. Despite this, we know relatively little about how carers use information about dementia or the effects that it has on their understanding of the symptoms of dementia. Recent studies indicate that providing facts about dementia to carers is not enough, as many carers may not understand that the symptoms they observe are related to the diagnosis (Paton et al, 2004), or may become anxious about medical information (Proctor et al, 2002). Poor knowledge about dementia can increase stress in carers who may attribute cognitive, behavioural and psychological symptoms to causes other than dementia, and believe that the person with dementia has control over their behaviour. Furthermore, carers vary greatly in how they respond to information about dementia, so what may be useful for one individual may only serve to increase anxiety in another. This is an area where there is a need for more research to inform clinical practice. In particular, further research from the perspective of carers who are receiving information would provide valuable insight into what carers feel their need for knowledge is at different stages of the caregiving career. Given what we know so far, it seems clear that education about dementia should not be delivered in a prescriptive way, but should focus on the carer's individual understanding. There should be space for information to be explored in a supportive environment, with an opportunity to discuss emotional reactions and individual meaning that is attached to the information provided.

Continuing to listen and learn: A crucial part of developing a care standard

In developing a care standard for dementia in Europe, it is crucial that we take the time to listen to those involved in the care process at all levels. It is only by listening to carers and people with dementia that we can start to fully understand the complexity of their needs and how these develop over time. Carers should play an active role in the development of care policy and practice, and should be represented in a meaningful way at all stages of health and social care delivery. The development of service user forums, consultation with community groups and the use of carers' accounts of health and social care will help to incorporate the carers' perspective into the development of service provision for the future.

References

Brown LJ, Potter JF, Foster BG. Caregiver burden should be evaluated during geriatric assessment. *J Am Geriatr Soc* 1990; **38**: 455–60.

Coen RF, Swanwick GRJ, O'Boyle CA, Coakley D. Dementia carer education and patient behaviour disturbance. *Int J Geriatr Psychiatry* 1997; **14**: 302–6.

Cooke DD, McNally L, Mulligan KT, Harrison MJG, Newman SP. Psychosocial interventions for caregivers of people with dementia: A systematic review. *Aging Ment Health* 2001; **5**: 120–35.

Department of Health *Caring about carers: A national strategy for carers.* London: Department of Health 1999a.

Department of Health. *National Service Framework for mental health: Modern standards and service models*. London: Department of Health; 1999b.

Donaldson C, Tarrier N, Burns A. The impact of the symptoms of dementia on caregivers. *Br J Psychiatry* 1997; 170: 62–70.

Henwood M. *Ignored and invisible?* Carers' Experience of the NHS. Carers' National Association.

Mittelman MS, Ferris SH, Shulman E, Steinberg G, Levin B. A family intervention to delay nursing home placement of patients with Alzheimers disease. A randomized controlled trial. *JAMA* 1996; 276: 1725–31.

Mittelman MS, Roth DL, Coon DW, Haley WE. Sustained benefit of supportive intervention for depressive symptoms in caregivers of patients with Alzheimers disease. *Am J Psychiatry* 2004; 161: 850–6.

Paton J, Johnston K, Katona C, Livingston G. What causes problems in Alzheimer's disease: Attributions by caregivers. A qualitative study. *Int J Geriatr Psychiatry* 2004; 19: 527–32.

Proctor R, Burns, Stratton Powell H, et al. Behavioural management in nursing and residential homes: A randomised controlled trial. *Lancet* 1999; 354: 26–9.

Proctor R, Martin C, Hewison J. When a little knowledge is a dangerous thing . . .: A study of carers' knowledge about dementia, preferred coping style and psychological distress. *Int J Geriatr Psychiatry* 2002; 17: 1133–9.

Teri L, Truax P, Pearson J. Caregiver depression and burden: What are the correlates? *Gerontologist* 1988; 28 (special issue): 199A.

Testad I, Aarsland D, Aasland AM. The effect of staff training on the use of restraint in dementia: A single-blind randomised controlled trial. *8th International Conference on Alzheimer's Disease and Related Disorders. Neurobiology of Aging.* July/August 2002; Vol. 23, NO1s.

Thompson EH, Futterman AM, Gallagher-Thompson D, Rose JM, Lovett SB. Social support and caregiving burden in family caregivers of frail elders. *J Gerontol* 1993; 48: S245–54.

chapter 34

The carer and the family facing Alzheimer's disease: The current state of affairs and future perspectives

Jacques Selmes Van Den Bril

The individual nature of the carer only became apparent as we approached the 1970s. It then became an essentially psychosocial research subject, without taking into consideration, in the majority of studies, the rest of the family unit.

Three important aspects must be highlighted concerning the involvement of the carer (the primary caregiver) in the illness of a relative:

- the carer takes responsibility for care in the home
- the carer and the sufferer from Alzheimer's disease (who we will refer to as patient) form a fused couple – it could be called an osmosis – and the knock-on effect of the moods and attitudes of one has important repercussions on the other
- the carer is not only the decision-maker and the care provider but also is very much a 'medical advisor'.

The importance of the carer's role leads us to the question of what will happen in a few years' time. Profound changes in society, family structures and the evermore important involvement of women in the workplace (they currently represent 70% of carers) allow us to foresee a fundamental question: 'Who will take care of the patient in 10 years' time?'

Some things to consider about Alzheimer's disease

Of course, Alzheimer's disease is, firstly, a brain disease, referring to the lesions which affect specific areas of the brain. However, this is far from being its only characteristic. It is also an individual's disease, and a family's disease.

It is an individual's disease in terms of the psychological reactions patients face with the changing of their memory and the disruption to their emotional life. In short, patients are not indifferent to what is happening to them.

It is a family's disease because the people around the patient react. The other family members, as much as the carer, are not passive witnesses in the face of the different manifestations of the disease. They suffer the consequences. They too react . . . and, in turn, their reactions condition those of the patient.

Thus, Alzheimer's disease can be considered, at the same time, a brain disease, an individual's disease and a family's disease. If these different aspects are more often than not interrelated, it is nevertheless important to distinguish them, for they interact and, above all, each requires a different treatment. The first aspect (Alzheimer's, a brain disease), clearly of a biological nature, involves drug-related treatment, the two others (Alzheimer's, an individual's disease and a family's disease), which are of a psychological and emotional nature, are to a great extent, improvable by a better understanding of the situation and by psychological help.

And this is where the role of the carer is fundamental to this approach.

Who takes responsibility?

Surveys show that:

- In couples, it is the spouse who, in more than 50% of cases, assumes the role of carer.
- In the absence of a spouse (be they divorced or deceased), it is the children, mostly daughters or daughters-in-law, who get involved. This group represents approximately 30–40% of the total amount of all carers. It must be highlighted that, in 20% of cases, the carer also looks after a third person (a child or an adolescent).
- Finally, it can fall to other members of the family, neighbours or volunteers.

Be that as it may, the burden predominantly rests on the women, who represent 70% of carers. If the average age of the carer is 57 years old, it must be highlighted that 10% of them are 75 years old or over, which limits their capacity for taking responsibility for the patient.

What does the responsibility involve?

When we analyse the hours that the carer dedicates to their relative, we must remember that 1 month has 720 hours, of which 160 are officially spent at work (less in France).

In a care home, a professional carer spends, on average, 36 hours a month per each Alzheimer patient.

The principal carer at home dedicates 286 hours a month to their relative, i.e. 8 times more than the professional carer.

How are these 286 hours divided up? What type of 'services' does the carer provide?

- Of this time, 32% is spent on key activities: looking after the house, cooking, shopping, taking the sufferer to the doctor, resolving administrative problems . . .
- Of this time, 23% is reserved for the basic activities of everyday life: washing, dressing, feeding the sufferer . . .
- Of this time, 13% corresponds to social activities and leisure pursuits shared with the relative.
- Finally, 32% comes under attention given to the behaviour of the sufferer: supervision, physical support, strategies for resolving behavioural trouble (including aggressive reactions) and mood-related problems. Hence, the importance of knowing them, anticipating them, and facing up to them.

Of course, all this involves patients whose dependence is already great. It is not the case at the beginning of the disease, carers must know what is ahead of them when they make the decision to take up their role.

How to organize oneself?

The diagnosis of Alzheimer's disease turns the life of the sufferer and their family upside-down. The crucial question is how to organize oneself . . . and the only way of doing it is through close collaboration with the other members of the family.

Three stages are to be considered.

Who will be the principal carer?

The disease is going to upset the balance and the division of the roles among the whole family. Carers find themselves forced to reorganize their time at work and map out their personal time, often having to sacrifice their own plans. In fact, when a relative develops Alzheimer's disease, all the members of the family, including the spouse, the adult children and the sons and daughters-in-law, are affected, regardless of geographical distance or the number of hours spent with the patient.

In general, the principal carer naturally emerges from the different members of the family. It is most often the spouse, the daughter or the daughter-in-law of the affected person. But with the progression of the disease, the carer cannot cope alone with the care, the custody and all the problems which arise.

It is important to go through with the other members of the family the division of tasks, the economic consequences and the possibility of arranging times for the carer to rest and have free time. It is clearly evident that families who have a heightened sense of solidarity are the ones who will best succeed in passing through this stage. Emotionally close, organized and practical families are in a better position to face the trials than more distant and conflicting ones.

The changing of roles

Each member of the family has distinct responsibilities, and plays a particular role, despite the fact that certain areas are shared, in particular between married couples.

If the person with the disease is a woman, a large part of her responsibilities in the home (such as culinary and domestic activities) will have to be taken on by her husband or by her daughter. If the patient is a man, the economic responsibilities and the management of the home will be assumed by his wife or by one of his children.

Changes of role are never simple and require, if possible, the help of other members of the family.

At a more advanced stage of the disease, a redefinition of the affected relative's identity takes place, in that from then on the carer will think of them as a child or a baby.

Taking decisions and assessing risks

Carers are confronted by all sorts of decisions concerning their relative in relation to the organization of their private lives.

These topics must be discussed, if possible, within the family, so that each person can participate . . . and so that decisions are made in agreement, without being the sole act of the principal carer.

In fact, decisions concerning the organization of private life very often include an evaluation of risk.

Let us consider, for example, the extent of freedom of movement left to the patient, as well as their ability to look after children if they are grandparents, or drive a car. In all these cases, the decision must include the consideration of the potential risks the patient runs, or that they pose to others. These depend to a large extent on the environment (it is not the same living in a town as it is living somewhere rural), and on the consequences that the decision may have upon everyday life (it is more difficult to forbid use of the car when that represents a substantial reduction of autonomy in doing the shopping, for example).

During all these stages, the family dynamic is essential. Each family will have to resolve these problems according to the possibilities open to them. However, a family dynamic exists, resulting from the family's history and its previous development, its ability to face up to situations of conflict and resolve the problems it is confronted with. Each family will solve these in its own way and according to its own means. Children may work and live a long way from their parents' home. There may be old family conflicts that have damaged communication between members of the same family, and which can resurface when the disease arises. Experience also shows that divided or normally indifferent families can, when this happens, sort things out and face things together.

For a long time, families have been alone in facing Alzheimer's disease and the problems it raises. This situation has radically changed with the development of Family Associations, which are civil society's response to the indifference and isolation experienced by the families of an Alzheimer's patient.

The emergence of a fourth power

Families have recognized the need to unite, work together and form a representative group that can be a voice when talking to political and administrative powers. The group of national Family Associations belonging to 27 countries comes together as Alzheimer Europe and Alzheimer Disease International.

Why contact a Family Association?

The Family Association responds to real needs:

- to combat feelings of isolation – one must be able to talk about problems and share them with people who are going through, or have been through, the same thing
- to inform oneself about the disease and its development
- to use the experience of others
- to find moral and psychological support
- to take part in finding collective solutions.

What are its aims?

The main objective of an Association is to help families improve their quality of life. To reach this goal, aims are:

- to inform and advise families (including in a legal and an administrative sense)
- to train carers in order to give them the abilities to provide quality care
- to provide emotional and psychological support
- to train volunteers
- to make the public, the influential groups, the medical profession and the politicians responsible for issues related to social health policies more aware of the responsibilities that families face
- to represent the interests of carers and patients.

What services does it offer?

Each Association has its own profile of services. In general, you will find:

- telephone help-lines (including advice in crisis periods)
- contact with other families via meetings and round table discussions
- training courses
- psychological help through support groups
- logistical support – legal, administrative and tax-related advice
- home-help, or perhaps day centres or even a reception centre
- exhaustive information on all aspects of the disease (reports, books, reviews etc.).

The development of the Associations movement, through its strength and its representative capacity, has made way for the emergence of a fourth power (that of the sufferers, the carers and the families) alongside the traditional political, scientific and administrative decision-making centres. Today, it is difficult to conceive of family representatives not being present in the working groups or the commissions charged with developing social health policy on Alzheimer's disease.

Darker perspectives

The significant increase over the coming years in the number of people developing the disease has become a topic attracting attention. But alongside quantitative changes, we must ask how to know what the qualitative changes affecting the patient and their carer will be, bearing in mind that no cure or preventative treatment will be available in the medium term.

The life expectancy of a patient? As for each one of us, the life expectancy of a patient increases by 15 minutes every hour, that is to say, 1 year for every 4. The first logical conclusion from this is that patients will live longer and that we will have to face up to not only more of them but also to a greater number of older patients.

Diagnosis at an earlier stage? It is a current trend to diagnose the disease at its outset, which leads us to assume that the number of 'young' sufferers risks increasing, along with the particular set of problems that the disease poses when it occurs under the age of 65 years old.

The change of women's role in society? If 70% of current carers are women, what will happen with their greater participation in the world of work? Who will take care of the patient at home? Have these perspectives, along with the increase in the number of patients and the drastic reduction in the amount of potential carers, been taken into consideration by those in charge of social health policy in the leading European countries? The answer, unfortunately, is no.

chapter 35

Carer organizations

Susan Frade

Dementia not only affects the person with dementia but it also affects the entire family, with the greatest burden being placed directly on family carers. Research indicates that many aspects of caring for a person with dementia are the same the world over; the majority of carers are women and caring is associated with substantial psychological strain resulting from grief, guilt, anger, embarrassment and loneliness (Prince, 2004; Murray et al, 1999).

Given that age is the biggest risk factor for developing dementia and with life expectancy rising in almost every country, the number of people with dementia in the world will increase dramatically. Alzheimer's Disease International (ADI), the worldwide federation of Alzheimer associations, estimates that there are currently 18 million people with dementia in the world; four million of whom live in Europe (Iliffe et al, 2003). ADI projects the number of people in the world with dementia to almost double to 34 million by 2025. Although much of this increase will be in rapidly developing and heavily populated regions, there are thought to be about 600 000 new cases of dementia developing in Europe each year (Iliffe et al, 2003).

Yet dementia remains a hidden problem because it is not often recognized as a disease. It is seen as a normal part of ageing or the strange behaviour of elders (Patel and Prince, 2000) and so families do not seek medical help. However, the lack of people seeking help does not imply a lack of need. In contrast to the developed world, people with dementia in developing countries commonly live in three-generational households, with their children and their grandchildren. Even with extended families, the pilot research work of the 10/66 Dementia Research Group shows that the main carer faces major caring commitments, high economic costs and psychological strain on the whole family (Prince, 2000).

And visiting a physician does not necessarily ensure a diagnosis; a US-based study found that half of all dementia cases were undiagnosed (Boise et al, 1999). Barriers identified included the failure to recognize and respond to the symptoms of dementia; perceived lack of need to determine a specific diagnosis; limited time; and negative attitudes toward the importance of assessment and diagnosis. These barriers keep physicians from diagnosing dementia and, consequently, from offering concrete help for the person with dementia or for their family.

The lack of awareness and understanding that dementia is an illness is just the first hurdle; in most countries, dementia is not a healthcare priority. Furthermore, in developing countries, health services are ill equipped to meet the needs of older people, and particularly those with dementia (Shaji et al, 2002). Health care, even at the primary care level is clinic-based; the older person must attend the clinic, often involving a long journey and waiting time. The assessment and treatment that they receive is orientated towards the identification and treatment of acute conditions rather than chronic conditions such as dementia. Like in the US study (Boise et al, 1999), even if the family were to seek help, it is unlikely that it would be offered to them.

Such research shows there is an urgent need to develop interventions designed to improve the quality of life for people with dementia and their families. Key interventions found to support carers and relieve their stress include:

- early identification of problems
- comprehensive assessment of social and medical needs
- availability of treatments
- information, advice and counselling
- continued support and review ideally from a known and trusted individual
- regular help with domestic and personal care tasks
- regular breaks from caring
- financial support and permanent residential care when it becomes necessary.

It is clear that people with dementia and carers need support and practical help. Priorities for action to meet their needs include the recognition that dementia is a disease, improved assessment, diagnosis and management of dementia, availability of information and advice and education and training for all involved in dementia care.

In many countries, it has been the formation and growth of carer-focused, not-for-profit organizations such as ADI and its member Alzheimer associations which has led the way in improving the quality of life for people with dementia and their carers. Canada, the USA, UK and Australia were the first countries to develop national Alzheimer associations about 25 years ago.

These associations are now well established, recognized and respected by their governments. They are run with large numbers of staff, large incomes and branches around the country.

These four associations were also the impetus for the formation of ADI in 1984. Since then, Alzheimer associations have been founded in every world region and new ones continue to be formed. In 2004, ADI welcomed Iran, Lebanon and Portugal, bringing the number of associations in this federation to 69. The continued growth of ADI and the development and formation of new associations is vital; Alzheimer associations are more closely aligned to service users, making them better positioned to identify need, understand barriers, propose solutions and help in the delivery of change. In addition, they provide somewhere helpful for professionals to refer people to, fill the gaps left by the health sector and can have a powerful influence on policy makers and professionals.

The degree to which Alzheimer associations are able to provide services depends on a number of factors, not least how long the association has been established. As a minimum, all associations raise awareness amongst members of the general public, policy makers and professionals about dementia and the impact it has on families. This can be achieved in a number of ways but the dissemination of accurate and sensible information underpins all associations' work. Most Alzheimer associations also run self-help groups and training courses, advocate on behalf of people with dementia and their carers and assist in the development of public policy issues.

Advocating on behalf of people with dementia and their carers has become a key priority for ADI and Alzheimer associations. World Alzheimer's Day, 21 September each year and coordinated by ADI, has provided ADI and Alzheimer associations with a platform to raise global awareness about dementia and the role of Alzheimer associations. The 2004 campaign 'No time to lose' came after findings from a pan-European Facing Dementia Survey in which 87% of carers and 71% of physicians felt their governments do not invest enough in treating dementia. The survey was conducted in over 2500 people, including those with dementia, carers, physicians, policy makers and the general population in France, Germany, Italy, Poland, Spain and the UK. In response to the findings, ADI wrote to all the world's health ministers alerting them to the economic consequences of an ageing population and calling on them to provide better services for people with dementia. Associations around the world joined ADI in their efforts. In Scotland, members of Alzheimer Scotland's Dementia Working Group met with the health minister to discuss the importance of early diagnosis, respite care and access to medication.

Alzheimer associations have also had considerable success in their own national campaigns. In 2000, the Alzheimer's Association of Israel succeeded in making drug treatments for Alzheimer's disease available free of charge. The 2-year campaign commenced by enlisting the support of the Deputy Minister of Health. However, the Minister of Health rejected the Association's proposal. When the Deputy Minister of Health was appointed Minister, the Association relaunched their campaign in parliament while the scientific committee prepared and circulated position papers on the drugs amongst public committees and the media. The new Minister of Health approved the Association's recommendations. The success of this campaign made the Association an important and powerful lobbying organization in Israel.

Alzheimer associations also lobby national and local governments to improve dementia services. In April 2000, the Japanese government introduced a new public long-term care insurance (LTCI) to tackle the challenges of providing care to their rapidly ageing population. This insurance provides care services for two groups of people, namely those 65 years old and over, and those between 40 and 64 years old. Care services are given in accordance to a care service plan made by a certified care manager. The programme covers community and residential services as well as the cost of equipping and renovating a person's home. The insured person makes a contribution of 10% of the total care cost and the remainder is paid by public insurances.

Prior to the introduction of the LTCI, Alzheimer's Association Japan set up a study committee for the new programme. The Association distributed information and collected its members' opinions, which were passed onto the Ministry of Health, Labour and Welfare. Shortly after the programme had been implemented, the Association carried out a second survey. Feedback identified several problems, including incorrect certification for dementia, restriction in the use of short-stay services and financial burdens, especially for low-income families. The Association took quick action by lobbying the Ministry to improve these conditions, which resulted in improvements in several parts of the programme. More significant though was the involvement of the Association's members with the programme's central and local committees. In this way, Alzheimer's Association Japan continues to check quality and quantity of care services from the viewpoint of the person with dementia and their carer.

More recently and after years of campaigning from Alzheimer's Australia, the Coalition Government led by Prime Minister Howard committed itself to making dementia a national health priority. At the launch of the Coalition's Election Policy in 2004, the Prime Minister made a 4-year commitment to support the following:

- AU$52 million to develop and monitor strategies to improve health outcomes for people with dementia
- AU$128 million to provide 2000 high-care packages in the home, specifically targeted to people with dementia
- AU$20 million to expand the Carer Education and Workforce Training Project to provide dementia-specific training.

Alzheimer associations play a critical role in helping reduce carers' stress. They do so directly by providing accurate and reliable information. Booklets such as ADI's *Help for carers* help carers cope with the personal and emotional stresses of caring, whereas information about dementia helps carers understand what is happening to the person they are caring for. Self-help groups provide an opportunity for carers to share their feelings, problems, ideas and information with others who are undergoing similar experiences. By lobbying on behalf of people with dementia, Alzheimer associations can help shape policy and service delivery, which will ultimately improve the quality of life for people with dementia and their carers.

References

Boise L, Carnicioli R, Morgan DL, Rose JH, Congleton L. Diagnosing dementia: Perspectives of primary care physicians. *Gerontologist* 1999; 39: 457–64.

Iliffe S, Manthorpe J, Eden A. Sooner or later? Issues in the early diagnosis of dementia in general practice: A qualitative study. *Fam Pract* 2003; 20: 376–81.

Murray J, Schneider J, Banerjee S, Mann A. EUROCARE: a cross-national study of co-resident spouse carers for people with Alzheimer's disease. *Int J Geriatr Psychiatry* 1999; 14: 662–7.

Patel V, Prince M. Ageing and mental health in a developing country: Who cares? Qualitative studies from Goa, India. *Psychol Med* 2001; 31: 29–38.

Prince M. Dementia in developing countries. A consensus statement from the 10/66 Dementia Research Group. *Int J Geriatr Psychiatry* 2000; 15: 14–20.

Prince M; 10/66 Dementia Research Group. Care arrangements for people with dementia in developing countries. *Int J Geriatr Psychiatry* 2004; 19: 170–7.

Shaji KS, Arun Kishore NR, Lal KP, Prince M. Revealing a hidden problem. An evaluation of a community dementia case-finding program from the Indian 10/66 dementia research network. *Int J Geriatr Psychiatry* 2002; 17: 222–5.

chapter 36

Elder abuse

Sean Lennon

Elder abuse is a violation of Human Rights and a significant cause of injury, illness, lost productivity, isolation and despair.
Confronting and reducing elder abuse requires a multisectoral and multidisciplinary approach.

(WHO, 2002a)

Introduction

The abuse of older people is the cause of considerable suffering. Although its nature is well described and many of its causes understood, action to prevent such abuse is still not producing responses in society and in services to older people which can give us confidence that the problem can be controlled.

What is elder abuse?

Elder abuse has been defined in a number of ways: in the UK, Department of Health guidance included older people within a category of vulnerable adults; such a person is one:

who is or may be in community care services by reason of mental or other disability, age or illness; and who is or may be unable to take care of him or herself or unable to protect him or herself against significant harm or exploitation. (Department of Health, 2000a)

The definition continues:

Abuse may consist of a single or repeated acts. It may be physical, verbal or psychological. It may be an act of neglect or an omission to act or it may occur when a vulnerable person is persuaded to enter into a financial or sexual transaction to which he or she has not consented or cannot consent. Abuse can occur in any relationship and may result in significant harm to or exploitation of, the person subjected to it.

(Department of Health, 2000b)

The Declaration of Toronto (WHO, 2002b) confined itself to abuse of older people and defined this as:

Elder abuse is a single or repeated act or lack of appropriate action occurring within any relationship where there is an expectation of trust which causes harm or distress to an older person.

Elder abuse is not simply confined to physical abuse or neglect and it may occur in any sort of care setting. It has various forms, physical, psychological, emotional, sexual, financial or it reflects intentional or unintentional neglect.

Who does it affect?

The reported rate of elder abuse has been found to be between 2% and 10% of the elderly population (Lachs and Pillemoer, 2004). It is likely that rates of abuse are similar across all countries (Tornstom, 1989). It also seems likely that these estimates may reflect 'the tip of the iceberg'. An estimate of the incidence of elder abuse in the United States suggested that only 16% of cases of abuse and/or neglect are reported (National Center on Elder Abuse, 1998). It is a problem affecting older people of all social and ethnic backgrounds. There may, however, be a gender difference. The National Elder Abuse Incident Study (National Centre on Elder Abuse, 1998) found increased rates for emotional and physical abuse amongst women and a higher proportion of abandonment for men. People with dementia may be more vulnerable than other older people. Although older people are victims of the same sort of abuse as other vulnerable adults, they may be particularly vulnerable because of a 'fundamental loss of respect for older people' (Bennett, 2002). Unlike many other vulnerable adults, older people may still be living on their own and they may have significant economic resources which may make them more vulnerable to financial abuse.

Abuse is associated with significant morbidity and mortality (Lachs et al, 1998). Much abuse occurs in institutional settings (Compton and Flanagan, 1998) and there is evidence that older people living in institutional care settings are at higher risk of abuse than those who live in the community (Glendenning, 1997; Garner and Evans, 2000). Those with depression and dementia are at particular risk (Royal College of Psychiatrists, 2004). Within the institutional setting abuse may take the forms already described but the institution may be, in itself abusive, where, for example, institutions may have a culture of 'warehousing older citizens' (Garner and Evans, 2000).

Risk factors

There is an interaction between factors leading to abuse and the characteristics of those who commit abuse. In the setting of a person's own home there is the potential for abuse to occur in what could be described as a private setting: i.e. where care may be provided on a one-to-one basis and where the older person may be dependent on the district nurse, a care worker or other paid carer who comes into the home. Much care for older people at home is provided by informal carers and the British Geriatric Society, in its submission to the Health Committee of the House of Commons (2003–2004) identified a number of potential risk factors. These were:

- Social isolation – those who are abused usually have fewer social contacts than those who are not abused;
- A history of poor quality long-term relationship between the abused and the abuser;
- A pattern of family violence (the abuser may have been abused as a child);
- Dependence of the person who abuses on the person they abuse (e.g.: the accommodation, financial and emotional support;
- A history of mental health problems or of personality disorder, drug or alcohol problem in the person who abuses.

Taken together with what is known about public policy to support people as far as possible to live in their own homes, it seems likely that abuse in one's own home is a common type of abuse but, because it is so little observed, it is perhaps the most difficult to address. Although it is likely that caregiver stress may be associated with some forms of elder abuse, there is no good evidence that this is a frequent association; more commonly, it is other factors in the abuser which play an important role, e.g. some families are more prone to violence and it has become a learned behaviour. In these circumstances, abuse is the response to tension or conflict. In other care relationships, particularly when an adult child is abusing their parents, the fact that they suffer from mental and emotional disorders, alcoholism, drug addiction and financial difficulty, are factors associated with abuse. On occasion, this occurs because the adult child is dependent on the elders for their support.

Within an institutional setting, there are a number of factors relating to the carer, to the patient characteristics and the organization which increase the risk of abuse of an older person. These issues are carefully explored by the authors of the Royal College of Psychiatrists Report (Garner and Evans, 2000) who point out that 'even in the grossest cases personal malevolence is not an adequate explanation although individual psychopathology cannot be ignored.' Clearly, there may be abusers who are bullying or aggressive but, for many carers, the caring role has been undertaken without any ill-will and it would appear that psychological factors such as job dissatisfaction, stressful personal life and low morale may all be associated with abuse. The organizational factors described by Garner and Evans demonstrate the essential roles of good management and staffing in preventing elder abuse. The culture of an institution which commends speed and efficiency rather than spending time with residents may be the sort of culture which does not recognize factors which might lead to abuse. A further report from the Royal College of Pychiatrists lays out very clearly institutional risk factors (Garner and Evans, 2002); see Appendix 1.

Prevention

Elder abuse in any of its forms cannot be tolerated and it should be emphasized that it is not just institutions and practitioners which should find it intolerable but also older people who suffer abuse should be helped to find it intolerable rather than accepting it or sometimes even blaming themselves for the abuse (Kahan and Paris, 2003). The response of services has a number of facets: the first of these is to prevent abuse. Prevention depends firstly on awareness of the problem and with awareness there must be training to make it possible for people who are in contact with an abused person to recognize both the risk factors associated with abuse and the signs of abuse. An example of a screening tool is given by Kahan (Appendix 2) (Kahan and Paris, 2003). There needs to be a public awareness so that informal carers, family members and others, if they suspect abuse, have some knowledge of where to turn for help but, also, the older person suffering abuse needs to be able to seek help personally. In the UK, Action on Elder Abuse is a voluntary sector organization producing advice of the highest standard and also campaigning to address the problem of elder abuse.

The Toronto Declaration (WHO, 2002b) states:

> It is not enough to identify cases of elder abuse. All countries should develop the structures that will allow the provision of services (health, social, legal protection, police referral, etc.) to appropriately respond and eventually prevent the problem.

In the area of public policy in the UK, reports such as the Department of Health report, *No secrets* (Department of Health, 2002a) and the Health Select Committee report make strong recommendations for public action. Improvements in services which can prevent, detect and manage elder abuse will come about through development of public policy and its implementation (House of Commons Health Committee, 2003–2004). Professional organizations must also lead this change – in the UK, the Nursing & Midwifery Council (2002) provides guidelines for practitioners. For psychiatrists, the Faculty for the Psychiatry of Old Age in the Royal College of Psychiatrists (2004) has produced a range of guidance. The particular role of the psychiatrist may be to take a lead in promoting an examination of ageism and the capacity for abuse in care homes and the wards in which they work. A psychiatrist is in a good position to understand and influence the institutions and also should have a good understanding of the inherent difficulties in caring for many of the older people who fall victim to abuse (Garner and Baldwin, 2001; Garner and Evans, 2002).

The effectiveness of training in management of elder abuse has been explored by a number of authors (McCreadie et al, 2000; Kahan and Paris, 2003) and this is clearly an essential element of the development of skills in staff who care for the elderly. However, despite these sorts of initiatives, there continues to be findings of failures in services and a failure to learn lessons (Tonks and Bennett, 1999; Commission for Health Improvement, 2003).

Conclusions

Elder abuse is underrecognized and the reported numbers may be less than one-fifth of the total number of cases. Much is known about the nature of abuse and its causes. Although public policy is developing and awareness is increasing, there continues to be a failure to produce changes in the care of vulnerable older people which would significantly reduce the suffering experienced. Professional organizations together with voluntary sector organizations must take a lead in reforming services.

References

Bennett G. Elder abuse. *Age Ageing* 2002; **31**: 329.

Commission for Health Improvement. Report on Rowan Ward. Commission for Health Improvement; 2003.

Compton SA, Flanagan P. Elder abuse in people with dementia in Northern Ireland: Prevalence and predictors in cases referred to a psychiatry of old age service. *Int J Geriatr Psychiatry* 1997; **12**: 632–5.

Department of Health. No secrets. TSO. Para 2–3. London: Department of Health; 2000a.

Department of Health. No secrets. TSO. Para 2.5–2.6. London: Department of Health; 2000b.

Garner J, Baldwin R. *Old age psychiatrist.* The Royal College of Psychiatrists, Faculty for the Psychiatry of Old Age, Winter 2001.

Garner J, Evans G. *Institutional abuse of older adults.* The Royal College of Psychiatrists Council Report CR 84, 2000.

Garner J, Evans S. An ethical perspective on institutional abuse of older adults. *Psychiatr Bull* 2002; **26**: 164–6.

Glendenning S. The mistreatment and neglect of elderly people in residential centres: Research outcomes in the mistreatment of elderly people. In: Decalmer S, Glendenning P, eds. *The mistreatment of elderly people* 2nd edn. London: Sage; 1997.

House of Commons Health Committee. Elder abuse. 2nd Report of Session 2003–4.

Kahan F, Paris B. Why elder abuse continues to elude the health care system. *Mount Sinai J Med* 2003; **70(1)**: 62–8.

Lachs M, Pillemoer K. Elder abuse. *Lancet* 2004; **364**: 1263–72.

Lachs MG, Williams CS, O'Brien S, Pillemer KA, Charlson ME. The mortality of elder mistreatment. *JAMA* 1998; **280**: 428–32.

McCreadie C, Bennett G, Gilthorpe MS, Houghton G, Tinker A. Elder abuse: Do general practitioners know or care? *J R Soc Med* 2000; **93**: 67–71.

National Centre on Elder Abuse. The National Elder Abuse Incidence Study, 1998.

Nursing & Midwifery Council. *Practitioner–client relationships and the prevention of abuse.* Nursing & Midwifery Council; 2002.

Royal College of Psychiatrists. *The Rowan Report: implications and advice.* London: Royal College of Psychiatrists; 2004.

Tonks A, Bennett. Elder abuse. *BMJ* 1999; **318**: 278–9.

Tornstom L. Abuse of elderly in Denmark and Sweden. *J Elder Abuse Neglect* 1989; **1**: 35–44.

WHO. *Active ageing, a policy framework.* Geneva: WHO; 2002a.

WHO. *The Toronto Declaration on the global prevention of elder abuse.* Geneva: WHO; 2002b.

Appendix 1: Institutional abuse risk factors

When considering whether units are at risk of institutional abuse, members are urged to consider the following:

The unit

- Wards caring for vulnerable elderly people (commonly continuing care units) are isolated – physically, clinically, educationally, managerially and from the community.
- Wards were not originally intended for the needs of older people. They are poorly designed, in poor physical condition and unsuitable for people with chronic, enduring mental health problems.
- Relatives, other professionals, voluntary groups and advocates rarely or never visit.

The residents

- Wards have a mixed population of residents with different needs, e.g. organic and functional disorders.

The staff

- There is a low staff to patient ratio.
- Staff are poorly trained and poorly paid.
- Staff have limited or no access to training, are not frequently or adequately supervised and have little support from clinical colleagues and managers.
- Staff can be 'burnt out', institutionalized and resistant to change, or there is a frequently changing staff population owing to high turnover.
- 'Bank' or agency staff are often used.
- Task-led rather than patient-centred care is prevalent.

The management

- The culture of the ward is inward-looking: little interest is shown in good practice, improving the quality of outcomes, or clinical governance issues.
- There are no clear policies within the unit for reporting incidents, protection of vulnerable adults and 'whistle-blowing'.
- Audit does not take place.

- Performance management measures (e.g. sickness rates, staff turnover, agency usage, etc.) are not collected, or, if they are, are not scrutinized, so that patterns suggesting problems are not recognized.
- Mental health in old age is not seen as a priority and there is no clear management responsibility or structure present. There is little investment in people, training or resources.

Appendix 2: Elder abuse/neglect screening assessment tool

1. Has anyone ever hurt you?
2. Does anyone ever talk or yell at you in a way that makes you feel bad about yourself?
3. Has anyone ever taken anything from you or used your money without permission?
4. Are you afraid of anyone or has anyone ever threatened you?
5. Has anyone ever refused to help you?
6. Do you feel that your food, clothing and medications are available to you at all times?
7. Are you able to go out of your house when you wish to do so?
8. Do you get to see other relatives and friends?
9. Do you have ready access to a telephone?
10. Do you live with anyone or have any close family members who abuse drugs and alcohol or have a psychiatric or emotional illness?

Source: adapted from: *Elder mistreatment guidelines for health care professionals: Detection, assessment and intervention.* New York: Mount Sinai/Victim Services Agency Elder Abuse Project; 1988: 6.

Services

chapter 37

The impact of memory clinics on the care of dementia patients

Hannes B Staehelin

The concept of memory clinics

The pioneer in the field of memory clinics was Exton-Smith, who established the first memory clinic in London as a diagnostic outpatient service. Soon thereafter the first memory clinics on the Continent were founded (Stahelin et al, 1989; Monsch et al, 1998) – Basel opened in 1986; Munich opened in 1985, at the same time as a research institution.

One of the driving forces to establishing memory clinics is the need to have access to clinical research, particularly in patients at an early stage of the disease. However, since the possible benefit to the patient with a dementing illness is difficult to predict, the memory clinic should offer additional services that improve the quality of life of patients and caregivers or ameliorate the management of the disease. The goals and the presumed benefits of a memory clinic are listed in Table 37.1.

Thus, the memory clinic yields an ideal platform for the management of the complex and, in early phases, often difficult to diagnose psychogeriatric illnesses.

Competences necessary in a memory clinic

Dementia is not a nosological entity but a defined cognitive disability operationalized by neuropsychological and social parameters. Thus, neuropsychological competence is indispensable. Since a correct differential diagnosis is essential for specific treatment, competence in geriatric medicine to detect

Table 37.1 Characteristics and benefits of a memory clinic

Characteristics	*Benefit*
Competence of the interdisciplinary team	Rapid assessment, comprehensive case management
Early diagnosis	Early start of therapy, social adjustment to the illness by patient and family, avoidance of inefficient diagnostic and therapeutic actions, treatable causes are detected and secondary dementias become rare
Support for patients and caregivers	Efficient case management and relief in a difficult situation
	Counselling of patients, family members and caregivers
Advice and support for referring physicians and primary care physicians	Enables the primary care physician to manage effectively dementia patients at home
Pre- and postgraduate teaching	Increasing the competence of the medical profession
Strong link to basic and clinical and neuropsychological research	Access to new treatment regimens, access to patients at an early stage of the disease, high diagnostic accuracy already early during the illness
Epidemiological and health services research	Support in effective health care planning
Increasing the awareness of the population and political representatives	Advocacy for the disadvantaged, reducing the fear of dementia in old age
Developing and setting quality assessment standards	Guarantees diagnostic and therapeutic standards under clinical governance
Promulgating minimal data sets	Exchange of compatible data improves performance, shared documentation facilitates the integration between health and social care

concomitant illnesses, competence in diagnosis and treatment of neurological disorders as well as competence in diagnosing and treating psychiatric disorders are required in a memory clinic. As outlined above, social factors are predominant in the management of dementia (Cattanach and Tebes, 1991; Vugt, 2004). Thus, the memory clinic needs competence in assessing social needs of patients, their family and the caregivers involved. A formalized cooperation with the social institutions caring for psychogeriatric patients in the community, e.g. Alzheimer Society, specialized nursing homes, etc., is important. If necessary the memory clinic should offer services such as memory training (Ermini-Fünfschilling and Meier, 1995; Zarit et al, 2004), and specialized treatment, e.g. in the context of new pharmacotherapeutic approaches. This requires competence in biomedical research. Thus, affiliation to academic institutions is advantageous.

Probably the most important competence is that of working effectively in an interdisciplinary way. This requires the respect of the other academic or non-academic team members, and the skill and the patience to listen and to communicate openly within the team and with the partners of the memory clinic.

To arrive at a coherent view of the problems presented by patients, diagnosis conferences that unite all specialists involved in their treatment have proved useful. In managing dementia patients, it is important to reach a consensus and agree on a treatment concept. Since one of the prime functions of most memory clinics is the cooperation and support of primary care physicians, it is essential to establish a protocol suitable to the needs of family physicians and the memory clinic.

True need or newly created need?

The emergence and spread of memory clinics leads to the question of whether the demographic change with increasing numbers of old people has induced the development or whether it corresponds to a true need. The numbers of the general population from which patients are seen at a typical memory clinic, the young old, has not increased dramatically over the past 40 years, by contrast with the very old, who are not the characteristic patients seen in memory clinics. Forty years ago the scientific interest in neurodegenerative diseases was low, but the pharmacotherapeutic options were not dramatically less than today, and the understanding that dementia management requires an interdisciplinary approach to successful management was less evident. The typical patient of the Basel memory clinics is 72–74 years old, has an MMSE of 22, is female (60%) and has received 12 years of education (Stahelin et al, 1997), rather similar findings to those observed in other locations (Stratford et al, 2003). Thus, it is clearly the wish of the patient and his family to frequent a memory clinic. The rapid deployment of memory clinics over the last 10 years demonstrates that the institutions respond to a demand and are seen as beneficial in the management of the devastating neurodegenerative disorders (van Hout et al, 2001; Gardner et al, 2004).

Access to memory clinics

Most memory clinics have a referral system for patients, most often by general physicians but also by specialists and hospital services. This raises several questions. Is the primary care physician competent in detecting dementia? Could it be that since the primary care physician has little training in psychogeriatrics and often has a rather negative view of old age that he attributes cognitive decline to ageing per se and tries to dismiss complaints by patients and caregivers. This would raise the barrier to the access of the services of memory clinics. Similarly, the triggers seeking advice for memory complaints may differ culturally and may be influenced by socioeconomic factors. A Dutch study suggests (van Hout et al, 2000) that they are able to make appropriate selection for referral. Our own experience with a two-step approach where the case finding is done by family physicians shows a comparable distribution as, for example, reported by an Australian team (Stahelin et al, 1997; Stratford et al, 2003). With regard to referrals by specialists compared to general practitioners there seems to be no significant difference in detecting and referring patients (Damina et al, 2003).

It is evident that public and professional awareness crucially affect referral to memory clinics. Analysing the factors leading to diagnosis-seeking at a memory clinic, it was found that changes in the patient accounted for 81% of the trigger events, cognitive changes dominating over behavioural alterations. In nearly the half of the cases, two or more changes were reported (Streams et al, 2003).

In an Italian study the authors observed a strong impact of physical function. In patients with normal physical function age, female sex and lower cognitive function were associated with longer time to diagnosis. In subjects with physical impairment, earlier stages of dementia had already led to a diagnostic work-up (Cattel et al, 2000). Furthermore, in comparing urban–rural differences in a memory clinic population, it was found that the typical urban clinic patient was significantly more likely to be living in a facility and more educated than the typical rural patient. Caregivers and family members of urban patients reported more memory problems, twice as many personality changes, more frequent behaviour problems as well as more adverse reaction to problems. Hence, families in urban settings are more sensitive to patients' cognitive and behavioural symptoms than rural families (Wackerbarth et al, 2001). Cultural factors impact too. Comparing patients in Australia of English- vs non-English-mother tongue, LoGuidice et al. (2001) observed in their memory clinic in Melbourne among the non-English-speaking patients (mostly of Italian descent) a higher number of either normal or depressed patients and if dementia was present, patients with more advanced cognitive impairment, than the patients from an English-speaking background.

Are memory clinics effective?

Memory clinics unite different specialties and thus offer a wide array of services. Nevertheless, the question remains whether they operate more effectively and lead to higher 'consumer satisfaction' than traditional services. A comparison of the memory clinic with traditional old age psychiatry services found that the memory clinic was frequented by significantly younger patients with lower levels of cognitive impairments leading to an earlier diagnosis by 2 years compared to the traditional service (Luce et al, 2001). Using optimized methods such as neuropsychology and imaging impacts significantly on the diagnostics, as shown by Hentschel et al (2004).

Consumer satisfaction was found in several studies. Thus, van Hout et al (2001) report positive opinions on the way the results were recorded and communicated. In an Australian study the general practitioners were most positive about the completeness and utility of the assessment and diagnostic information provided, but less positive as in the study by van Hout about the advice regarding the family's coping and community support services for the patient (van Hout et al, 2001). This indicates that the academically more rewarding disciplines such as medical and neuropsychological competences are stronger and better established in the current memory clinic setting than the psychosocial competence (Gardner et al, 2004). Clearly, the cooperation among memory clinics and the adoption of assessment and treatment protocols as well as the interdisciplinary cooperation offers the possibility to improve on quality in this respect.

The memory clinics are here to stay. They offer the health professional and thus also to the general public an efficient access to assessing and coping with complex cognitive disorders. Clinical governance is important to maintain and improve quality, ensure equal access and to implement new developments.

Conclusion

Together with increasing scientific interest, progress in elucidating the causes of the psychogeriatric illnesses and public awareness, the memory clinics became a success. It is probably difficult to prove beyond any doubt that the memory clinic approach is superior to a less-focused more individualized management of dementia patients. It may also be that progress in establishing the differential diagnosis of dementia by simple technical procedures and simple and effective therapeutic options such as vaccination, for example, may make many memory clinics unnecessary. However, for the time being and in the foreseeable future, the concept of the memory clinic offers the most focused and most effective approach to a comprehensive management of patients with dementia. Even if great progress is made, a multidimensional assessment is required that covers the cognitive, behavioural and functional aspects of the disease as well as the effect on family caregivers, the use of formal and informal care, quality of life and patient and family satisfaction. To this end, the memory clinic is best suited.

References

Cattanach L, Tebes JK. The nature of elder impairment and its impact on family caregivers' health and psychosocial functioning. *Gerontologist* 1991; 31: 246–55.

Cattel C, Gambassi G, Sgadari A, et al. Correlates of delayed referral for the diagnosis of dementia in an outpatient population. *J Gerontol A Biol Med Sci* 2000; 55: M98–102.

Damina M, Kreis M, Krumm B, Syren M, Hentschel F. Is there a referral bias in the diagnosis of patients of a memory clinic? *Z Gerontol Geriatr* 2003; 36: 197–203.

Ermini-Fünfschilling D, Meier D. Memory training: An important constitutent of milieu therapy in senile dementia. *Z Gerontol Geriatr* 1995; 28: 190–4.

Gardner IL, Foreman P, Davis S. Cognitive dementia and memory service clinics: Opinions of general practitioners. *Am J Alzheimers Dis Other Demen* 2004; 19: 105–10.

Hentschel F, Damian M, Kreis M, Krumm B. Effects of extended clinical diagnostics on the diagnostic spectrum of an outpatient memory clinic. *Z Gerontol Geriatr* 2004; 37: 145–54.

LoGuidice D, Hassett A, Cook R, Flicker L, Ames D. Equity of access to a memory clinic in Melbourne? Non-English speaking background attenders are more severely demented and have increased rates of psychiatric disorders. *Int J Geriatr Psychiatry* 2001; 16: 327–34.

Luce A, McKeith I, Swann A, Daniel S, O'Brien J. How do memory clinics compare with traditional old age psychiatry services? *Int J Geriatr Psychiatry* 2001; 16: 837–45.

Monsch AU, Ermini-Funfschilling D, Mulligan R, et al. Memory clinics in Switzerland. Collaborative Group of Swiss Memory Clinics. *Ann Med Interne (Paris)* 1998; 149: 221–7.

Stahelin HB, Ermini-Funfschilling D, Grunder B, et al. [The memory clinic]. *Ther Umsch* 1989; 46: 72–7.

Stahelin HB, Monsch AU, Spiegel R. Early diagnosis of dementia via a two-step screening and diagnostic procedure. *Int Psychogeriatr* 1997; 9: 123–30.

Stratford JA, LoGiudice D, Flicker L, et al. A memory clinic at a geriatric hospital: A report on 577 patients assessed with CAMDEX over 9 years. *Aust N Z J Psychiatry* 2003; 37: 319–26.

Streams ME, Wackerbarth SB, Maxwell A. Diagnosis-seeking at subspecialty memory clinics: Trigger events. *Int J Geriatr Psychiatry* 2003; 18: 915–24.

van Hout HP, Vernooij-Dassen MJ, Hoefnagel WH, Grol RP. Measuring the opinion of memory clinic users: Patients, relatives and general practitioners. *Int J Geriatr Psychiatry* 2001; 16: 846–51.

van Hout H, Vernooij-Dassen M, Poels P, Hoefnagel W, Grol R. Are general practitioners able to accurately diagnose dementia and Alzheimer's disease? A comparison with an outpatient memory clinic. *Br J Gen Prac* 2000; 50: 311–12.

Vugt D. *Behavioural problems in dementia: Caregiver issues.* Maastricht: NeuroPsych; 2004.

Wackerbarth SB, Johnson MMS, Markesbery WR, Smith CD. Urban–rural differences in a memory disorders clinical population. *J Am Geriatr Soc* 2001; 49: 647–50.

Zarit SH, Femia EE, Watson J, Rice-Oeschger L, Kakos B. Memory Club: A group intervention for people with early stage dementia and their care partners. *Gerontologist* 2004; 44: 262–9.

chapter 38

Promoting independence through design of the environment

Mary Marshall

Throughout Europe there is widespread recognition that the environment has an impact on people with dementia and that special efforts need to be made to make that impact a positive one. The father of environmental gerontology, M Powell Lawton (1982) coined the term 'environmental press' to explain the fact that the more disabled you are the greater the impact of the environment. Most of us can understand the buildings in which we find ourselves and we are able to find our way. For those with cognitive impairment, this can be very difficult and the buildings can effectively disable them.

Most people with dementia have a set of impairments which include:

- impaired memory
- impaired reasoning
- impaired learning.

These result in high levels of stress and, like any other impairments, increased dependence on remaining ways of understanding and coping with environments. For people with dementia this means that they use their senses increasingly as their cognition deteriorates. The aim of design is to compensate for these impairments and thereby to enable people with dementia to remain as independent as possible. If you have to ask the way to the toilet, for example, or wait until somebody takes you there, you are in effect disabled by the environment in which the toilet is hard to find.

With dementia, these impairments can be complicated. Impaired memory, for example, usually starts with recent memory. Well-established memory can remain until the condition is well advanced. It seems that the memory for spaces is laid down when we are young adults, so that these memories will be strongest. The implication of this is that design will make most sense if it relates to this time of life, which for most people with dementia aged 80+ will be the 1930s and 1940s. In those days, people were not constantly refurbishing their houses so the house they lived in at that time would not look too different right into the 1950s and 1960s.

Another complication is that most people with dementia are older and will have many of the disabilities of old age: yet, they will not understand this and will fail to make allowances. Their eyes, for example, will be less and less able to discriminate between colours, so hindering their ability to make sense of the environment through colour. Designers have to use very strong colour contrast for important features (such as the toilet door). The ability to see three dimensions also deteriorates in many ageing eyes. People with dementia will not be able to adjust to this, which makes it important not to change floor colours, which can be then seen as steps. Glare and reflections are particularly difficult for the ageing eye (Brawley 1997).

Many people with dementia will have hearing impairment, not just hearing loss. One of the most difficult conditions is selective frequency hearing loss, or presbycusis, which impairs the ability to separate out sounds. It can be very overwhelming. A quiet environment is essential if people with dementia are to make sense of any sound, and to reduce their stress levels.

The consensus on design features which are helpful to people with dementia is common throughout Europe (Judd et al, 1997). It includes:

- *Small scale.* People with dementia cannot cope with too much stimulation, so small units with small numbers of people are crucial. Ideally, any unit should have fewer than 8 people. Many of the Swedish care houses have 6. Many new developments are a cluster of small units to allow for economies of scale for central kitchens and laundries and for staff. The sector which has yet to really understand the importance of small scale is the day-care sector. Many day centres and hospitals cater for 20 or 30 people, which can be very disabling for people with dementia, especially at meal times (Calkins, 1988). This can prevent people with dementia from eating because they are so stressed.

- *A domestic environment.* In order to maintain past skills and to provide meaningful, familiar activities it is now widely understood that a domestic environment is important. It should make possible all the day-to-day activities such as washing dishes, washing and hanging out clothes, working in the tool shed, washing the car and so on. Ideally, all these facilities should be age-appropriate.

- *High levels of visual access.* People with dementia have to rely on their eyes because they cannot learn where rooms are or remember where to go. They need to be able to see where they need to go. This means that most up-to-date dementia environments throughout Europe have an open-plan design as far as possible. Counter kitchens, bedroom doors opening onto the lounge/dining areas and highly visible toilet doors are commonplace. This understanding also results in glazed walls and glass panels in doors, so that people can see what is in the room. It can even extend to glass doors on cupboards so that people can see what is in the cupboard and do not have to remember. An important feature for many people with dementia is being able to see the toilet from the bed. A low light may be required at night. If they can see it, they can find their way to it and incontinence will be reduced.

- *Good signage.* Clear signs that incorporate pictures and words can be very helpful to people with dementia. The best words have a capital at the start and then lower case, and use a font without a serif. The picture needs to look familiar. The clearest sign is black on yellow which is best for people with impaired sight (Barker and Fraser, 2000). These general rules for signage will not help everybody and it is important to be more sensitive to individual requirements with personal front doors. Signage here needs to be individually recognisable. For some it will be a photograph, others a drawing, others a number or name and some will even require a three-dimensional object to assist them to find their own door.

- *Landmarks not colour aid orientation.* There is a great deal of misunderstanding about the importance of colour to older people, which results from a failure to understand what happens to the ageing eye. As we get older, we are usually less and less able to discriminate between colours. Objects, pictures, hangings, curtains, trellises and carefully placed furniture are likely to be much more effective in helping people with memory problems to remember where things are. Many will not be able to learn at all and some will require a lot of coaching. But no amount of learning will help them to see colour differentiation, except for sharp contrast.

- *Concealing doors that are not important.* To assist people with dementia it is helpful to make unimportant doors invisible by continuing décor, handrails and skirting boards over them. Ideally, they should be in areas of units where people with dementia seldom go, but this is not always possible.

- *Lots of light.* Older people need a great deal more light to see effectively than younger people and there is research to show how additional light aids orientation (Nelten, 1993). There is very little literature to assist in deciding what kind of light is best beyond avoiding light which gives sharp shadows, which can be frightening. Lighting types are therefore highly variable in dementia units.

- *Quiet.* Hiatt (1995) points out that noise to people with dementia is the equivalent to steps for people in wheelchairs, because it is so totally disabling. The quickest route to stress reduction is to reduce noise. Yet, · many units are very noisy, with radios blaring, trolleys rattling, vacuum cleaners roaring and staff talking. Much of this is not a design issue, but design can help with sound-absorbing ceiling tiles, fabrics and carpets.

- *Age-appropriate décor and furnishing.* This is a real challenge to many designers. Choosing paintwork, carpets, curtains, chairs, tables and so on which are able to withstand constant use and frequent incontinence while being familiar to the people living in the unit is not easy (Pollock, 2003). Much work is still required with the manufacturers. However, staff can make a huge difference if they try for a 1940s look to bed covers, tablecloths and ornaments. They often fail to provide pictures on the walls, which make sense to the people with dementia in terms of style and content. Ensuring the furniture contrasts with the floor is important given the difficulties the ageing eye has with colour contrast. However, much good work is achieved when staff understand the reasoning. Most units now would understand the need for plates to contrast with table-cloths and to provide a contrast with the food. Few places would now provide white fish in white sauce with potato on a white plate on a white cloth. Most staff now understand that, in these circumstances, the food is invisible.

- *Avoid a sense of confinement.* People with dementia are very sensitive to a feeling of imprisonment and will make determined efforts to escape, perhaps to return to their own familiar home. Much can be done to make units feel less like prisons. First, the fire door: fire doors are often located at the end of corridors and have a window in them. People with dementia are drawn to the light and then push open the door. There is no need to put these doors at the end of corridors. Some of the best units have them in small sitting rooms at the end of corridors or to the side of the corridor. Maximizing autonomy and control is important, (Cohen and Weisman, 1991), which means that opportunities to open doors and go somewhere provides this. Doors to a safe garden, where there is a path which brings them back to another door, can be very helpful. It may be necessary to conceal fences around gardens with planting, so that they do not add to the feeling of being confined.

This list makes the whole design process seem easy but it is far from that. There are real challenges, not least with hygiene and fire regulators who get anxious when people with dementia are allowed to use kitchens, or when there is open plan, which raises fire safety concerns. There are always challenges with costs. Very often, designers fail to put themselves in the shoes of someone with cognitive impairment and they provide super-modern taps that are unusable for people with dementia, or fail to provide access to the garden (Pollock, 2001) in a way that helps people to find their way back in.

Technology will help in the future to make design easier. Sprinkler systems to put out fires can make open-plan design easier. Safety devices on cookers can make them safer. Systems using movement detectors can help staff to feel more relaxed about single rooms and en-suite facilities, since detectors can be programmed to alert staff when something exceptional occurs.

There are now a great many buildings, both domestic houses and more commonly care homes and health facilities throughout Europe, that are 'dementia friendly'. They are all built to the same principles. They will be small, domestic in style, quiet, well-lit, old-fashioned in terms of décor and furnishings and very easy to navigate. Two concluding points are required:

1. Good design does not make good care happen, but it makes it easier.
2. What is good for dementia is good for all of us.

It would be good to know that all buildings will increasingly take note of what is good for people with cognitive impairment, so that all of us can feel more comfortable in them.

References

Barker P, Fraser J. *Sign design guide: A guide to inclusive signage.* London: JMU; 2000.
Brawley EC. *Designing for Alzheimer's disease.* New York: John Wiley and Sons, 1997.
Calkins MP. *Design for dementia planning: Environments for the elderly and the confused.* Maryland, USA: National Health Publishing; 1988.
Cohen U, Weisman GD. *Holding on to home: Designing environments for people with dementia.* Maryland, USA: The Johns Hopkins University Press; 1991.
Hiatt LG. Understanding the physical environment. *Pride Institute J Long-Term Care* 1995; **4**: 12–22.

Lawton MP. Competence, environmental press, and the adaptation of older people. In: Lawton MP, Windley P, Byetss T, eds. *Ageing and the environment: Theoretical approaches*. New York: Springer; 1982.

Judd S, Marshall M, Phippen P. *Design for dementia*. London: Hawker Publications; 1997.

Netten A. *A positive environment*. Aldershot: Ashgate Publishing; 1993.

Pollock A. *Designing gardens for people with dementia*. Stirling: Dementia Services Development Centre; 2001.

Pollock R. *Designing interiors for people with dementia*. Stirling: Dementia Services Development Centre; 2003.

chapter 39

Dementia services development centres in the UK

Caroline Cantley

Introduction

This chapter briefly describes the nature and activities of dementia services development centres (DSDCs) in the UK and discusses some of the ways in which these centres have contributed to improving standards of dementia care.

Background

The model of a DSDC, described in more detail below, was pioneered in Scotland where the first centre at Stirling was set up in 1989. The needs of people with dementia and their families had been a policy issue for some time before this. However, the issue had been largely subsumed within the broader policy contexts of developing old age psychiatry services, of shifting the balance of care from institutional to community settings and, linked to this, of addressing the needs of family carers (Cantley, 2001). The setting up of the first DSDC was a significant step in the recognition of 'dementia care' as an underdeveloped area that deserved specific, dedicated resources to develop knowledge, and to promote improvements and innovation in professional practice and service organization.

Such was the early success of the Stirling DSDC, directed by Professor Mary Marshall, that it attracted much interest from service providers and other interested groups elsewhere in the UK. By the mid-1990s, work was under way to develop similar facilities in a number of the English regions. The idea for regional centres was informed by the experience of the DSDC in

Scotland that a population of around 5 million was large enough to create the level of demand required to sustain a centre, while remaining small enough for centre staff to be responsive to local service needs.

By 1997, largely as a result of the efforts of local 'champions' of dementia care, centres were established in Bristol, Newcastle and Oxford. Further spread of the DSDC model was assisted by support from a senior adviser to the Department of Health who facilitated informal meetings of interested people with a view to achieving comprehensive coverage by DSDCs across the UK. These meetings eventually evolved into the national DSDC Network (described below). Ten DSDCs have now been established to serve all regions of the UK except Northern Ireland.

Aims and values of dementia services development centres

DSDCs aim to promote better dementia care by working with policy makers, service planners and commissioners, and service providers, in a specified geographical area. Centres have a multi-disciplinary and multi-agency approach to working across professional and agency boundaries in health and social services. They also work at all levels within services, from front-line care staff to senior management.

All DSDCs share a value base that they have summarized as:

. . . the belief that people with dementia, their relatives, friends, staff and volunteers who care for them, are all people who make a special and unique contribution to society, have the potential for growth and change and are deserving of the highest quality research, training, information and expertise.

Structure and organization of dementia services development centres

Although DSDCs each cover a population of a similar size, their geographical catchment areas vary hugely according to differences in population density in different parts of the country. Also, since there was no central commissioning of regional DSDCs, their organizational structures have developed in an ad hoc way, depending upon local circumstances and funding opportunities and the background of the individuals who in each region 'championed' the setting up of the centre.

In principle all DSDCs are committed to being 'not for profit' organizations with management arrangements that reflect a range of 'stakeholders' interests, including those of service users with dementia and their families and carers. Some DSDCs have independent voluntary sector (charitable) status, some are university-based units, some are hosted in service provider organizations and some have combined charitable and university status. Most, if they are not located within a university, have links with a university department. The centres generally have some core funding, which may come from statutory or voluntary sector sources, and which is usually modest and time limited. All centres have to work continuously to raise funding and generate income to support the continuation and expansion of their work.

The DSDC Network provides a forum for existing and developing DSDCs in the UK. Its purpose is to promote and facilitate information sharing, collaboration and joint working amongst the DSDCs, to reduce possible areas of duplication and competition, and to enable the coordination of resources and funding. As well as the UK DSDCs, the membership of the Network has included a DSDC for Ireland, based in Dublin.

The Network, which for some years received funding support for its meetings from the Department of Health, has met regularly since its inception. Representatives from the Department of Health have attended meetings, as have representatives from other organizations with complementary roles and interests, including the Alzheimer's Society and the Bradford Dementia Group. One of the complications for the Network has been the establishment of devolved government to Scotland and Wales and, with this, a growing need to relate to rather different policy, organizational and funding contexts in different areas of the UK.

Services provided by dementia services development centres

Central to the concept of a DSDC is the aim of offering a combination of services that are needed to bring about change and improvement in dementia care:

- information, education and training
- practice and service-related research
- support for service development through the provision of advice, facilitation and consultancy.

In practice, there is some variation in the range and nature of services provided by the centres, depending on staff capacity, the skills and interests of the staff and the centre's organizational base. Thus, for example, although all DSDCs respond to information enquiries from practitioners and service managers in their region, they do not all have a dedicated information specialist on their staff. Information provision is one of the areas in which the Network has been important, for example, in facilitating the development of shared service and bibliographic databases. The rapid growth that has been taking place in service providers' access to electronic information sources has required the DSDCs to keep their approach to information services under review and one recent development has been the uptake by a number of centres of an electronic current awareness bulletin produced by the Stirling DSDC.

Impact of dementia services development centres on standards of dementia care

DSDCs work in a wide variety of ways to influence standards in dementia care. Although some activities have mainly local impact, other work that individual DSDCs undertake is relevant beyond the regions that they primarily serve. Examples of some of the ways and areas of service provision in which the centres have variously been significant include:

- *Identifying and documenting the nature of good practice* by drawing upon research and experiential evidence to produce a wide range of care practice guides.
- *Identifying and documenting good models of service delivery* by drawing upon research and experiential evidence to produce service development guides, for example, in relation to care home management, housing with care and advocacy.
- *Developing practice tools*, for example, in relation to assessment and to activities with people with dementia.
- *Developing the dementia care practice and management workforce*, for example, by producing resources to support trainers, by delivering training, by piloting the use of learning sets and learning networks for practitioners and managers and by developing academic programmes.
- *Focusing attention on neglected or inadequately addressed issues* by raising awareness of, and promoting action on, for example, dementia care in acute hospital settings, in palliative care and for marginalized groups including younger people and minority ethnic communities.

- *Promoting innovation in care practice and service provision*, for example, in dementia-friendly building design, in the use of smart technologies in dementia care, in the role of the arts in dementia care and in spirituality in dementia care.
- *Challenging ideas and assumptions*, for example, about the extent to which people with dementia can communicate their views and feelings and, more specifically, be involved in service planning and development. DSDCs, also, by their commitment to interdisciplinary working, challenge traditional professional and agency boundaries.
- *Providing feedback on service performance*, for example, by providing service reviews and evaluations of both long-established and innovative services.
- *Promoting the development of change management and service improvement expertise*, for example, by developing and promoting uptake of quality management systems for use in dementia care and by supporting the adaptation of a generic service improvement method to dementia care (the Dementia Services Collaborative).
- *Influencing local and national policy development*, for example, by undertaking projects for government departments and through staff membership of advisory groups and official committees.
- *Promoting research in dementia care* by undertaking studies that have practical relevance for practitioners and managers and also by working with academic colleagues on more conceptual, 'blue skies', research.

Further information about many of the above activities can be obtained through the DSDC website contacts listed after the References.

There has been no evaluation of the extent of the impact of the DSDCs in the UK; it would in any case be difficult to disentangle the impact that the DSDCs have had from other influences. For example, over the same period that the DSDCs have been in existence, demographic and scientific developments have undoubtedly had an impact on expectations about dementia care and service standards. In addition, the work of other dementia care organizations, including the Alzheimer's Society, Alzheimer Scotland – Action on Dementia and the Bradford Dementia Group, has also been influential.

Recently in the UK we have seen government policy for health and social care place an increasingly strong emphasis on setting and improving standards and on making performance against standards explicit. For example, in England (there is some variation in Scotland and Wales), there have been a range of government initiatives relevant to dementia care. These initiatives include national minimum standards and new inspection arrangements for care homes (Department of Health, 2003) and a National Service Framework (NSF) for Older People (Department of Health, 2001). The NSF has one section dealing specifically with mental health services for older people, including a service model for the identification and management of dementia. The DSDC Network was one of very many influences in the policy processes that resulted in the standards for dementia services set in the NSF. And in the smaller-scale policy arenas of Scotland and Wales, the local DSDCs can have an influential voice. However, the role of DSDCs is not primarily the development or monitoring of such 'top down' standards, although the work of the centres often assists service providers in achieving their requirements. Rather, the DSDC role is based on the assumption that such centrally set minimum standards must be accompanied by a culture of continuous learning and improvement, with a substantial 'bottom up' component to ensure the commitment of practitioners and managers to the best possible service provision (Cox, 2001).

The future

Much has changed since the first DSDC was set up, and changes in the policy and organizational context in which DSDCs operate continue apace. One of the greatest challenges facing DSDCs is how to adapt their work as the development of dementia care services moves increasingly from the margins to the mainstream of health and social services concerns.

References

Cantley C. Understanding the policy context. In Cantley C, ed. *A handbook of dementia care*. Buckingham: Open University Press; 2001.

Cox S. Developing quality in services. In Cantley C, ed. *A handbook of dementia care*. Buckingham: Open University Press; 2001.

Department of Health. *Older people: National Service Framework for Older People*. London: Department of Health; 2001.

Department of Health. *Care homes for older people. National minimum standards*, 3rd edn. London: The Stationery Office; 2003.

Contact details for dementia services development centres

Dementia North
http://www.dementianorth.org.uk

North West Dementia Centre
http://www.pssru.man.ac.uk/NWDC.htm

Trent DSDC
http://www.trentdsdc.org.uk/

Dementia Plus (West Midlands)
http://www.dementiaplus.org.uk

London Centre for Dementia Care
http://www.ucl.ac.uk/~rejumli

Oxford Dementia Centre
http://www.ipc.brookes.ac.uk

Dementia Voice
http://www.dementia-voice.org.uk

DSDC South East
http://www.dementiacentre.cant.ac.uk

Stirling DSDC (Scotland)
http://www.dsdc.stir.ac.uk/

Wales DSDC
http://www.bangor.ac.uk/dsdc

Dementia Services Information and Development Centre (Ireland)
http://www.dementia.ie

chapter 40

Norwegian Centre for Dementia Research, Service Development and Education

Knut Engedal

Background

Norway is a large country with a small population of 4.5 million inhabitants, of whom 700 000 are 65 years old and above 200 000 are 80 years old and above (Central Bureau of Statistics, 2001). The public sector plays the major role in providing health and social care to the inhabitants. Until recently, the public healthcare system was the only option offering healthcare services in Norway, ideally according to patient need, independent economic status and place of residence. The private market for health and social care services is growing, but still plays a modest role.

The state is responsible for specialist healthcare services, whereas 435 municipalities are responsible for primary healthcare and social care services that include the care for the elderly at home (home help and home nursing) and in various residential care facilities. It is estimated that about 60 000–70 000 people suffer from dementia, and that the incidence rate/year is 10 000 (Engedal and Haugen, 1993; Bjertness, 1995) About 40% of all people with dementia are cared for in institutions (Engedal and Haugen, 1993).

The establishment of the Centre

To support and educate social and healthcare personnel, the Norwegian Ministry of Social and Health Affairs in 1990 gave funding to a 5-year development programme on dementia, and in 1992 a 3-year development programme on old age psychiatry. Both programmes were successful in the sense that new services for the elderly suffering from dementia and other mental disorders were established in specialist health care and in the municipalities. Educational programmes were offered to a variety of health and social care personnel, and textbooks and other learning material were produced.

In connection with the Norwegian Parliament's Communication No. 50 (1993–94) 'Cooperation and management – aims and means for a better health service', the Standing Committee on Health and Social Affairs discussed separate measures for the oldest old, and especially for the patients suffering from dementia. As a result of this discussion and the information that the Standing Committee received from the two development programmes, the Ministry of Social and Health Affairs appointed a subcommittee to examine the question of funding a centre of excellence (knowledge) on dementia. The Norwegian Centre for Dementia Research, Service Development and Education was established, and began to operate in September 1997, with funding from the Government.

The assignments of the Centre

In agreement with the Ministry, the Centre should develop new services to people suffering from dementia and their caregivers through research and experimental activities. This should be attained by an interaction between the development of new expertise and instruction, advice and guidance to the health sector. The Centre has been given four priority areas:

1. Carrying out research and experimental activities towards a better health and social care service, including treatment for people suffering from dementia and their caregivers. According to the Ministry, about half of the funding should be used to develop new services and to implement them in the care systems either in the municipalities or specialist health care. The development activities should preferably be designed according to standard research criteria.
2. Providing advice and guidance to primary and specialist healthcare authorities regarding the development and evaluation of new care programmes. This assignment should preferably be carried out in cooperation with local authorities, and on requests.
3. Developing and distributing teaching materials for a variety of health and social care personnel and for the public. The Ministry especially wanted the Centre to establish an information centre and act as an

information bank with library services for the public and social and healthcare personnel with no tradition of searching literature themselves (i.e. personnel with no formal or little education).

4. Offering educational programmes in the field of dementia by means of courses, conferences and meetings.

Organization, manpower and funding

The Centre is organized in close connection to clinical activities and is affiliated to two hospitals: one part of the Centre is located at Ullevaal University Hospital, Oslo, Department of Geriatric and Psychogeriatric Medicine; the other part of the Centre is located at the psychiatric hospital in Vestfold County (about 1 hour drive south of Oslo), Section of Old Age Psychiatry. Although the Centre is located in two different hospitals, it works as one unit with one scientific leader, the Professor of Old Age Psychiatry at the University of Oslo, and two day-to-day managers, one at each hospital. The three of them form the executive group.

In 2003, 21 persons were employed comprising physicians, psychologists, nurses, occupational therapists, librarians, a journalist, an economist and clerical personnel.

The government funds the Centre with about 900 000 Euros/year. In addition, about 300 000–500 000 Euros/year come from other sources such as the Norwegian Research Council, the Norwegian Health Organization and the European Commission, among others.

Development and research projects

During the 7 years that the Centre has been in existence, various development and research projects have been carried out, covering different aspects: examples are:

- implementation of models for diagnosing dementia in an early phase in specialist and primary healthcare
- a nationwide study of housing facilities for people with dementia
- development of a comprehensive municipality care programme
- development and evaluation of sense gardens for people with dementia.

In 2004 the Centre is responsible for and runs 11 research projects, including

- 'Enabling technology for persons with dementia', an EU-funded research project coordinated at the Norwegian Centre, but with contributions from Ireland, England, Finland, Lithuania and Norway. New technological devises are tried out in trials.
- 'Dementia in the family' is a multicentre controlled trial studying the effect of psychoeducation given to family caregivers.
- 'Use of constraints in nursing homes' is a study of the use of constraints towards patients with dementia in a random sample of nursing home residents.
- 'The efficacy of short mental tests in suspected dementia' is a project to study the efficacy of three short mental tests as confusional state evaluation (CSE) detection tools.
- 'The prevalence of dementia in younger persons and their life situation' is a study of all possible people with a dementia disorder aged 64 and under, living in three Norwegian counties.

Other projects deal with the development of day-care programmes in the countryside and how to involve farmers in such programmes, the needs and service provision to people with dementia in the municipalities and how to develop an educational programme using broadband (internet) and video conferencing.

Advice and guidance to local healthcare administrators and specialist health care

The Centre has regular contact with county health officers, who cooperate in meetings and in educational programmes. There is a close collaboration also with departments and sections of old age psychiatry throughout the country, both for common educational programmes and for advising the departments in question about delivering new services to demented patients and their caregivers, e.g. establishing a memory clinic. The Centre is responsible for a continuing educational programme in old age psychiatry. An intranet solution is chosen in order to reach all the departments in the country, every second Tuesday throughout the year.

Social and healthcare administrators in municipalities often contact the Centre for advice on how to build new institutions and implement new technology in the buildings for elderly demented patients. Personnel from the Centre often visit municipalities to run educational programmes.

Doctors, nurses, students, professionals and family caregivers contact the Centre every day to discuss problems regarding treatment, care and diagnostic work-up of individual patients. Second-opinion examinations of patients are part of this service.

Development and distribution of teaching materials

The Centre has a publishing house. Books (textbooks), leaflets, reports and videos are produced, printed and sold at the market, mainly through the Centre's own distribution net, but some books can also be purchased in bookshops throughout the country. In 2003, 4000 copies of textbooks and 13000 copies of various leaflets were sold. This activity gives the Centre a surplus that can be used for research projects.

The Centre offers library services to health and social care personnel, students (especially) and caregivers from all over Norway. The home page (www.nordemens.no) is frequently used by the public.

The Centre publishes the periodical *DEMENTIA*, with four issues a year; it is the only periodical in the Nordic countries that deals only with dementia. The readers of the journal are nurses and primary care physicians.

Educational activities

The Centre organizes about 25 courses and conferences a year, and 2000–2500 participants attend these courses. There are special courses for doctors, for nurses, for occupational therapists and for personnel with no formal education, but most courses are run as interdisciplinary courses. All courses and conferences give formal credits for continuing education for physicians, psychologists, nurses, nurse aids and occupational therapists. The courses are organized in different parts of the country, making it easier for the participants to attend. There are two big events every year: 'The Dementia days' with 700 attendees, and 'Days of old age psychiatry' with 200 specialists working in sections of old age psychiatry. In addition, the personnel at the Centre give lectures at the University of Oslo and at different colleges throughout Norway – about 500 lectures/year both at graduate and postgraduate level.

One special course has to be described, the 'ABC in Care for the Elderly', which is an educational programme developed by the Centre. It is a self-studying course that is implemented at the participants' working places in the municipalities. It consists of a basic education in gerontology and psychiatry, and a special education in geriatric medicine, old age psychiatry and dementia. The target group for this programme is personnel with no formal or little education working in nursing homes and in home care. The programme gives credits in continuing education for all health personnel, except for doctors and psychologists

Other activities and spin-off effects

All personnel at the Centre are given the opportunity to improve their own qualifications. Some staff attend international conferences presenting their research, and some take part in formal continuing education. In 2004, three of the employees worked on their PhD theses and four on masters degree theses.

The Centre also organizes international meetings, and is part of a European network for service development centres in Europe. The participants of this network meet annually.

During the last 4 years, the Centre has been invited by the Norwegian Ministry of Social Affairs to take on new assignments. In 1999, the Centre started a development programme under the title 'Physical Disability and Ageing', funded by the Government with 250 000 Euros/year. In 2003, another assignment was given to the Centre. Funded with 350 000 Euros/year a developmental programme on 'Learning Disabilities and Ageing' started. Both these two new programmes are carried out in the same way as the Dementia Centre, by an interaction between research, development of new expertise and instruction, advice, guidance and through educational activities. Moreover, the Centre has become a centre of excellence for ageing and disabilities of various causes.

Conclusions

The Norwegian Centre for Dementia Research, Service Development and Education has the aim of improving the quality of care for people suffering from dementia. This is achieved by an interaction between research, the development of new expertise and instruction, advice and guidance, and through educational activities for personnel in the health sector, at both specialist and primary care level. The work so far has been successful and has led to new assignments using the same model of work in the fields of ageing and physical disabilities and ageing and learning disabilities.

References

Bjertness E. Forekomst av demens – hvilke tall kan man stole på? In: Nygaard AM, ed. *Ja, tenke det, ønske det, ville det med*. Sem: Info-banken; 1995: 31–45 [In Norwegian].

Central Bureau of Statistics. *Statistical yearbook 2001*. Oslo; 2001.

Engedal K, Haugen PK. The prevalence of dementia in a sample elderly Norwegians. *Int J Geriatr Psychiatry* 1993; 8: 565–70.

chapter 41

Economics of dementia care

Anders Wimo

Introduction

The immense economic consequences of dementia disorders are one of the most important issues when the situation of the health and social sectors are under discussion (Johnson et al, 2000). The OECD (Organization for Economic Cooperation and Development) has, in a recently published report, emphasized that dementia is a major health and social policy issue in its member states (Moise et al, 2004). Dementia is also regarded by the World Health Organization (WHO) as one of the major reasons for disability. In 2000, there were approximately 7.4 million people in Europe suffering from dementia (Table 41.1), which was about 30% of the worldwide dementia population (Wimo, 2002). A forecast based on demographic prognoses (UN, 1998) and known age-specific dementia prevalence (Fratiglioni et al, 2001) shows that the number of demented people in Europe will increase to about 9 million in 2010 and to 12.3 million in 2030 (Figure 41.1).

Table 41.1 Dementia in Europe in 2000

	Total number of demented people (millions)	Demented 65+ year olds of all 65+ years old
Eastern Europe	2.42	6.1%
Northern Europe	1.17	7.9%
Southern Europe	1.63	6.9%
Western Europe	2.22	7.6%
All Europe	7.43	6.9%

Source: adapted from Wimo et al (2003).

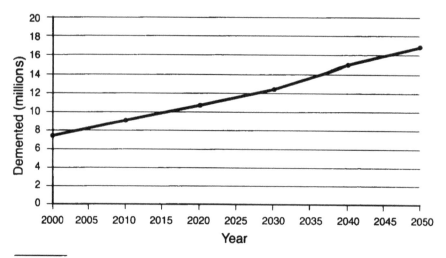

Figure 41.1 Prognosis of the number of demented people in Europe 2000–2050.

The very high costs of dementia care in combination with the demo-graphic changes and an economic crisis in the welfare systems in many countries highlight the fundamental questions in any health economic analysis about how costs are distributed among different payers and the cost-effectiveness of dementia care. Therefore, the Swedish Council on Technology Assessment in Health Care is working on a dementia report which also includes an extensive health economic section.

The available scientific database in this field is rather small and there are also several methodological issues that need to be highlighted (Winblad et al, 1996; Wimo, 2004). It is also important to emphasize that not only drugs (such as the cholinesterase inhibitors) should be evaluated from a health economic viewpoint. Different kinds of 'programmes', e.g. day-care, care-giver support, case management approaches, new forms of living arrangements), should also be the focus for such evaluations.

Costs of dementia

As seen in Table 41.2, the costs of dementia are extensive. However, the great variation in cost figures from different European countries also illustrates the methodological problems in this field. It is hardly likely that the costs of dementia care are six times higher in Italy than in Denmark. It is fundamental that any health economic analysis must define its perspective (Jonsson et al, 2000). The implications of a societal health economic per-

Table 41.2 Cost of illness studies of dementia in some European countries.

Country	Annual costs per demented patient	Cost categories included	Reference source
England	25,000	D, IC	(Lowin et al., 2001, Bosanquet et al., 1998)
Sweden	26,900	D (gross costs)	(Wimo et al., 1997)
Sweden	17,500	D (net costs)	(Wimo et al., 1997)
Germany	12,500	D	(Schulenberg and Schulenberg, 1998)
Denmark	9,200	D	(Kronborg Andersen et al., 1999)
Italy	55,400	D, IC	(Cavallo and Fattore, 1997)
Italy	8,600	D	(Cavallo and Fattore, 1997)
The Netherlands	10,300	D	(Koopmanschap et al., 1998)
Ireland	13,900	DC, IC	(O'Shea and O'Reilly, 2000)

D = directs costs; IC = costs of informal care.
Recalculations are made from original papers, expressed as 2003 euros (currency conversions to euros via US dollars) by PPPs (purchasing power parities), time transformations by CPI (consumer price index).
Source: for PPP and CPI: OECD (Organization for Economic Cooperation and Development), data on file: www.oecd.org

spective, which is often recommended, is that the costs of informal care should be given a cost. The inclusion of informal care or not in the presented cost of illness figures is probably the main reason for great cost differences between countries, which is illustrated by the Italian cost figures in Table 41.2. Another methodological issue is whether gross costs (all costs of people with dementia) or net costs (costs related to the dementia disorder) are presented, which the Swedish figures illustrate. It must also be clarified whether costs of dementia or solely Alzheimer's disease are presented.

Based on results from the Kungsholmen project (Fratiglioni et al, 1992), we have calculated costs of different levels of cognitive decline. As seen in Table 41.3, there is a linear relationship between costs and cognitive deterioration in terms of the mini mental state examination (MMSE) (Folstein et al, 1975).

The need for transparency in how costs are calculated stresses the need for standardized methods. We have developed a framework for the assessment of resource use, RUD (resource utilization in dementia), which aims to serve as a source for calculations of costs from a societal perspective (Wimo et al,

Table 41.3 Annual costs per mini mental state examination (MMSE) stage.

Severity	Annual cost (Sweden)[a]
MMSE 21–26	10,500
MMSE 15–20	25,300
MMSE 10–14	29,100
MMSE 0–9	38,600

[a] Figures are rounded off and expressed as 2003 euros.

1998). With complete RUD, the resource utilization by caregivers is also included. There is also a short version, the RUD Lite (Wimo and Winblad, 2003). The components of RUD are shown in Table 41.4.

Major cost drivers

The major cost drivers in dementia care from a societal perspective are the costs of institutional long-term care and unpaid informal care. Both these concepts are, however, a bit vague. An institution can be a huge building

Table 41.4 Components of the resource utilization battery in RUD and RUD Lite

Patient	Caregiver
Accommodation/long-term care	Informal care time (for patient)
Work status[a]	Work status[a]
Respite care	Respite care[a]
Hospital care	Hospital care[a]
Outclinic visits[a]	Outclinic visits[a]
Social services/home help	Social service/home help[a]
Home nursing care	Home nursing care[a]
Day care	Day care[a]
Drug use[b]	Drug use[a]

[a] Not in RUD Lite.
[b] In RUD Lite and clinical trials: only study drug.
Source: Wimo and Winblad (2003).

with hundreds of patients, but it can also be a small, home-like unit with 6–9 residents with staff around the clock (Wimo et al, 1995). Due to how 'institutions' are characterized (staff ratio, medical equipment, etc.), there may be great variations in the costs.

Informal care provided by family members, friends and neighbours is of great interest from several aspects. Informal carers are part of a 'dementia family'. In that sense, their situation is often very stressing and it can be described in terms of, for example, burden, coping and morbidity. However, they are also producers of unpaid care. The amount of informal care is extensive. We found in a study of non-institutionalized demented in Sweden that the ratio between informal and formal care was about 4–5:1 in terms of support in personal and instrumental activities of daily living (ADL) (Wimo et al, 2002). If, also, the need for supervision and surveillance is included, the ratio is about 8–9:1. The informal carers spent about 10 hours/day on caregiving activities! This amount of informal care has been highlighted in many other studies (Rice et al, 1993; Stommel et al, 1994; Clipp and Moore, 1995; Cavallo and Fattore, 1997; Albert et al, 1998).

Costing informal care is, however, a complicated topic (McDaid, 2001). The replacement cost approach and the opportunity cost approach, which are two frequently used methods, have drawbacks when they are applied on dementia (Jonsson et al, 2000).

The need for research and representative data

In the light of the economic impact of dementia, the research expenditures on dementia are very limited in comparison to other major groups of diseases in society, such as cancer and cardiovascular diseases (Lowin et al, 2001). One important question is how representative are results from health economic studies? Even if resource utilization data are collected prospectively, it may be questioned whether such figures are generalizable to the common dementia population. This is of particular interest for those who pay for the care, irrespective of whether the payer is the state, a local authority (e.g. a municipality) or a private company. Furthermore, it is also important to analyse how costs are distributed among payers of different social sectors, and also how an intervention of any kind (e.g. day care, drugs) might cause a reallocation of resources and costs both in the short- and long-term.

Thus, from a policy point of view it is of great importance to have basic representative data. Longitudinal, population-based studies that include information about resource utilization are the best sources for such information. The Kungsholmen Project in Sweden, which started in 1987, is an example of such a longitudinal, population-based cohort study (Fratiglioni et al, 1992). A new and larger project, the Swedish National Study on Ageing and Care (SNAC) with about 10000 elderly, includes an extensive data collection of resource use and background data on non-demented and demented patients (Lagergren et al, 2004). It also allows analyses of users and non-users of various formal and informal resources.

Different types of health economic studies

To get valid information about costs of dementia and cost-effectiveness of treatment, it is important to use established health economic methods. Health economic studies are of two major types: descriptive studies and evaluation (normative) studies (Drummond et al, 1997).

Descriptive studies

In a cost description (CD), costs are presented without any comparisons with alternative treatments, neither are outcomes analysed. Therefore, CD is not a complete health economic analysis but it is the basis for such analyses, since the cost components that are included in any health economic study are based on the principles of CD.

From a theoretical health economy point of view, costs should be presented in terms of opportunity costs, which are based on the assumption that any resource has an alternative use to a certain cost. The opportunity cost should in theory reflect the market value of a resource. Example: for an informal caregiver at working age, the opportunity cost is the value of the work on the market that this caregiver has given up.

There are different ways to categorize types of costs. It is common to present costs as direct costs and indirect costs (although this is under debate). Simplified, direct costs are derived from 'resources used', such as costs in the formal healthcare and social service systems (e.g. hospital care, nursing home care, medications, home support, etc.), whereas indirect costs reflect 'resources lost' (e.g. loss of production due to morbidity and mortality).

Cost of illness studies (examples are presented in Table 41.2), are descriptive: thus, they cannot serve as a basis for priorities between different types of treatment although such studies describe the amount of costs and how costs are distributed among different payers.

Evaluation studies

Evaluation studies can serve as a support in policy discussions and decisions; in that sense they are normative. In a complete evaluation study at least two different treatment strategies should be compared. In a cost minimization analysis (CMA), the effects of different treatments are shown or assumed to be equal (although easy in theory, this may be difficult in practice) and the analysis is aimed at identifying the therapy with the lowest cost.

In the cost-effectiveness analysis (CEA), the effect is expressed as a quantifiable (but non-monetary) outcome (e.g. the cost to postpone a shift from one stage of severity to a worse one). In a cost–benefit analysis (CBA), costs and outcomes are expressed in monetary units. The modern theory of CBA is complex, including willingness-to-pay approaches, and there are few applications of CBA on dementia. In a cost-utility analysis (CUA), quality adjusted life years (QALYs) are often used as outcome.

Even if the number of publications in this field is increasing, the number of papers with a complete health economic evaluation approach is limited. In a recently published review about the cholinesterase inhibitors, very few pharmacoeconomic papers with prospectively collected data on resource use and costs were identified (Wimo, 2004).

Conclusion

Issues concerned with dementia care are of great importance among policy makers, reimbursement authorities, clinical researchers, drug companies and patient/caregiver organizations. The immense societal costs of dementia disorders and the increase in the number of demented and economic problems in the welfare system highlight the need for basic knowledge and research on cost-effectiveness in the treatment of dementia. However, the scientific health economic database in this field is limited.

References

Albert SM, Sano M, Bell K, et al. Hourly care received by people with Alzheimer's disease: Results from an urban, community survey. *Gerontologist* 1998; 38: 704–14.

Bosanquet N, May J, Johnson N. Alzheimer's disease in the United Kingdom. Burden of disease and future care. London: Imperial College School of Medicine; 1998.

Cavallo MC, Fattore G. The economic and social burden of Alzheimer disease on families in the Lombardy region of Italy. *Alzheimer Dis Assoc Disord* 1997; 11: 184–90.

Clipp EC, Moore MJ. Caregiver time use: An outcome measure in clinical trial research on Alzheimer's disease. *Clin Pharmacol Ther* 1995; 58: 28–36.

Drummond MF, O'Brien B, Stoddart GL, Torrance GW. *Methods for the economic evaluation of health care programmes*. Oxford: Oxford University Press; 1997.

Folstein MF, Folstein SE, McHugh PR. 'Mini-mental state'. A practical method for grading the cognitive state of patients for the clinician. *J Psychiatr Res* 1975; **12**: 189–98.

Fratiglioni L, Viitanen M, Backman L, Sandman PO, Winblad B. Occurrence of dementia in advanced age: The study design of the Kungsholmen Project. *Neuroepidemiology* 1992; **11**: 29–36.

Fratiglioni L, Rocca WA. Epidemiology of dementia. In: Boller F, Cappa SF, eds. *Handbook of neuropsychology*, 2nd edn. Amsterdam: Elsevier; 2001: 193–215.

Johnson N, Davis T, Bosanquet N. The epidemic of Alzheimer's disease. How can we manage the costs? *Pharmacoeconomics* 2000; **18**: 215–23.

Jonsson B, Jonsson L, Wimo A. Cost of dementia. In: May M, Sartorius N, eds. *Dementia. WPA Series Evidence and Experience in Psychiatry*. London: John Wiley and Sons; 2000: 335–63.

Koopmanschap MA, Polder JJ, Meerding WJ, Bonneux L, van der Maas PJ. Costs of dementia in the Netherlands. In: Wimo A, Jonsson B, Karlsson G, Winblad B, eds. *The health economics of dementia*. London: John Wiley and Sons; 1998.

Kronborg Andersen C, Sogaard J, Hansen E, et al. The cost of dementia in Denmark: The Odense Study. *Dement Geriatr Cogn Disord* 1999; **10**: 295–304.

Lagergren M, Fratiglioni L, Hallberg IR, et al. A longitudinal study integrating population, care and social services data. The Swedish National Study on Aging and Care (SNAC). *Aging Clin Exp Res* 2004; **16**: 158–68.

Lowin A, Knapp M, McCrone P. Alzheimer's disease in the UK: Comparative evidence on cost of illness and volume of health services research funding. *Int J Geriatr Psychiatry* 2001; **16**: 1143–8.

McDaid D. Estimating the costs of informal care for people with Alzheimer's disease: Methodological and practical challenges. *Int J Geriatr Psychiatry* 2001; **16**: 400–5.

Moise P, Schwarzinger M, Um M-Y, et al. *Dementia care in 9 OECD countries. A comparative analysis*. OECD Health Working Paper No. 13. Paris: OECD; 2004.

O'Shea E, O'Reilly S. The economic and social cost of dementia in Ireland. *Int J Geriatr Psychiatry* 2000; **15**: 208–18.

Rice DP, Fox PJ, Max W, et al. The economic burden of Alzheimer's disease care. *Health Aff (Millwood)* 1993; **12**: 164–76.

Schulenberg J, Schulenberg I. Cost of treatment and cost of care for Alzheimer's disease in Germany. In: Wimo A, Jonsson B, Karlsson G, Winblad B, eds. *The health economics of dementia*. London: John Wiley and Sons; 1998.

Stommel M, Collins CE, Given BA. The costs of family contributions to the care of persons with dementia. *Gerontologist* 1994; **34**: 199–205.

UN. *World population prospects: The 1998 revision. World population 1950–2050*. New York: United Nations; 1998.

Wimo A. Pharmacoeconomics and dementia. In: *8th International Conference on Alzheimer's Disease and Related Disorders*. Stockholm; 2002.

Wimo A. Cost effectiveness of cholinesterase inhibitors in the treatment of Alzheimer's disease: a review with methodological considerations. *Drugs Aging* 2004; **21**: 279–95.

Wimo A, Karlsson G, Sandman PO, Corder L, Winblad B. Cost of illness due to dementia in Sweden. *Int J Geriatr Psychiatry* 1997; **12**: 857–61.

Wimo A, Mattson B, Krakau I, et al. Cost-utility analysis of group living in dementia care. *Int J Technol Assess Health Care* 1995; **11**: 49–65.

Wimo A, von Strauss E, Nordberg G, Johannsson L. Time spent on informal and formal care giving for persons with dementia in Sweden. *Health Policy* 2002; **61**: 255–68.

Wimo A, Wetterholm AL, Mastey V, Winblad B. Evaluation of the resource utilization and caregiver time in anti-dementia drug trials – a quantitative battery. In: Wimo A, Jonsson B, Karlsson G, Winblad B, eds. *The health economics of dementia.* London: John Wiley and Sons; 1998.

Wimo A, Winblad B. Resource utilisation in dementia: RUD Lite. *Brain Aging* 2003; 3: 48–59.

Wimo A, Winblad B, Aguero Torres H, von Strauss E. The magnitude of dementia occurrence in the world. *Alzheimer Dis Assoc Disord* 2003; 17: 63–7.

Winblad B, Ljunggren G, Karlsson G, Wimo A. What are the costs to society and to individuals regarding diagnostic procedures and care of patients with dementia: *Acta Neurol Scand Suppl* 1996; 168: 101–4.

chapter 42

Government perspectives in England

Andrew Barker

Introduction

Since its inception in 1948, healthcare in the NHS has been influenced heavily by the interests of powerful professional groups and individuals' interests, with service development skewed by politico-vocal pressures. Older people, and those with dementia and their carers, were not strong voices. Old age psychiatry only started to emerge as a specialty in the 1970s onwards, and the Alzheimer's Society as a national organization in 1980. In health policy terms, the 1980s saw an experiment with competitive forces in a managed market as a way of ensuring that the 'consumer' got the best out of services. This was seen to shift the focus of service development from a top-down provider perspective to more patient-centred services. However, it did little for equity of access to services, and there were what was seen as unacceptable variations in service levels and standards across the UK.

Dementia care in the UK is provided by a number of agencies – health and social care state systems, privately funded and provided services, voluntary organizations and family caregivers – in a range of settings. This complexity makes government intervention to drive up quality of care through regulation equally complex. For conditions such as dementia, with wide-ranging needs and service requirements, the separation of health and social care in the UK has probably also worked against the coordinated organization of services. There have, however, been some significant advances over the past decade in getting health and social care services to work more closely, around the needs of service users, with nationally set standards of care.

Recent policy development

The present government's attempts to develop the public sector have been founded on four principles:

- setting national standards and inspection processes with regulatory bodies
- ensuring devolution and delegation to the front line
- promoting plurality of providers and flexibility
- giving choice for users.

In 1997, 'The new NHS' (http://www.archive.official-documents.co.uk/docu ment/doh/newnhs/forward.htm) replaced the internal market as an attempt to modernize services, with centrally determined integrated care. This paper introduced National Service Frameworks (NSFs) as a method to improve the quality and consistency of services in a number of key areas. NSFs set national standards and identify key interventions for a defined service or care group, with strategies to aid implementation, and milestones and targets by which progress can be determined.

The NHS Plan, in 2000, re-emphasized the importance of NSFs in delivering consistent, high-quality care through national standards. A new independent regulatory body, the Commission for Health Improvement would regularly inspect all local health bodies for achievement against these standards. Alongside a sustained increase in funding, the NHS Plan gave an explicit national prioritization for service development by national target setting, again matched by enhanced performance management. The National Institute for Clinical Excellence (NICE) was to ensure that availability of expensive drugs was not dependent on where you live, but by their cost-effectiveness. A Modernization Agency was set up to spread best practice.

National Service Frameworks

The Mental Health NSF, in 2000, was one of the first to be produced (after frameworks for paediatric intensive care, cancer and coronary heart disease), although it addressed adults of working age only. The NSF for Older People (NSFOP) was published in 2001 and included mental health services for older people and the care of people with dementia of all ages.

Standard 7 which relates to mental illness proposes:

Older people who have mental health problems have access to integrated mental health services, provided by the NHS and councils to ensure effective diagnosis, treatment and support, for them and for their carers.

The targets to be met relate to the development of local health and social care protocols for the care and management of older people with mental health problems.

Standard 7 encourages GPs to be trained in the use of a screening tool for detection of dementia, good information-giving to patients and carers and advises when to refer to specialist services. The delivery of seamless care, as close to peoples' homes as possible, by community teams with specified professionals in the use of antidementia medications, day and inpatient care, the sharing of information and common care planning are all described.

Compared to the Mental Health NSF, the NSFOP was seen as a weak document for promoting older people's mental health services, with rather vague targets, little performance management and no additional resources. This is a shame, since there was little to criticize in the descriptions of care and service models that should be considered core NHS business, and some standards are visionary. Standards on antiageism, person-centred care and general hospital care would, if implemented, markedly change the way all older peoples' health · and social care services work together, tailoring services to an individual's needs.

The trouble was, that in a financially restrained health economy with other more pressing priorities (access to GPs and accident and emergency services, and waiting times for operations have dominated the healthcare agenda), service development went elsewhere. The lack of detailed descriptions of what was considered an integrated mental health service or what should be included in the protocols, and the lack of robust performance management against these targets, certainly did not help. In 2003, health and social care inspection bodies reported that older people's mental health services were dropping between services for older people and mental health, and attracting little new investment.

The NSFOP was originally introduced as a 10-year plan. We are half way through this now and, at the time of writing, a formal review of progress is underway, by a combined inspection of the Healthcare Commission, the Commission for Social Care Inspection and the Audit Commission. This coordinated approach may give opportunities to examine dementia care across health, social care and local government. There is a commitment to ongoing reviews against standards of care, as outlined in the NSF.

Modernization agency

The culture of strong, centrally driven performance management has receded latterly, partly because it was seen to result in services gaming the system to meet targets, and distorting clinical priorities. The Modernization Agency, effectively a governmental health and social care change management organization, has taken a greater role in supporting service development towards good practice, as outlined in the NSFs. Although this agency is also to be reorganized in the near future, its approaches will continue to be influential. For dementia care, a checklist was produced to help identify the particular needs of people with dementia to plan appropriate care during and after discharge from acute general hospitals (Discharge from hospital: getting it right for people with dementia, http://www.dh.gov.uk/assetRoot/04/06/82/70/04068270.pdf) and there is a whole programme of work underway supporting the development of older people's mental health services through the National Institute for Mental Health (England) and the Change Agent Team, both branches of the Modernization Agency (http://www.nimhe.org.uk/priorities/olderpeople.asp). This work-stream is still based on standards outlined in the NSFOP.

National Institute for Clinical Excellence

NICE supports the NHS in producing guidance for clinicians and service providers based on best-available evidence. There are currently three forms of guidance:

- technology appraisals, which look at new and existing medicines and treatments using clinical and economic evidence to advise on whether something is good value for money in the NHS
- clinical guidelines, which look more generally at appropriate treatment and care of people with a particular disease or condition
- guidance on interventional procedures (operations or invasive investigations), to comment on their safety and effectiveness for routine use.

Although all NICE guidance is expected to be fully taken into account when clinicians are exercising their clinical judgement, there is a specific requirement for the relevant funding and resources to be provided within 3 months of publication of a technology appraisal guidance.

Of particular relevance for dementia care is the technology appraisal for cholinesterase inhibitors, which sets the national requirement to make these drugs available under the NHS for people with mild to moderate Alzheimer's disease according to a specified assessment and treatment protocol, and the clinical guideline under development for the management of dementia, including the use of antipsychotic medication in older people. For the first time, this guideline is being developed jointly by the NICE and the Social Care Institute for Excellence (SCIE). This presents great opportunities for evidence-based standards of care across health and social care organizations in England.

With over 150 sets of NICE guidelines being produced by the end of 2004, there have been concerns about the capacity of services to introduce such changes, and NICE is now taking a more active role in promoting the implementation of its guidance.

Regulation of private care agencies and national minimum standards

The NSFOP describes standards of core services that should be provided by state health and social care organizations. However, large numbers of people with dementia are cared for by services provided by private care organizations, either funded privately or by the state.

To regulate the quality of care provided by these agencies, the Care Standards Act 2000 (http://www.legislation.hmso.gov.uk/acts/acts2000/20000014.htm) extended the scope of regulation beyond care homes to cover services not previously registered, including domiciliary care agencies, and introduced national minimum standards for care homes for older people (http://www.dh.gov.uk/assetRoot/04/05/40/07/04054007.pdf) and domiciliary care (http://www.dh.gov.uk/assetRoot/04/01/86/71/04018671.pdf). To illustrate this, the range of standards for care homes covered: choice of home; health and personal care; daily life and social activities; complaints and protection; environment; staffing; and management and administration. A new independent regulatory body was set up to oversee the implementation of standards and regulations (The National Care Standards Commission, now dissolved and responsibilities transferred to the Commission for Social Care Inspection (CSCI)).

Proprietors of care homes must apply for registration to provide residential or nursing home care and, equally, domiciliary care agencies must legally be registered to provide personal care for people in their own homes who are unable though illness or disability to manage independently. The standards for care homes or domiciliary care are included in the criteria by which these services are assessed by the CSCI, and ultimately the CSCI have the power to de-register the care home or agency if they cannot satisfy these standards.

Care homes specify their purpose and must be seen to be delivering appropriate care for their residents' needs: for example, through specified levels of psychiatrically trained staff for people with dementia. However, there still remains the problem of underdiagnosis of dementia and the lack of recognition of the needs of people with dementia. The NSFOP described the training that was needed for GPs in delivering the protocols for the care and management of older people with mental health problems, although there are educational needs of non-medical personnel also.

Education and training

Other than the obvious potential in getting dementia issues in curricula for the training of qualified health and social care professionals, there are two other developments worthy of mention. In the National Minimum Care Standards for care homes, there is a requirement for a minimum ratio of 50% of non-nursing care staff to be qualified to National Vocational Qualification (NVQ) level 2 or equivalent by 2005. Although this will undoubtedly improve the training level of all care staff, there is no requirement for the curriculum for this qualification to include knowledge or skills related to dementia. With estimates of dementia in residents even of non-specialist care homes in the UK as high as 70%, there is scope to include some basic skills such as an awareness of communication issues with people with dementia as part of the core syllabus.

The other development of potential relevance is the 'Ten essential shared capabilities', produced by the National Institute for Mental Health England and the Sainsbury Centre for Mental Health (http://www.dh.gov.uk/assetRoot/04/08/71/70/04087170.pdf). The purpose of this document was to set out the abilities that all staff working in mental health should achieve as part of their prequalifying training. A set similar to this, specifically for staff working with people with dementia, could be used across agencies and care settings to define what the essential elements of care staff training should be to maximize quality of care for people with dementia.

Conclusion

The Department of Health in England has tried to use standards to drive up quality of care for people with dementia through implementation of NSFs, guidelines from NICE and SCIE, through education, and through National Minimum Standards for care homes and domiciliary care. Effective implementation requires close monitoring and incentivization, although it can work across state-run or privately owned agencies.

Nationally determined standards carry weight and so may European ones. With different healthcare systems across Europe, both in terms of funding and delivery of care, it would be difficult to determine standard service models in the way that the Department of Health in England has tried to with its NSFs and regulation of agencies. The underlying principles of care will be the same, however: that of person-centred care, anti-ageism, improving communication skills and respecting capacity for self-determination wherever possible. A common agreement about these elements in best management of people with dementia would be well worth achieving.

chapter 43

Government perspectives in Germany

Petra Weritz-Hanf

Initial position

Like all other industrial countries, the Federal Republic of Germany is currently undergoing a profound social restructuring process. We are on the way to an 'age-changed society'. In particular, the over 80-year-old age group will be growing in the future.

However, a very old-age population also means an increasing number of cases of dementia. All in all, the number of persons suffering from moderate to serious dementia is estimated at over 900 000, and when mild forms of the disease are included, the number rises to 1.2 million. The number of dementia patients will continue to rise. By the year 2020, the number is likely to be some 1.4 million, or even some 1.7 million if we include the milder stages of the disease. If no breakthroughs are made in prevention and therapy, a total of over 2 million patients can be expected by 2050.

Two-thirds of the persons affected by dementia are being cared for at home by relatives. The willingness of spouses and children to assume responsibility for care is, in principle, quite high. Of the age group 90 years old and over, some 57% live in private households. Given the way in which current trends – the trend towards single households, the gainful employment of women and the lack of children – are expected to play out, a reduction in this caregiving potential within families is to be reckoned with. This challenge can only be met if neighbourhood assistance networks can be formed to support a nursing service that is close to home and to everyday life. Community involvement will have an increasingly significant role to play in this area in the future.

Dementia disorders are usually the foremost reason for moving patients to a home since, even with outpatient support, home care more often than not comes up against limiting factors as the disease progresses.

Of the people who move to residential accommodation or a home for the elderly, the percentage of residents suffering from dementia is less than 20%, whereas, in the case of nursing homes, the proportion of people with advanced dementia disorders is approximately 60%.

In some establishments, dementia patients account for up to 80% of the residents.

Overall, a total of some 400000 dementia patients are estimated to live in homes of various types. Between 10 and 20% of them require special care, as they exhibit a serious behaviour disturbance, i.e. so-called 'challenging behaviour'.

Despite intensive research, no way has been found to date to treat the causes of this disorder. This is, however, no reason to give in to therapeutic nihilism. There are specific medicines that are able to slow down the progression or alleviate the effects of the disorder, but these are either not being used consistently or not at the right time.

The reasons range from shortcomings in early detection, a lack of knowledge on the part of non-hospital doctors, the fact that insufficient account is taken of the necessary benefits and services in the context of the fee system, to concerns about claims for compensation by the Association of Panel Doctors if the costs claimed surpass the average costs of comparable doctors' practices.

Moreover, in recent months, the effectiveness of these preparations has basically been challenged in press reports, which, it must be added, were based on studies that used controversial methodology.

Other substances are being used to alleviate possible secondary symptoms such as anxiety, depression, restlessness and problem behaviour. However, the proper medication of very old patients displaying multimorbidity is not always guaranteed, also owing to the fact that the treatment conditions are more difficult. Above all, medical treatment and care in homes presents a problem if every resident brings his or her own doctor in for treatment.

From the panel doctors' perspective, consensus-based national guidelines on the diagnosis and therapy of dementia-related diseases could help to improve the provision of care. To date, three medical scientific societies have published treatment guidelines.

The most helpful elements, however, are:

- the environment is appropriately designed
- the manner in which the patient is treated is sufficiently appreciative and adapted to the person's biography and needs
- offers for useful activity which are oriented on the course of the disease are provided. In other words, a therapeutic environment is created.

What is needed is a holistic approach to care which requires special qualifications but, above all, requires a specific basic attitude on the part of caregivers. People suffering from dementia need sensitive and understanding companions through life and on a day-to-day basis in order to guarantee quality of life.

An increasing number of facilities offering assistance to the elderly are taking into account the special needs of dementia patients and have developed a variety of their own concepts. Corresponding support and development programmes exist at federal and Land level.

The huge number of dementia patients incurs very high costs – €43 767 per patient and year – whereby 2.5% are met by the statutory health insurance and another 29.6% by the social long-term care insurance. The affected families bear 67.9% of the costs.

Over the past 10 years, the social long-term care insurance has been playing a major role in ensuring that dementia patients receive proper care.

However, the all-round guidance or continuous supervision which dementia patients need on a regular basis cannot possibly be considered here. Consequently, underlying the determining concept of 'activities of daily living', is a somatically very narrow concept of what constitutes a need for long-term care. This makes the long-term care insurance blind to the special needs of people suffering from dementia.

Efforts to achieve comprehensive reform have, thus far, failed because of cost considerations.

The Act Supplementing Domiciliary Care Services renders supplementary services for people with an impaired ability to perform the activities of daily life only possible if they have already been placed in a care category.

Development

It was only over the past 15 years, that the challenge of providing a proper care for people suffering from dementia came within the focus of the 'planners and doers' in the area of health policy and policy for the elderly.

For a long time, the dimensions and urgency of the problem went unnoticed or were denied.

Nevertheless, as early as 1975, the publication of the German Parliaments Report on the State of Psychiatry in the Federal Republic of Germany (*Bundestagsdrucksache* 7/4200) resulting from the Study Commission on Psychiatry (1971–1975) instituted by the Bundestag, triggered a development process which included gerontopsychiatry and assistance for the elderly in the reform of nursing care.

However, the Federal Government's Psychiatry Pilot Programme (1980–1985), which was based on this process, focused predominantly on modifying psychiatric care, especially the creation of a system of differentiated and graduated aids in a finely meshed, complementary network of care services.

Finally, in its recommendations on the basis of the pilot programme, the Expert Commission of the Federal Government on the Reform of Care in Psychiatry and Psychotherapy 1988 also touched on the problem of mentally ill older people (*Bundestagsdrucksache* 11/8494).

With its response to the major interpellation on the 'Situation of the Mentally Ill in the Federal Republic of Germany' (*Bundestagsdrucksache* 12/4016), the Federal Government rendered its account in 1992 of the state of gerontopsychiatric care.

The response to the major interpellation on the 'Situation of Dementia Patients in the Federal Republic of Germany' (*Bundestagsdrucksache* 13/3343) in 1996 was the first time that reference was explicitly made to the target group of dementia patients. It has come to constitute what was the starting point for a series of projects and measures that aimed to improve the life situation of people suffering from dementia.

A special milestone on the path to elaborating a policy for people with dementia was the Fourth National Report on the Elderly of 2002. These reports on the elderly result from the implementation of a mandate given by the Bundestag. For each legislative period, one general and one special report on the situation of the older generation is drawn up, alternately, by an independent expert commission, supplemented by a statement from the Federal Government and submitted to the Parliament.

The 'Fourth Report on the Situation of the Older Generation in the Federal Republic of Germany: Risks, Quality of Life and Care for the Elderly – taking special account of dementia diseases' (*Bundestagsdrucksache* 14/8822) deals with the living conditions and needs in a societal group which is slated for rapid growth in the future – that of the 80 year olds – and takes a close and detailed look at the impact of a very high age and dementia. Of special importance is the fact that it does not treat the dementia issue as being predominantly the task of the medical profession but supplements the analysis with a look at the social repercussions and the resulting demands on society.

Moreover, the Final Report of the Study Commission on 'Demographic Change' (*Bundestagsdrucksache* 14/8800, 2002) also makes explicit reference to the growing number of elderly dementia patients in Germany.

Both reports present clear and determined ideas about quality improvement and quality assurance in nursing care. Above all, the drawing up of nursing standards by an independent national committee or expert standards, precisely for dementia patients, was called for in the light of the special demands which this group places on nursing and care services.

The perusal of political documents allows us to trace the protracted and arduous path which the issue of dementia has trod, moving from the shadows as a subgroup of psychiatry, into the focal point of policy and the sights of policy makers.

Alongside the advances made in research, various other factors contributed decisively to this development.

These include the creation and structuring of specialized scientific societies and self-help groups such as the German Alzheimer's Society, whose qualified suggestions and demands are increasingly being heard. Since 1999, the Society's work has received financial support from the Federal Ministry of Family Affairs, Senior Citizens, Women and Youth.

However, it was the experience of being affected in one's own family or circle of friends and acquaintances, and being confronted with the shortcomings in care services, that has changed the political awareness of the situation.

Finally, the increasing financial impact on the health and long-term care insurance system also served to increase the pressure to tackle the development of quality-assured care for dementia patients so as to make optimum use of existing resources.

Slowly but surely, the realization is dawning that dementia patients need a special type of care and attention and that this can by no means be provided everywhere. The need for and urgency surrounding the improvement of care on the whole, and care for dementia patients in particular, remains uncontroverted. Various players are working on the issue in different ways.

Quality is generated as a result of the many influences which come to bear on a complex development process.

In such a process, a Federal Ministry is only one of many players in a complex construct.

In the current and past legislative periods, the Federal Government has introduced a number of legislative measures to improve the quality of care. These have been accompanied by diverse research and pilot projects.

Long-term Care Quality Assurance Act

The aim of this law is to ensure and secure further improvements in the quality of care and to strengthen consumer rights in the inpatient domain. Here, we are convinced that quality cannot 'inspect its way' into care facilities from the outside but must develop from the inside out, from the facility managers' innate sense of responsibility and that of the institutions which pay for the benefits. Alongside the reform of quality inspection procedures, the Act has therefore also targeted the strengthening of these facilities' own internal quality assurance strategies.

Act Supplementing Domiciliary Care

For the very first time, this law has envisaged additional benefits and improved care services not only for confused elderly patients but also for the mentally disabled and the mentally ill in need of long-term care and with a considerable need for general long-term care. Within the framework of a supplementary budget, quality-tested benefits and services can be purchased individually.

In this context, home care takes priority – an approach which is also in line with the needs of most of the affected who prefer home care to residential care. Consequently, the Act envisages, for example, providing financial support for low-threshold offers (relatives' groups and the like). These offers are mainly directed at relieving the strain on caregiving relatives.

Both of the above-mentioned Acts form part of the Social Code Book XI (Social Long-Term Care Insurance).

Act on Residential Accommodation

The new Act on Residential Accommodation entered into force on 1st January 2002. With it, the Federal Government implements its objective of continuing to improve the quality of care and nursing services and to ensure that residential accommodation provides a life which respects the principles of human dignity. The amended Act focuses on the following priorities:

- increasing transparency in contracts with residential facilities
- furthering (patient) participation
- strengthening the supervision of residential institutions
- improving the cooperation between the supervisors of residential institutions, the Medical Advisory Service of the Social Health Insurance, the long-term care insurance funds and the bodies responsible for social assistance
- differentiation of residential accommodation and assisted living facilities.

Furthermore, the amended Ordinance on Resident Participation in Home Management entered into force on 1st August 2003.

Act on the Care of the Elderly

The Act on the Care of the Elderly, which entered into force on 1st August 2003 established, for the first time, uniform national standards governing training in geriatric care. This Federal Act replaces the varying provisions hitherto in force in the 16 Federal Laender. The aim of the Act is to achieve a uniform level of training throughout the country, to make the profession's image more attractive and to give the profession as a whole a clear profile. This is achieved by standardizing the regulations governing training structures, training contents/curricula and examination requirements, at national level. Caring for persons suffering from dementia will be given special attention in the Training Ordinance.

Round Table on Care

In addition to the laws and ordinances, the Round Table on Care also constitutes an instrument in which we place great hopes. This Round Table was the joint creation of the Federal Ministry of Family Affairs, Senior Citizens, Women and Youth and the Federal Ministry of Health and Social Security, and all of the players in the field of care provision – the Laender, municipalities, charitable organizations, private bodies running facilities and the agencies providing the funds – were asked to collaborate in it. Its task is to identify best practice and to facilitate the swift implementation of improvements without making a detour via the legislative process. The rights of people in need of assistance and care are more clearly stipulated in a charter.

Research and pilot projects sponsored by the Federal Government

In recent years, several subject concepts have already been successfully tried 'on the ground' with the support of the Federal Ministry of Family Affairs, Senior Citizens, Women and Youth and the Federal Ministry of Health and Social Security and with the collaboration of well-known scientists and specialist institutions.

To give an example: the Federal Ministry of Health and Social Security's Pilot Programme on the Promotion of Care Facilities yields information about the organization of care facilities, hospice work, the care of dementia patients, the networking of assistance offers or the counselling of people in need of long-term care.

The same applies to the Pilot Programme 'The Structures of Caring for the Elderly in the Future' sponsored by the Federal Ministry of Family Affairs, Senior Citizens, Women and Youth which delivers important contributions towards the further development of the existing care structures.

A range of projects deal with quality improvement in care:

- establishing expert standards on decubitus, patient transfer management, preventing falls, pain management and incontinence
- developing national quality levels (eating and drinking with impaired daily living skills, safety and motility, personal lifestyle and participation)
- developing quality assurance and control instruments for the specialized care of dementia patients (QSP)
- developing standardized framework recommendations to further develop and secure qualified care for dementia patients
- developing instruments for the praxis and intervention-oriented measurement of the quality of life enjoyed by mentally altered residents of nursing homes.

Furthermore, within the framework of the Government's programme: 'Health Research: Research for People' initiated by the Federal Ministry of Education and Research, the competence network 'Dementia' is being supported. This project is meant to produce uniform and progressive guidelines for the diagnosis and treatment of dementias in Germany and thereby ensure the highest degree of quality in care.

A current focus is the inclusion of quality aspects in the care of dementia patients within the priority area of nursing care research.

Conclusion

'The legislator has laid down the statutory framework conditions for quality, quality assurance and quality inspection in nursing and health care. The Act on the Long-Term Care Insurance (Social Code Book XI), the Act on the Statutory Health Insurance (Social Code Book V), the Act on Residential Accommodation, the Act on the Care of the Elderly, the Federal Social Assistance Act, and various other statutory regulations (e.g. health and safety at work, fire protection, hygiene and sanitation regulations) commit those who are involved in the provision of care, in different ways, to improving and controlling quality in nursing care. However, these regulations have hitherto operated, to a great extent, isolated from one another. The task now at hand is to bring them together into a comprehensive, consistent quality assurance concept.'

(Final Report of the Study Commission on Demographic Change)

We have, as yet, gone only a short distance along this path.

Precisely for the proper care of the target group of dementia patients there is a great paucity of clear care and nursing standards. Uncertainty often exists as to how quality care and nursing for dementia patients can be successfully and effectively provided. Dialogue between the nursing sciences and nursing practice must provide reliable, scientific findings, the implementation of which in caregiving praxis can be guaranteed and evaluated. At the same time, we are faced with the task of finding ways and means of enabling those affected – relatives, interested lay people and residential facility supervisors – to evaluate the quality of the care which is provided. An important aspect here is, to my mind, using the quality of the outcomes as the primary criteria.

It is the task of policy makers to further this development, to follow it carefully and to create the necessary framework conditions for it to thrive.

This is, however, no easy undertaking in light of the diversity of day-to-day work in the field, the shortcomings which exist in communication and networking and the division of powers between the Federal Government and the Laender.

This is a process which will profit from the inclusion of the experiences of and suggestions from our European neighbours. I hope that the work of the North Sea Dementia Research Group founded in 2000 can help us to make progress. This notwithstanding, it will undoubtedly be some time before joint European standards in the care of dementia patients can become a reality.

References

Deutscher Bundestag. Unterrichtung durch die Bundesregierung 'Vierter Bericht zur Lage der älteren Generation in der Bundesrepublik Deutschland: Risiken, Lebensqualität und Versorgung Hochaltriger – unter besonderer Berücksichtigung demenzieller Erkrankungen' und Stellungnahme der Bundesregierung. *Bundestags-Drucksache* 14/8822; 2002.

Deutscher Bundestag. Schlussbericht der Enquête-Kommission 'Demographischer Wandel – Herausforderungen unserer älter werdenden Gesellschaft an den Einzelnen und die Politik'. *Bundestags-Drucksache* 14/8800; 2002.

Further reading

Deutscher Bundestag. Antwort auf die Große Anfrage der Abgeordneten Regina Schmidt-Zadel, Ingrid Becker-Inglau, Dr. Ulrich Böhme (Unna), weiterer Abgeordneter und der Fraktion der SPD 'Situation der Demenzkranken in der Bundesrepublik Deutschland'. *Bundestags-Drucksache* 13/5257; 1996.

Hallauer JF, Kurz A, Hrsg. Weißbuch Demenz. Versorgungssituation relevanter Demenzerkrankungen in Deutschland. Stuttgart: Thieme Verlag; 2002.

OECD Health Working Papers No. 13 Dementia Care in 9 OECD Countries: A Comparative Analysis Perre Moise, Michael Schwarzinger, Myung-Yong Um and the Dementia Experts' Group 28 July 2004-11-19 including Country Report: Germany.

Kurz A, Bickel H, Hartmann J. Technische Universität München.

Ethical and Legal Issues

Legal and ethical issues – promoting the autonomy and dignity of people with dementia

Jean Georges

People with dementia belong to one of the most vulnerable groups of society. As such, their rights need to be particularly respected and reinforced in situations where their condition has deteriorated and where they may no longer be able to understand or take decisions affecting their daily lives. Respect for fundamental human rights, such as the right to self-determination, the freedom of the individual and the integrity of the human body, remains paramount and must dictate any approach to finding pragmatic legal solutions to the problems faced by people with dementia.

This chapter presents some of the recommendations that Alzheimer Europe developed in the framework of an EC-funded project. These recommendations aim at improving the legal protection and rights of people with dementia. This was accomplished in collaboration with its member associations, as well as with the direct assistance of legal experts and other concerned individuals. The recommendations focus on three main areas – guardianship measures, restriction of liberty of movement and bioethical issues.

Guiding principles

When drafting the recommendations, several guiding principles emerged. These included the promotion of autonomy, the adoption of the least-restrictive care environment with minimum intervention in the affairs of the adult for the minimum time necessary and the importance of maintaining support and acknowledging existing friendships and family ties that the person has developed as a means of understanding his/her well-being and personhood.

Legal capacity

In order to promote the rights of people with dementia, an early diagnosis is extremely important, if not essential, for numerous decisions which must be taken in these three areas. Everyone should have the right to decide how s/he wants to lead his/her life. Yet people with dementia find this increasingly difficult due to the consequences of the disease, which gradually lead to incapacity and in many cases dependence on others.

However, it is not only the disease but also other people's attitudes that make it difficult for people with dementia to manage their own lives. It must also be borne in mind that participation is not an all or nothing experience. In the past, most countries had a legal system which concentrated on the protection of the person's financial assets. Protection of the person was in some cases inadequately addressed; in others it was based on a paternalistic approach, often linked to a loss of legal capacity.

Diagnosis disclosure

Nowadays, it is generally recognized that a combination of the two approaches is necessary, although in some countries the situation has still not changed. In a growing number of countries there is a much greater emphasis on empowering as opposed to simply protecting the individual. It is essential that people with dementia are given the opportunity to take their lives in their own hands while they are still in a position to do so. This means that every person diagnosed with dementia should have the right to be informed of the diagnosis as soon as possible.

This is consistent with respect for the individual and his/her right to self-determination. Disclosure of the diagnosis should obviously be done tactfully and in a way that the person can understand. Non-disclosure solely on the grounds that it may be disturbing for the person can no longer be tolerated, although a clear refusal to be informed should be respected. Disclosure of the diagnosis should be accompanied by information about the consequences and progression of the disease, as well as any possible treatment, care facilities or useful contacts. This information should be given orally and provided in writing if requested or appropriate (taking care to avoid causing unnecessary anxiety and suffering).

The autonomy of the person with dementia should be respected at all times. As long as s/he maintains the ability to make decisions concerning his/her life, such decisions should be sought, respected and given priority over any proxy decision maker. Indeed, irrespective of the level of capacity of the person with dementia, his/her interests must always come first. There should always be an assumption in favour of capacity and of involvement and choice.

Advance directives

Unfortunately, cognitive abilities steadily decline and there generally comes a time when the person with dementia can no longer manage entirely alone. S/he may need help making decisions of varying importance to his/her life, e.g. regarding residential care, organ donation and participation in research, etc. Assistance could be provided by a guardian/lawful representative, although combining this with an advance directive would better ensure that his/her wishes were respected.

People with dementia should be informed about the advantages of writing an advance directive and appointing a guardian/lawful representative (preferably, but not necessarily together). The necessary structures or facilities should be put into place by governments to ensure that this is possible.

Alzheimer Europe recommends, however, that people seek guidance from a doctor in order to ensure that the advance directive is clear and in line with modern practice. It is also necessary to ensure that the adult with incapacity is aware of the consequences of his/her choices and that s/he has sufficient capacity to write such a document.

In order to ensure that advance directives are respected, legal representatives and medical professionals should be obliged to take into consideration wishes expressed in such documents. Failure to do so should require valid justification. Furthermore, national registers of advance directives should be set up and details about advance directives should be included in existing computerized medical files (subject to respect for national laws on data protection).

Guardianship systems

An advance directive can give people with dementia the opportunity to personally choose a suitable guardian or guardians/lawful representatives well in advance of major incapacity. However, even if this is not the case and the guardian/lawful representative is appointed at a later stage, people with dementia should be involved as much as possible in the procedure to establish the guardianship measure and for the duration of it, including choosing the guardian/lawful representative and deciding on his/her duties.

As it is now apparent that incapacity due to dementia is not an all or nothing affair, guardianship measures must be sufficiently flexible to be able to respond to the person's actual needs, which might be related to property, financial assets and/or personal well-being. The guardianship measure should enhance a person's autonomy in the sense that the appointed guardian/lawful representative should only act on behalf of the person with dementia if and when s/he cannot act alone.

As stated earlier, there should be an assumption of capacity. It should not result in any automatic loss of legal capacity. Guardians/lawful representatives should always consult the person with dementia and keep him/her informed of decisions being made on his/her behalf. It should be the guardian's/lawful representative's duty to take into consideration the person's wishes (insofar as this is possible and taking into consideration his/her difficulties in communicating them and any difficulties understanding him/her) even if the person is considered to be incapacitated, particularly when trying to determine what would be in his/her best interests. This includes not only the person's present wishes but also any previously expressed wishes – hence the importance of the advance directive.

People should make arrangements in advance for the appointment of a guardian/lawful representative with specific responsibility for care and treatment decisions. In order to allow relatives and carers to play an active role in this domain, an easy procedure should be established to empower them and enable them to be appointed as a guardian/lawful representative for such decisions. On the other hand, the appointment of a guardian/lawful representative (who is not related to the person with dementia) should not rule out the necessity of consulting the person with dementia and his/her carer and/or relatives/close friends.

Placement of people with dementia

Many people with dementia reach a stage when they can no longer carry on living alone and need assistance. In many cases, it is possible to provide the necessary assistance at home either through family, friends or independent service providers and this approach should be given priority. However, this is not always possible and it may sometimes be necessary to place a person with dementia against his/her will in an establishment where the appropriate care can be provided. In certain cases, it may be necessary for a person with dementia to be admitted into an establishment against his/her will (or without his/her consent) for the purposes of receiving medical treatment. In either case, this involves a restriction of his/her liberty.

Alzheimer Europe recommends that non-voluntary placement for the purpose of medical treatment should involve a formal and legal/administrative process to determine the appropriateness, location and kind of placement required. In the case of non-voluntary placement solely for care, a guardian/lawful representative should be appointed with responsibility for deciding on the place where care should be provided.

The place where the treatment is to be carried out should be that which is most suited to the needs of the person with dementia, i.e. not necessarily a psychiatric institution as is the case in many countries. As already stated, non-voluntary placement for treatment or care purposes involves a restriction of liberty of movement.

Personal advocates

For this reason, in addition to the safeguards provided by the relevant legislation and procedure and irrespective of whether a person has been non-voluntarily placed for the purposes of treatment or simply for care, Alzheimer Europe recommends that a personal advocate be appointed to guide and advise him/her in all matters relating to placement both during and after the process to establish it, and also whenever a measure intended to further restrict his/her liberty of movement is applied. The personal advocate should not be linked to the establishment in any way. S/he should be responsible for informing the person of his/her rights, helping with complaints or appeals and regularly checking on his/her personal welfare.

In many countries, people with dementia are non-voluntarily placed in care establishments or non-psychiatric institutions where various forms of restraint may be applied and where legislation on compulsory detention does not apply. Although the use of restraint is not always unjustified, any restriction of liberty (which includes the use of restraint) should be carefully monitored and controlled in accordance with appropriate legislation. Such legislation should be applicable, irrespective of the kind of establishment where the person has been placed.

In addition, the personal advocate should be informed whenever any form of restraint is applied. This includes the use of physical and mechanical means of restraint, but also less obvious forms such as technological or psychological restraint and in some cases drug therapy.

End-of-life decisions

It is important to ensure that at all stages, as well as when the person with dementia approaches the end of his/her life, his/her rights are respected and his/her dignity maintained. Certain decisions which need to be taken at the end of a person's life cannot be easily taken by someone else, e.g. concerning resuscitation, life-prolonging treatment, the use of certain forms of harsh or invasive treatment or painkillers and the provision of palliative care. Such decisions should therefore ideally be noted in an advance directive. This should be clearly recorded in his/her medical file.

People with dementia who are nearing the end of their lives should have the right to receive palliative care either at home or in hospital (depending on their wishes). In all cases they should be assisted by specially trained medical staff and should be granted the right to have the company of at least one person of their choice (e.g. a friend or relative) for as long as they wish.

As an organization which represents the families and carers of people with dementia, Alzheimer Europe is also concerned about the rights of those accompanying the person with dementia at the end of his/her life. They should also be treated with respect and provided with adequate understanding and assistance to relieve their suffering. Furthermore, if necessary, governments should ensure that family members and/or close persons responsible for the care of the dying person are granted sufficient time off work to care for and accompany him/her.

The legal protection of people with dementia remains an important topic and calls for multidisciplinary approaches that bring together not only legal experts and ethicists but also medical professionals. As people with dementia are diagnosed earlier, they will be more able to take an active part in decisions affecting their lives, and Alzheimer associations worldwide will need to identify ways of consulting people with dementia, as well as carers in the development of their policies. Any successful strategy to enhance the legal rights of people with dementia ultimately depends on people with dementia playing an active part in policy development and advocacy for change. The recommendations that Alzheimer Europe developed are but a first step in that direction.

chapter 45

End-of-life care and medical decision-making in patients with dementia

Cees MPM Hertogh

Introduction

Medical decision-making at the end of life of patients with dementia is a complicated matter, both medically and morally. First of all, a lot is still unknown on the natural course of the dementia process and its prognostic indicators. Also, it is often difficult to assess the reactions of dementia patients to diagnostic and therapeutic procedures because of difficulties in communication and uncertainty as to the adequacy of their expressions and the consistency of their opinions. In general, most demented patients in the more advanced stages of the disease lack the decisional capacity to contribute to decisions regarding their care and treatment, so physicians often have to resort to proxy decision-making, which has its own dilemmas and pitfalls.

Next, there is – at least in the Netherlands – the societal debate on dementia. In a greying population such as ours, the number of people with dementia is rapidly increasing. Today, virtually everyone knows someone in his near surroundings who suffers or died from dementia. The subject receives wide coverage in newspapers, TV documentaries and an increasing number of novels. Many people, especially the elderly, are fearful of becoming demented and generally the disease is viewed upon as a humiliating affliction that affects self and personality. With no therapeutic breakthrough to be expected in the near future, more and more people are drawing up a living will, in which they refuse treatment and/or request for active euthanasia in case of dementia. In contrast, another fear that exists in the general public is that doctors – just because dementia cannot be cured – will do little to keep them alive and improve their quality of life.

All these anxieties and opinions are reflected in medical practice and have their influence on medical decision-making. The pivotal issues here are to find the optimal treatment option between the two undesirable extremes of under- and overtreatment and to balance respect for the wishes and opinions of the formerly competent person on a life with dementia against the respect we equally owe to the actual person with dementia. In order to resolve these issues scrupulously in each individual case, a policy framework is needed that can offer practical and moral guidance in this field. The concept of palliative care can offer such a framework but, before entering into more detail on that subject, a brief overview will be presented of the several types of end-of-life decisions and their ethical status.

However, in order to put the whole discussion on the goals and limits of medical interventions in dementia a bit into perspective, it must be said from the outset that the most relevant life-prolonging or life-sustaining 'treatment' concerning patients with dementia does not belong to the realm of medicine, but to that of the typical human activity we call 'care' with its inherent dynamic of caregiving and -receiving. In view of this primordial social practice, when it comes to the (quality of the) survival of demented persons, medical treatment has relatively little to add.

One final orienting remark: because many patients with dementia are admitted to a nursing home during the last phase of their life, this contribution is primarily written from the standpoint and perspective of (Dutch) nursing home medicine.

Typology of end-of-life decisions

The Netherlands has won a degree of international renown on the subject of euthanasia and physician-assisted suicide (PAS). Unfortunately, there are a lot of semantic and conceptual misunderstandings with regard to the definition of euthanasia. In many countries the term 'euthanasia' covers all life-terminating acts performed by physicians, irrespective of whether termination of life has been requested by the patient. In others, the term covers both active termination of life (active euthanasia) and decisions to stop or forgo life-sustaining treatments (passive euthanasia). Finally, some also hold the opinion that a shortening of life as an intended or unintended side effect of symptom relief must also be considered an act of euthanasia (indirect euthanasia). This latter 'opinion', however, is mainly based on ignorance and misconception with regard to the effect and potential of opioid drugs in end-of-life care.

In the Netherlands the definition of euthanasia is very strict: only the active and intentional termination of a patient's life at the explicit request of the patient is considered as an act of euthanasia. Correspondingly, PAS is defined as deliberately helping a patient to terminate his life at the patient's explicit request. Under current Dutch law both euthanasia and PAS are only legally justified if performed by a physician and if that physician acts properly in accordance with the criteria for prudent euthanasia/PAS. Central to these criteria are the following prerequisites:

- the physician is satisfied that the patient's request is voluntary, sustained, well-considered and well-informed and that he/she was fully competent at the time of the request
- the physician is satisfied that the patient perceives his/her situation in terms of unbearable and hopeless suffering
- an independent physician has been consulted to assess the patient's condition, competence and prognosis and to check that his request was truly voluntary.

It is clear from this definition of euthanasia that intensive discussions with the patient are necessary before any request can be granted. It is also clear that in case of a patient with a clinical diagnosis of dementia this kind of contact and in-depth discussions will rarely be possible due to the impaired cognitive skills of the patient. This is one out of several reasons why euthanasia in case of dementia is practically almost an unthinkable option.

Euthanasia/PAS are always an ultimum refugium in palliative care and are only administered in exceptional cases, amounting to less than 3% of all deaths per year in the Netherlands (Van der Wal et al, 2003). They have to be clearly distinguished from the following end-of-life decisions:

1. non-treatment decision – stopping or desisting from treatment at the explicit request of the patient
2. medical futility – withholding or withdrawing medical treatments that are or have become futile
3. relief of symptoms – acting for the purpose of relieving symptoms of suffering while accepting the hastening of death as a possible, though unintended side effect.

On an international level, there is an ongoing debate on the exact definition and validity of the concept of medical futility and on the validity of the double-effect doctrine that hides behind the third type of end-of-life decision. As already said, some contend that the latter is a form of indirect euthanasia. As to the concept of futility, it is suggested that this has medical as well as ethical aspects, because the question of whether a treatment presents a benefit worth pursuing or a harm that needs to be avoided also entails a value judgement to be made at least together with the patient or his surrogate. In the Netherlands, however, these types of end-of-life decisions are widely accepted as normal medical acts and all three have a legitimate place within the context of palliative care (Hertogh and Ribbe, 1996). A fourth type of end-of-life intervention, namely the so-called practice of terminal sedation or deep sedation, arouses more controversy. Terminal sedation is propagated by many antagonists of euthanasia/PAS as a 'natural' alternative for euthanasia/PAS. Some even hold the extreme opinion that in due time euthanasia/PAS will become obsolete. On the other hand, others contest the 'naturalness' of terminal sedation and state that there really is not a large difference between the deep sedation and euthanasia. Their argument is, that in case of deep sedation, a coma is induced until the patient dies a foreseeable and inescapable death from dehydration, because artificial (re)hydration is withheld (Royal Dutch Medical Association, 2004). An intensive debate on these issues is beyond the scope of this chapter. Suffice it to say that no medical decision in the face of death is without moral conflict. Nonetheless, the framework of palliative care can help physicians, patients and their relatives to make a tailored care plan that respects the patient's values as well as the physician's professional and personal norms.

Palliative care in dementia

Originally, the concept of palliative care was strongly related to and focused on cancer patients. Also, at least in the Netherlands, the so-called 'palliative care movement' or 'hospice movement' acted as a sort of anti-euthanasia lobby party. During recent decades, the scope of palliative care has gradually expanded to include other categories of patients. Today, it is no longer exclusively linked up with the hospice movement and the original controversy on palliative care versus euthanasia, although not entirely overcome, has moved from the fore to the background of discussions. But most importantly, palliative care is no longer restricted to the terminal phase of a disease trajectory, but is considered of relevance to all patients whose disease does not or no longer responds to curative treatment, as is evident from the following definition adopted from the WHO:

> Palliative care is integral multidisciplinary care for patients with incurable diseases, aimed at reaching and maintaining optimal quality of life for both patients and their relatives. More specifically, palliative care:
> Regards dying as an integral part of life;
> Does neither intend to hasten or postpone death;
> Aims to relieve pain and other symptoms of discomfort;
> Offers supportive care to help patients to remain as active and autonomous as possible;
> Offers supportive care to help family in coping with the disease of their loved one.
>
> (WHO, 1990)

This concept is central to the perspective of nursing home medicine, on medical treatment and caregiving in dementia (Dutch Association of Nursing Home Physicians, 1997). But although intuitively clear, two elements of this definition are in need of some further clarification: namely, the concept of *quality of life* and its applicability in the care for people with (advanced) dementia and, secondly, the place of *life-prolonging medical treatment* within the context of palliative care (Hertogh and Ribbe, 1996; Dutch Association of Nursing Home Physicians, 1997; Hertogh, 2001).

Quality of life (QoL)

QoL as a concept is still a debatable issue. Health-related QoL can be defined as the subjective way in which a person appraises his present state of life on several health-related domains. Researchers have tried to make QoL measurable through the development of several multidimensional questionnaires, but the question remains: Are the values of researchers, which have led to these questionnaires, comparable to the values of the person with dementia? It is well known that patients suffering from chronic diseases gradually shift their values and change their priorities in life, a phenomenon known as response shift, resulting in a so-called disability paradox (Rapkin and Schwartz, 2004). Research has shown that – in patients with mild to moderate dementia – direct assessment about their quality of life is preferable to proxy assessment, because caregivers have a tendency to report lower scores on QoL than patients themselves. This discrepancy is probably the combined effect of a patient's response shift and caregiver's bias as a result of their care burden: the higher the level of care burden experienced by the caregiver, the lower they seem to rate the patient's QoL (Sands et al, 2004). Another problem is, that in the more advanced stages of dementia, reliable self-reports on QoL are no longer obtainable and thus only estimate evaluations of discomfort and state of well-being are possible. These estimations strongly depend on (formal and/or informal) caregivers' observations and appraisals of behaviour and non-verbal communication, which are always more or less influenced and biased by their own situation and care burden. Also, the emotional ties between caregivers and the patient often make it difficult for them to distinguish between their own wishes and opinions and the wishes formerly held by the patient. This dilemma needs to be addressed openly and empathically as an integral part of palliative care.

Prolonging life

From the definition of palliative care, it follows that prolonging life is not its primary objective. But this does not mean that life-prolonging effects of palliative treatments are by definition contraindicated. Here it is morally relevant to consider the difference between *objectives* and *effects* of medical interventions. In palliative care, patients will often be treated for diseases which they have on top of their chronic illness, such as intercurrent urinary or respiratory tract infections or co-morbid conditions such as diabetes, thyroid disorders or cardiac failure. The objectives of such treatments are to reduce physical discomfort and maintain or improve well-being, but the side effect can and will also be that life is prolonged. The more the dementia process advances however, the more often the question comes to the fore whether treatment of concurrent illnesses with a possible life-prolonging effect is still morally justified, since every substantial extension of life will also expose the patient to a further progression of the debilitating dementia process. Thus, the focus gradually shifts from QoL to the quality of death and, at a certain moment, life-prolonging side effects of medical treatments with a primarily palliative intention are no longer morally acceptable. Then, time has come to shift from a palliative care policy to a symptomatic care policy (Dutch Association of Nursing Home Physicians, 1997). The crucial difference between both policies lies in the consideration that with a symptomatic policy further prolongation of life is considered worse than adequate relief of symptoms. In other words and in sum:

> With a palliative care policy, medical treatments are primarily directed towards optimal quality of life and relief of pain and other symptoms of discomfort, while prolongation of life as a secondary effect of such

treatments is acceptable or even co-intended. With a symptomatic care policy, relief of symptoms and distress remain paramount goals, but a life-prolonging effect of the therapeutic means to realize these objectives is no longer acceptable.

The question as to what type of interventions or treatments have to be considered futile is thus answered on the basis of the chosen treatment policy, so the concept of medical futility always derives its specific content and relative meaning from a covering care policy. For example: with a palliative policy, pneumonia can be treated with an antibiotic; with a symptomatic policy, however, this method of treatment is considered to be futile and treatment is restricted purely to relieving symptoms, for instance with oxygen or morphine to relieve breathlessness (Dutch Association of Nursing Home Physicians, 1997; Olde Rikkert and Rigaud, 2004).

These distinctions between specific decisional frameworks are of importance in defining individual goals and limits of medical treatment and they are of specific importance in dealing with living wills.

Defining individual treatment goals and limits

The choice of a palliative or a symptomatic care policy is determined on the grounds of (1) medical–professional considerations and (2) norms based on the views and wishes of the patient. In general, these are the two categories of norms that guide medical decision-making.

Professional norms and medical criteria

As indicated above, the general goal of medical policy is to optimize the patient's well-being within the limits set by the disease and its course. It is important to be aware that each treatment decision in dementia is a decision in a disease trajectory that is irreversible and accompanied by a decreased life expectancy. In early stages of the natural course, a palliative care policy is indicated, but there is always the question at what moment in the course of the disease we can say, following the old Hippocratic saying, that the patient 'has been overmastered by his disease' and further medical treatment has become futile.

The domain of meaningful medical treatment is not only restricted by questions concerning the moral justification of life-prolonging treatment. The possible harmful effects of treatment options on the physical as well as the psychological well-being of the patient have also to be considered carefully here. This latter consideration deserves extra attention in demented patients, because – due to their limited cognitive and communicative skills – they often lack the understanding of what is happening to them and they may experience medical treatments as intrusive events, resulting in confusion, anxiety and resistiveness. These psychological effects, which are stronger in the more advanced stages of the disease, limit the domain of medically appropriate interventions while expanding the domain of medically futile treatments. These issues often become acute in situations where hospital admission is under consideration, where tube feedings or (subcutaneous or intravenous) infusions are indicated to correct dehydration or malnutrition, etc. Then it is of great importance to weigh the prognostic influence of several treatment options on the course of the dementia and their effect on the patient's well-being, before a balanced decision can be made. This is still a field of decision-making where there is a huge grey area and research is urgently needed (Hertogh and Ribbe, 1996; Hertogh, 2001).

One out of many questions in this respect is how to distinguish between an intercurrent illness with a fair chance of improvement through treatment and a possible terminal complication that – with a symptomatic policy – will procure the patient a dignified death.

For instance, ever since Sir William Osler made his famous statement that pneumonia was considered to be a friend of old age, a saying that is still widespread among the general public, many believe that abstaining from treatment in case of pneumonia in a demented patient will automatically result in a peaceful death. Research in Dutch nursing homes, however, has unmasked this belief as erroneous in many cases and demonstrated the clinical importance of differentiating between the type of respiratory tract infection that needs to be treated and the one in which treatment with antibiotics is medically futile. Clinical intuition is often a valid factor here, but there is a need for more objective prognostic factors. The above-mentioned study, for example, yielded some clinical signs that are predictive for a bad prognosis, such as the absence of coughing, low body weight and dysphagia (Van der Steen et al, 2002a, 2002b). Future research in this direction is required to give more substance to the concept of medical futility as a protective devise against overtreatment in order to spare patients from useless, but burdensome, interventions and vice versa.

Patient-derived criteria

Respect for autonomy is an important ethical norm to be considered in medical decision-making in demented patients. Here we should distinguish between several situations, depending on the degree of decision-making capacity of the patient.

1. The patient is competent with regard to the decision in question

In the Netherlands the terms competence and capacity are used interchangeably as equivalents and both are seen as task- or decision-related. The more complicated a decision and its consequences, the higher the threshold in terms of decision-making capacity for a consent or dissent to be valid. An important implication of this task-related concept of competence is its so-called 'asymmetry': just because a patient is competent to consent to a treatment, it does not follow that he is also competent to refuse it. Consent to a medical treatment is thus weighed differently and requires a relatively lower level of capacities than the refusal of that same treatment (Berghmans, 2000; Schermer, 2001).

Respect for autonomy first of all refers to the current wish of a person who has become demented and it is the responsibility of the physician to interpret the current wish of the person as accurately as possible. In this respect, it is imperative that his questions and information are in attunement with the patient's level of comprehension.

2. There is doubt about the competence of the patient regarding the decision in question

In this situation an assessment of decision-making abilities seems to be required. An ethically preferable alternative would be to assess the consequences of respecting the patient's view or wish, in spite of the existing doubt, and to see if care plans can be rearranged in such a way that the wish of the patient can be respected without harming his health. The rationale for this approach is that a judgement of incompetency has far-reaching moral consequences for a person's right to self-determination (Berghmans, 2000). Furthermore, executing a treatment against the patient's present wish can also result in resistive behaviour, which in turn will lead to sedative medications or other restrictive measures. For these reasons, often 'second best' treatment options have to be chosen (e.g. enteral instead of parenteral administration of antibiotics, because a patient refuses intravenous infusions or pulls out the needle after an initial consent).

If an assessment of capacities proves necessary and the patient is judged to be incompetent with regard to the decision at stake, then the third situation is at hand.

3. The patient is incompetent with regard to the decision in question
In this case, the patient's representative – most of the time his partner, children or other relatives – acts as interpreter of the patient's views. When the patient has made a living will, then – under Dutch law – the views expressed in the will carry more weight than the views of proxies.

Living wills are a valuable instrument to assist proxies and physicians to decide what is best for the patient from his former viewpoint as laid down in writing. Yet they also create new moral problems, which will be discussed in the next section.

Living wills

In recent years, increasingly more elderly people have been formulating a living will or advance directive. By means of this instrument, decisionally capable adults give written instructions that pertain to future medical treatment preferences and values of the party executing the document. With the implementation of the Medical Treatment Act (WGBO) in the Netherlands, the living will has been imbedded in jurisdiction. As to its validity, this law differentiates between positive and negative living wills. Whereas in a positive living will a patient explicitly requests specific forms of action from the physician, in a negative living will the patients requests that a certain treatment should be withheld. Morally and legally, negative living wills have more validity than positive living wills, because of a person's fundamental right to say no to infringements on one's anatomy and physical integrity. By contrast, positive living wills always involve an action from another person, in case a physician who has his own professional norms and moral values and who can never be forced to act against these. The Medical Treatment Act only regards the negative living will: in case of incompetence, the physician is obliged to comply with its contents.

In general, advance directives take effect only if the patient is decisionally incapacitated at the time the specific decisions need to be made. In such a case, the text of the living will always requires careful interpretation based on the following guidelines:

1. The text of a living will is, in principle, a valid expression of the wishes of the person who made it, provided that this person was competent at the time he drew up his declaration. Nonetheless, interpretation of the literal text is always mandatory. It may be that new developments in medical care and treatment that the patient was unaware of at the time may have changed the situation. There is also a problem when a literal interpretation of the text offers the patient insufficient care and protection, as is the case in the so-called 'refusal of treatment' declaration (vide infra). In such circumstances, the physician must deviate from the literal wording of the living will and act in accordance with the intention thereof.

2. In the interpretation of a living will, the patient's representative plays a central role: in principle he or she will assess whether or not the situation has arrived that the patient had in mind when he made up his will (Hertogh, 2004).

Recent (qualitative) research indicates that the medical condition of the patient, the wishes of the family and the interpretation of the patient's QoL often appear to be more important factors in decision-making than living wills. Further research is needed into the exact reasons for this, because if this proves to be a more general practice, then physicians and representatives, in their strivings to realize optimal palliative care, are acting in conflict with the law (The et al, 2002).

Negative living wills

Examples of a negative living will are the non-resuscitation declaration and the non-treatment declaration: the Medical Treatment Act stipulates that a physician must comply with them, unless there are serious reasons for deviation. This could occur if the wording of the text is contradictory to the apparent intention, e.g. with the 'non-treatment declaration' in case of dementia. Many people who have made such an advance directive had the old saying of Osler in their head when they made an advance refusal of antibiotic drugs. As a result, they manoeuvred themselves into a position of insufficient care by binding the hands of their caregivers, because their refusal also implies a non-treatment of a number of ailments, such as urinary tract infections, erysipelas, and most forms of pneumonia, that will seriously deteriorate their condition and QoL, without procuring for them the dignified death they so much desired for themselves. In these cases, it is relevant to explain to proxies and – if still possible – to the patients themselves, that a palliative policy as described above will do much more justice to the intention of the living will than complying with the literal text. In addition, mere existence of an advance refusal sometimes also causes tensions between proxies and physicians, especially when the patient currently consents to treatments he formerly refused in writing and discrepancies arise among proxies or between proxies and caregivers on the patient's level of decisional capacity (Hertogh, 2004).

Positive living wills

The most prominent example of a positive living will is the euthanasia declaration in case of dementia. In the Netherlands a growing number of seniors draw up an advance directive in which they express the wish to have their lives terminated in case of dementia. The societal debate on this subject reached a new stage with the adoption in 2002 of the Euthanasia Act, because this law stated that a living will can replace an oral request for euthanasia in case of incompetence.

But a living will in itself does not suffice here, because euthanasia – as stated earlier in this contribution – can only be legally justified when a patient also suffers unbearably and hopelessly from his condition. Up until now, most experts in the field don't see how dementia can meet this criterion for justified euthanasia. In their opinion most demented people don't really suffer under the condition they previously feared and often seem to accept a situation they formerly despised.

So, at present there appears to be a yawning gap between the opinion of the pre-demented authors of advance directives and the actual practice of caregiving. In the eyes of many, this state of affairs is unsatisfactory, because of the extensive public support for the case of active termination of life in dementia. For that reason pleas are made, for instance by the Health Council, to continue the public debate on this subject and to find ways to meet the desires shared by so many citizens, although it seems very difficult as yet to see how this can be realized (Health Council of the Netherlands, 2002).

A relatively new approach to this debate is to introduce the voice of a third party, the party that is actually most involved and concerned here, and to ask the question: What do people with dementia think of their situation themselves? Of course not every demented person can participate in a discussion on this subject, certainly not those people who are in the more advanced stages of their disease. But the question of whether dementia in itself causes unbearable suffering is most relevant in the first and middle stages of the disease, when most patients are still more or less aware of their situation and still have a part in a common shared world of meaning and communication. Until very recently, however, it was taboo to talk with demented patients about their condition and their views were seldom actively sought (Cheston and Bender, 1999; Pinner and Bouman, 2002). Taking their views seriously involves a new and more phenomenological approach to the subjective world of people with dementia and necessitates us putting some crucial concepts and distinctions of traditional medical ethics in brackets. One of them is surely the concept of competence in its traditional rationalistic fashion and its privileging of cognition (Jaworska, 1999).

Although research in this field has only just begun, there is already growing evidence, that – contrary to traditional clinical opinion – people with dementia remain active agents up into the advanced stages of their disease. Just as most of the rest of us, they struggle to make sense of their world, but for them this struggle is harder because their capacities get weaker and weaker (Dröes, 1991; Miesen, 2004). Many of them seem to end up in a situation in which they appear not to realize the full implication of their disease. From a clinical–neurological point of view, this is called 'lack of awareness' or 'lack of insight'. But from a psychological perspective, there are good reasons to value these subjective reactions as perhaps the only viable way of coping with the onslaught of the disease in which the person with dementia is entitled to all the support he can get, beginning by acknowledging him as a person (Cheston and Bender, 1999; Clare, 2002). In line with the objectives of palliative care mentioned earlier in this chapter, this supportive care should be directed towards assisting patients in maintaining a positive self-image as in offering them a social environment in which they feel safe and secure (see also Chapter 48).

At this moment it is far too early to draw definite conclusions about the degree of suffering of people with dementia. There is an urgent need for more specific research into their experiential world before we can decide on the role and place of advance directives in dementia care in general and of euthanasia declarations in particular.

Final remarks

People with dementia are entitled to high-quality care – also in the last phase of their life. Goals and limits of medical care near the end of life in dementia are best defined in terms of a palliative policy, but a lot of research has to be done in this relatively neglected domain of medicine; the research is complex, conceptually, methodologically and morally. For that reason, in addition to quantitative studies, qualitative research can yield relevant additional information in this field.

In addition to much-needed empirical data on the natural course of dementia and the role and influence of co-morbid conditions and inter-current ailments, QoL research is needed, specifically in relation to the more advanced stages of dementia. We still know far too little of the subjective world of people with dementia and to what degree they suffer – or not – from their situation. Finally, more empirical data are required on the actual end-of-life care, with all its pitfalls and dilemmas, in order to explore and improve care practice in this field.

References

Berghmans RLP. *Bewkaam genoeg? Wils(on)bekwaamheid in geneeskunde, gezondheidsrecht en gezondheidsethiek.* Utrecht: Dutch Association for Bio-ethics; 2000. [*Competent enough? Competence in medicine, health care law and health care ethics*, report in Dutch.]

Cheston R, Bender MP. *Understanding dementia.* London: Jessica Kingsley; 1999.

Clare L. We'll fight it as long as we can: Coping with the onset of Alzheimer's disease. *Aging Ment Health* 2002; 6: 139–48.

Dröes RM. *In beweging. Over psychosociale hulpverlening aan demente ouderen.* PhD thesis, Free University Amsterdam, Amsterdam, 1991. [*Get moving. Psychosocial care for elderly people with dementia*, in Dutch.]

Dutch Association of Nursing Home Physicians. *Medische zorg met beleid.* Utrecht: Dutch Association of Nursing Home Physicians; 1997. [*Policy statement on end-of-life care in demented patients in nursing homes*, in Dutch.]

Health Council of the Netherlands. *Dementia.* Publication No. 2002/04. The Hague: Health Council of the Netherlands; 2002.

Hertogh CMPM. Palliatieve zorg. In: Jonker C, Verhey FRJ, Slaets JPJ, eds. *Alzheimer en andere vormen van dementie.* Houten/Diegem: Bohn Stafleu Van Loghum; 2001: 282–97. [*Palliative care in dementia*, in Dutch.]

Hertogh CMPM. Autonomy, competence and advance directives. In: Jones GGM, Miesen BML, eds. *Caregiving in dementia. Research and applications*, Vol. 3. New York: Brunner/Routledge; 2004: 391–403.

Hertogh CM, Ribbe MW. Ethical aspects of medical decision-making in demented patients. A report from the Netherlands. *Alzheimer Dis Assoc Disord* 1996; 10: 11–9.

Jaworska A. Respecting the margins of agency: Alzheimers's patients and the capacity to value. *Philos Public Aff* 1999; 28: 105–38.

Miesen BML. Towards a psychology of dementia care: Awareness and intangible loss. In: Jones GGM, Miesen BML, eds. *Caregiving in dementia. Research and applications*, Vol. 3. New York: Brunner/Routledge; 2004: 183–213.

Olde Rikkert MGM, Rigaud AS. Hospital-based palliative care and dementia, or what do we treat patients for and how do we do it? In: Purtilo RB, Have AMJ ten, eds. *Ethical foundations of palliative care for Alzheimer disease.* Baltimore: London, Johns Hopkins University Press; 2004: 80–96.

Pinner G, Bouman WP. To tell or not to tell: On disclosing the diagnosis of dementia. *Int Psychogeriatr* 2002; 14: 127–37.

Rapkin BD, Schwartz CE. Toward a theoretical model of quality-of-life appraisal: Implications of findings from studies of response shift. *Health Qual Life Outcomes* 2004; 2: 14.

Royal Dutch Medical Association. *Knelpunten bij levensbeïndiging.* Utrecht: Royal Dutch Medical Association; 2004. [*Problems in medical end of life care.* Conference report.]

Sands LP, Ferreira P, Stewart AL, Brod M, Yaffe K. What explains differences between dementia patients' and their caregivers' ratings of patients' Quality of Life? *Am J Geriatr Psychiatry* 2004; 12: 272–80.

Schermer MHNS. *The different faces of autonomy.* PhD thesis, University of Amsterdam, Amsterdam; 2001.

Steen JT van der, Ooms ME, Mehr DR, et al. Severe dementia and adverse outcomes of nursing home-acquired pneumonia: evidence for mediation by functional and pathophysiological decline. *J Am Geriatr Soc* 2002a; 50: 439–48.

Steen JT van der, Ooms ME, Wal G van der, et al. Pneumonia: The demented patient's best friend? Discomfort following starting or withholding antibiotic treatment. *J Am Geriatr Soc* 2002b; 50: 1681–8.

The AM, Pasman R, Onwuteaka-Philipsen B, Ribbe M, van der Wal G. Withholding the artificial administration of fluids and food from elderly patients with dementia: Ethnographic study. *BMJ* 2002; 325: 1326.

Wal G van der, Heide A van der, Onwuteaka-Philipsen BD, Maan PJ van der. *Medische besluitvorming aan het einde van het leven.* Utrecht: De Tijdstroom; 2003. [*Medical decision making at the end of life,* research report on the practice of euthanasia, in Dutch.]

World Health Organization (WHO). *Cancer pain relief and palliative care.* WHO Techn Rep Ser 1990; No. 804.

chapter 46

Legal issues: Developments in the law relating to mental incapacity in England and Wales

Steve Luttrell

Over the past decade in England and Wales, as in many other jurisdictions, there have been substantial developments in the legal rules relating to mentally incapacity. These include both an increased clarity about the way in which incapacity is determined and fairer and more sophisticated guidance on the way in which decisions should be made for those who are deemed to be mentally incapable.

These developments have been within the common law and have come about as a result of judicial decisions relating to individual legal cases. Whereas growth has been incremental and not as rapid as many might wish, this approach has allowed time for a more considered view of necessary changes. Unfortunately, however, the rules contained within the common law are often difficult to interpret and relatively inaccessible to those who are not lawyers. Nevertheless, they have had important implications for those people with dementia who are either at risk of losing or have lost the capacity to make some decisions for themselves.

The English Law Commission, in its 1995 report on mental incapacity, highlighted many weaknesses in the current law and recommended legislative change. After a lengthy interim period, which has included further public consultation, many of the Law Commission's recommendations have now been incorporated in a recently published Mental Incapacity Bill (2004). It is envisaged that this will be debated by Parliament in the near future and result in a Mental Incapacity Act which will reinforce many of the recent changes in the common law and introduce further rules to address those gaps which still exist.

Determining when a person is mentally incapable

The present common law test for mental incapacity is set out in re MB (1997), a Court of Appeal case involving a 23-year-old woman who was 40 weeks pregnant and who suffered a fear of needles. The case confirmed that a person lacks capacity if some impairment or disturbance of mental function renders that person unable to made a decision whether to consent to or refuse an intervention, either because he or she is unable to comprehend or retain information which is material, or is unable to use the information and weigh it in the balance as part of the process of arriving at a decision. This approach to the assessment of mental incapacity has now become widespread in medical practice. However, the determination can be time consuming for doctors who take on the task of assessment. It also requires skills and knowledge that hitherto have not been developed as part of medical training. There are obvious implications for those who organize medical training and for those who organize the provision of care.

Making decisions for those who are mentally incapable

While the legal changes in relation to the determination of mental capacity have been widely recognized by health professionals, there has been less professional acknowledgement of changes relating to the way in which decisions should be made for mentally incapable adults. This is certainly an area where the development of the common law has been slower than many would have wished and where there is a lack of clarity about how it should be interpreted and implemented on a day-to-day basis.

In the 1990 case Re F, the House of Lords took a very narrow view of best interests, relating it to saving life or ensuring improvement in health. This approach was supplemented by statements made in subsequent legal cases, such as *Airedale NHS Trust v. Bland* (1993), where the invasiveness of the intervention or the indignity to which the person might be subjected were considered relevant to a determination of best interests and in re J (1991), where quality of life after treatment was a relevant consideration. However, in all these cases the judicial test of best interest was based on the common law test for negligence – the approach set out in the *Bolam* case (1957) – in that if a responsible body of medical opinion were of the view the action was in the person's best interests then this would satisfy the courts.

Perhaps the most comprehensive review of the approach to be taken in determining best interests is set out in the more recent case of re S (2000), where it was highlighted that there was much more to a determination of best interests than those issues that might ordinarily be considered by the medical profession. The case highlighted that the *Bolam* test was only the starting point and that broader ethical, social, moral and social welfare considerations were important.

Although it is fair to say that the courts have increasingly taken a more sophisticated approach to the determination of best interests, it has not been clear how health and social care professionals should apply the new rules in day-to-day practice. The common law is difficult to access and there has been little practical guidance on how such decisions should be made.

It is particularly in this area that the clarity set out in the Mental Incapacity Bill is to be welcomed. The Bill states that in determining what is in a person's best interests the decision-maker must consider all the circumstances appearing to him to be relevant. In particular, the decision-maker must:

- consider whether it is likely that the person will at some time have capacity in relation to the matter in question
- permit and encourage the person to participate in the decision
- consider the person's past and present wishes and feelings and the beliefs and values that would be likely to influence his decision
- take into account the views of anyone named by the person as someone to be consulted on the matter in question or anyone engaged in caring for the person or interested in his welfare.

This much more detailed and rigorous approach to making best-interest decisions will help to ensure a less paternalistic approach by health and social care professionals and should encourage them to take into account those broader ethical, social, moral and social welfare considerations emphasized as important by the courts. However, the success of this change, as with those rules relating to the determination of mental incapacity, will be dependent on front-line staff having the time, skills and knowledge to participate in this new way of making decisions.

Making advance decisions

A mentally capable adult has the right to refuse all treatments even if this refusal will lead to his death. This right, which is captured in English common law (see Lord Goff in *Airedale NHS Trust v. Bland*), reflects the Human Rights Act 1998 which incorporates the European Convention on Human Rights into English domestic law. Article 8 of the Convention provides for a right to respect for private and family life, an interference of which includes compulsory medical treatment even if it is of minor importance, see *X v. Austria* (1980).

Although the validity of a contemporary refusal of treatment has been established for many years, it is only more recently that there has been legal clarity that an advance refusal of treatment (living will) can also be valid. For example, in re AK (2000), a 19-year-old boy with motor neuron disease indicated that he would wish his ventilation stopped if he was no longer able to communicate. He told his carers this by way of eyelid movements. His doctor explained to him what would happen if the ventilator was switched off and that he could be given drugs which would allow him to die without suffering. AK confirmed his wishes on several occasions. The court granted a declaration that it was lawful to discontinue artificial ventilation, nutrition and hydration 2 weeks after AK lost all ability to communicate. This case confirmed the legal view that an advance refusal of treatment will be recognized if it was made at the time the person was mentally capable and is clearly applicable to the circumstances which subsequently arise. However, the need for precision in creating such advance statements has limited and will probably continue to limit the wider use of living wills as a method of planning for the future. Patients at risk of mental incapacity often find it difficult to envisage and accurately set out the circumstances in which they might find themselves and the treatments they may wish to refuse.

Health and social care attorneys

The Mental Incapacity Bill introduces a new tool, a lasting power of attorney, which may prove to be much more popular with those at risk of future mental incapacity than living wills. Presently, in England and Wales, a person can nominate an attorney to make decisions about his/her property and affairs should he/she become mentally incapable. The new Bill changes this to allow a person to nominate another to make health, social welfare and/or financial decisions. More than one attorney can be appointed and it need not be the same person who makes both financial and health decisions. The attorney under such a power must make decisions in the best interests of the donor and any person making a decision for a donor must if it is practicable and appropriate consult the attorney. I envisage that the appointment of such attorneys will become a popular and practical way of planning for the future for people at risk of future mental incapacity. However, to ensure their success, health and social care professionals will need to understand the authority of such attorneys and work with them in decision-making.

Conclusion

A decade of changes in the common law relating to mental incapacity have done much to replace a system of decision-making which was in many instances paternalistic and lacked transparency and fairness. However, many of the common law changes in relation to decision-making for mentally incapable adults can be difficult to interpret and are poorly understood by health professionals. The future legislation envisaged within the Mental Incapacity Bill for England and Wales does much to improve this situation, clearly setting out the way in which decisions should be made and allowing individuals to nominate another person whom they trust to make health or social welfare decisions for them if they become mentally incapable. In a society committed to ensuring that the rights of all of its citizens are respected and upheld, these legal changes have much to commend them. For healthcare professionals, there is a need to ensure that skills and knowledge are developed and that time is made available to ensure that those who are mentally incapable and those who are at risk of mental incapacity are in a position to benefit.

References

Airedale NHS Trust v. Bland (1993) AC 789.
Bolam v. Frien Hospital Management Committee (1957) 1 WLR 582.
English Law Commission. *Mental incapacity*. Law Commission No. 231. London: HMSO; 1995.
Mental Incapacity Bill, Bill 120. London: The Stationery Office; 2004.
Re AK (2000) 58 BMLR 151.
Re MB (Medical Treatment) (1997) 2 FLR 426.
Re F (Mental Patient: Sterilization) (1990) 2 AC 1.
Re J (1991) 1 FLR 366.
Re S (Sterilization: Patient's Best Interests) (2000) 2 FLR 389.
X v. Austria (1980) 18 DR 154.

chapter 47

Ethical and legal questions on hospital-based care for patients suffering from dementia

Marcel GM Olde Rikkert and Wim JM Dekkers

Introduction

Reflection on the ethical and legal issues in the care for dementia patients in general and academic hospitals brings into mind a series of questions and dilemmas. Everyday practice of health care for frail older people with cognitive decline has the stigma of being boring, not rewarding and not spectacular for many physicians, medical students and other health professionals. The contrary is true, if one is prepared to be astonished by the overwhelming complexity of the overlapping dementias, if one is willing to broaden one's scope from the medical model to the biopsychosocial model and if one is prepared to discuss which diagnostic or treatment procedures really help the patients and, consequently, bypass clinical guidelines. In short, the healthcare worker who is sensitive to the medical, ethical and legal questions that are frequently met in health care for demented elderly patients in hospital will have an exciting time. The excitement may start with the question of how to manage extreme human frailty in the modern hospital organization, which is well adapted to the latest medical technology and the demand for quick production of diagnoses, but not to cognitive decline and enduring physical frailty.

In this chapter we will present a short and quick overview of important questions that dementia care in hospitals raises in the field of ethics and legislation. The aim is not to present elaborate in-depth reviews of topics such as withholding tube feeding and end-of-life decisions in dementia: we refer to an excellent book that serves this goal (see Purtilo and ten Have, 2004). Here we only want to present question marks that can be regarded as orange traffic lights at the dangerous crossroads of hospitals' clinical paths and the patients' journey along the stages of Alzheimer's disease.

The order in which these issues will be presented is the order of the subsequent stages of dementia and the reasons for a clinical encounter in hospital in those stages. Without being exhaustive, we distinguish five themes to which the questions and dilemmas are related:

1. Needs and preferences of care.
2. Disclosure of diagnosis.
3. Symptomatic treatment of dementia.
4. Social system breakdown.
5. Complications of dementia.

This helicopter view on dementia practice is primarily based on and fuelled by personal experiences. These experiences come from working in a geriatric department in an academic hospital, in which an outpatient memory clinic is located as well as a day clinic and an inpatient geriatric ward, and in which many patients are seen by means of a consultation team running throughout the hospital (MOR).

Needs and preferences of care in dementia

The first and perhaps most intense question to address is: 'Does a geriatrician, or in general a medical specialist, really have to offer something for patients who are suffering from cognitive decline, and who may be in the first stage of dementia? Are specialist diagnostic procedures to assess the diagnosis of dementia worthwhile for the patients' efforts and burden?'

General practitioners (GPs) in the Netherlands and Flanders are rather reluctant to refer their patients in early stages of cognitive decline for diagnostic aims. In practice, they refer approximately only one-half of the patients with cognitive decline, in whom the presence of dementia is uncertain, to specialist memory diagnostic services (de Lepeleire et al, 2004).

In talking to GPs about the question whether or not to refer their patients, the second explanatory question, which is often asked, is: 'What is the benefit of referral to a memory clinic for a patient, when you cannot offer a treatment that can really change the course of the disease?'. A family physician, being close to the patient, is right in being critical about specialist referrals. Elderly patients may not always benefit from the positivistic modern trend to get as much certainty as possible and to get specialist medical information about changes in mental or physical health. Sometimes this even seems an aim of its own.

Our answer to these critical questions usually is that the nihilistic approach, which often is the result from not starting the process of formal diagnostics, may also deny the patient and his or her family access to early and careful diagnosis of care needs, educational needs, behavioural problems, psychological burden and caregiver stress. Moreover, nihilism, doing nothing because of the absence of a medical cure, still enforces the stigma of dementia. Apart from a formal diagnosis, and curative drug treatment, we can also offer a number of diagnostic, monitoring and therapeutic non-drug treatment options, whose efficacy is already evidenced or being currently assessed in medical and psychological research. Recent Dutch standards of care (NHG standard for dementia; Wind et al, 2003) also advice GPs to take an active attitude towards early diagnosis.

However, for many reasons it is very good to be asked that very critical question by GPs at the start of individual diseases courses: 'What can you really offer my patients?' It is a strong stimulus to develop a memory service in the direction of the patient's needs and preferences. Secondly, it is a stimulus to really investigate the individual needs and preferences of the patients and families. So far, there is not a simple instrument to check the patient's needs and preferences. The development of such an instrument to support patients and carers in this process may be valuable, but the topic can also be addressed in a qualitative interview of the patient. This requires time, place and interest to reflect on individual goals and wishes, after the patient–physician relationship has become sufficiently confidential. Implementation of a patient's preferences is in fact a cornerstone of individualized evidence-based practice, but probably is one of the most difficult things to reach, because of the patient's declining mental capacities, intrinsically connected to dementia (Olde Rikkert et al, 2004). However, only by being aware of the needs and preferences of individual patients and their families, can medical specialists give a valid answer to that challenging and penetrating question: 'What can you really offer this patient with serious cognitive decline?'

Diagnostic disclosure

In a case where a patient was referred and the diagnostic criteria of dementia are met, the next striking question to be answered is whether one should or should not tell the patient the diagnosis of dementia. Disclosing the diagnosis of dementia to a patient is not common in clinical practice (Pinner and

Bouman, 2002). There are presumed advantages of disclosing the diagnosis at an early stage including opportunities to:

- improve the quality of life of patients and caregivers
- blame the disease and not the patient for behavioural changes (Doraiswamy et al, 1998)
- make preparations for future care planning.

Evidence about the preferences of the patients themselves is scarce (Bamford et al, 2004).

In our practice many physicians do not mention the diagnosis to the patient, and regularly family asks not to disclose the diagnosis to the patient. This is confirmed in literature, although with high variability. Geriatricians and old age psychiatrists disclose the diagnosis in 38–96% of their patients (Bamford et al, 2004). Unfortunately, one has to conclude that the existing evidence regarding diagnostic disclosure is both inconsistent and limited and does not give a clear answer to the question which benefits and risks may be expected in diagnostic disclosure (Bamford et al, 2004).

Recently, we found that both elderly people suspected of having dementia and their caregivers, in general, wished to be informed of the diagnosis (van Hout et al, 2001). Looking towards legislation in this field, physicians, generally speaking, have the duty to disclose the diagnosis, because patients simply have the right to know (Article 10, European Convention on Human Rights and Biomedicine). Dutch Health Law is fundamentally based on patients' rights and self-determinism (Article 22 of the Dutch Constitution). The Netherlands took a leading position in a law on medical contract and patients' rights. This law also formalizes the right of patients with Alzheimer's disease to be told the diagnosis, in a way that addresses their mental impairments. Only in restricted cases, doctors may withhold the diagnosis. The right to know has only rare so-called therapeutic exceptions, e.g. if the awareness of the disease would cause serious harm in patients or family.

Symptomatic treatment of dementia

Family practitioners may also refer patients, in whom dementia is already diagnosed, for treatment trials or regular therapeutic options (e.g. cholinesterase inhibitors, memantine). In essence, when cholinergic drugs are given, this only means that symptomatic treatment is given for cognitive decline. Some authors clearly describe a cholinergic drugs regimen as (part of) palliative care (Moss et al, 1999); however most do not. Because of the limited clinical effects of the anti-Alzheimer drugs that are currently available, one may ask oneself whether the prescription of these drugs, with a responder percentage of 10–30%, is ethically justified compared to the burden of gastrointestinal side-effects and the financial burden for both individuals and society. Again, we are only able to answer this question of potential clinical relevance by looking carefully at the individual patient. Individualized prescription should start with the general knowledge of efficacy, effectiveness and efficiency and the balance of potential benefits and adverse reactions (Post and Whitehouse, 1998). Next, a qualitative evaluation should be carried out of the wishes still expressed by the patient, the complications of dementia and other co-morbidity, the joy and quality of living of the patient, advance directives and valuation of these factors by the patient's proxy or representative.

In the literature it has been suggested that anti-dementia drugs could have overall negative effects by creating false hope, elongation of suffering, problems in stopping the drug again and in the patient re-experiencing the anxiety and depressive feelings of the early stages of dementia (Post, 1997). A recent qualitative study of caregivers' experiences showed that these potential problems were not met in the drug treatment of patients in early or moderately severe dementia (Huizing et al), 2002, which is in line with our own experiences.

Social system breakdown

Dementia patients may also be presented in hospital with acute care problems due to social network breakdown. For all kind of reasons (somatic disease of the patient, of a spouse or caregiver; dementia progression; limited availability of professional caregivers; burnout of primary caregiver, etc.), professional or non-professional care may stop or may become insufficient. Shortage of care often cannot be acutely solved by GPs, for instance because of waiting lists for nursing homes. The only solution one sometimes finds is to send these patients to the hospitals' emergency wards, with or without some sort of an acute care diagnosis. From the hospital-based point of view, there is enormous reluctance to take care of these patients and they are often sent home without even proper examination or history-taking. In this group of patients (sometimes pejoratively abbreviated as 'GOMERs': Get Out of My Emergency Room), a large number of untreated diseases can be diagnosed.

A difficult question is whether we should or should not admit frail demented patients with such a social system breakdown, without new somatic or psychiatric diseases. Family, carers and the patient will be often deeply helped by admission; however, the perceived 'risk' is that the patient may have to be indicated for long-term institutionalization and will become a so-called 'bed-blocker' in hospital for several months. Such bed-blocking patients are valued as inefficient by hospital managers and they will also have a higher in-hospital risk for iatrogenic problems. In general, all parties involved (patient, family, professionals, institutions and the community) should feel a shared responsibility to restore the balance of caring. There cannot be one solution here, but healthcare professionals in general cannot walk away from their share in the struggle for adequate and safe care and caring for demented patients. At least, the risks of sending patients home must be carefully evaluated and discussed.

Similar questions arise when it could be medically appropriate to discharge a demented patient from hospital after treatment for concurrent illnesses, but the family or caregiver system, under serious stress, refuses to take up caring for the older person again. From the intense emotions around these issues, conflicts may easily arise that hinder creative and reliable compromises. Guiding a team, a patient and a family towards a restored balance in caring may be a very rewarding operation, and make a strong appeal to all the competencies and skills of a medical specialist. Healing a broken leg usually is far less complex.

Complications of dementia

In different stages of dementia, different complications may occur (Hogan et al., 1999). As far as we know, only the study of Nourashémi et al (2001) presents empirical data on the prevalence of all possible reasons of patients with cognitive impairment for referral to emergency departments and acute Alzheimer care units. Complications such as behavioural problems (26.3%) and falls (18.6%) were the most important, followed by co-morbid gastrointestinal problems (14.4%), fever (11%), neurological disorders, including disturbed consciousness (11.8%), and social grounds (2.5%). These data were collected in a study on geriatric admission policy, in which a group of 118 patients was admitted in a period of 4 months (Nourashémi et al, 2001). The distribution of reasons for referral of course differs between (sub-)acute and non-acute admissions (Thorpe et al., 1994).

Behavioural complications are very important in disease management and mostly occur in the stages of moderate and severe dementia, although they are not confined to these stages, because of the substantial differences among individuals and differences in the natural history of Alzheimer's disease. There are peaks in incidence for different behavioural problems. First, one may encounter psychomotor activity disorders; and diurnal rhythm disorders; later on in natural history, depression and paranoia may occur, followed by an increasing incidence of wandering and aggression (Eastwood and Reisberg, 1999). These conduct disorders are called behavioural and psychological symptoms in dementia (BPSD). They have a large impact on the quality of life and need for care of patients, families and carers.

Because of the nature of these complications, however, patients may not want to move to a hospital, or, inside hospital, patients may be reluctant to accept (best) therapies. Apart from the careful medical analysis of the health problems, in which often several diseases play a role and interact, complex ethical and legal issues enter the arena, such as limits of autonomy, declined capacity to consent to treatment decisions, need for interpretation of the value and meaning of refusal, possibilities and desirability of treatments against one's will, the limits of acceptable intrusiveness of treatments, the burden of behavioural disturbances for the patient and the family, etc. In general, healthcare legislation does not give the physician solutions for these issues. Key characteristics of the process of decision-making in such cases should be the acquisition of sufficient objective medical and relevant non-medical details, collecting evidence of treatment options, subjective viewpoints of all who are involved, a multidisciplinary team meeting to discuss all reasonable alternatives and the intention to have the patient and family play an important role in the selection of the best treatment even though they may not understand all the details. Often a careful process of decision-making in the end stages of life is as (or even more) valuable as the outcome per se of the discussion. Principally, the demented patients should have access to the whole spectrum of medical diagnostics and treatments as well as to all modern tools of palliative care. Next, the question of what care is most appropriate has to be answered very carefully.

The substantial worsening of the prognosis in serious complications of patients with advanced stages of dementia often begs the question of whether palliative care or curative care is the best option. Living wills with statements concerning treatment of complications play an important role in the Netherlands at these points, but do not have to or should be followed blindly.

Conclusion

In our experience, working with patients suffering from dementia inside general or academic hospitals usually requires 'intensive care'. Within the Netherlands we have a well-equipped system of health care, with modern and well-equipped hospitals, nursing homes and family practices for which most elderly people are sufficiently insured. Moreover, the Netherlands has a reputation for well-developed health-related legislation and high-quality standards or guidelines on ethically important issues. However, these laws and guidelines do not and cannot make the everyday practice of medical care for frail elderly subjects with cognitive decline easier. We must keep struggling to provide the best care. The importance of good communication skills and well-developed medical and communication competencies cannot be overvalued in the challenges that dementia care in hospitals present. Keeping one's mind open to the ethical questions that arise is a precondition not to become separated too far from the heart of this matter.

References

Bamford C, Lamont S, Eccles M, et al. Disclosing a diagnosis of dementia: A systematic review. *Int J Geriatr Psychiatry* 2004; 19: 151–69.

De Lepeleire J, Vernooy-Dassen M, Moniz-Cook E, Aertgeerts B. Diagnosing dementia in primary care. *Age Ageing* 2004; 33: 321.

Doraiswamy P, Steffens M, Pithumoni S, Tabrizi S. Early recognition of Alzheimer's disease: What is consensual? What is controversial? What is practical? *J Clin Psychiatry* 1998; 59: 6–18.

Eastwood R, Reisberg B. Abnormal behaviour in Alzheimer's disease. In: Gauthier S, ed. *Clinical diagnosis and management of Alzheimer's disease.* Malden: Blackwell Science; 1999: 197–210.

Hogan DB, McCracken PN. Associated medical conditions and complications. In: Gauthier S, ed. *Clinical diagnosis and management of Alzheimer's disease.* Malden: Blackwell; 1999: 279–86.

Hout van H, Vernooij-Dassen M, Hoefnagels W, Grol R. Measuring the opinions of memory clinic users: Patients, relatives and general practitioners. *Int J Geriatr Psychiatry* 2001; 6: 846–51.

Huizing AR, Berghmans RLP, Widdershoven GAM, Verhey FRJ. Ethical aspects of anti-Alzheimer drugs: Experiences of caregivers. *Tijdschr Gerontol Geriatr* 2002; 33: 246–51. [In Dutch.]

Moss DE, Berlanga P, Hagan MM, Sandoval H, Ishida C. Methanesulfonyl fluoride (MSF): A double-blind placebo-controlled study of safety and efficacy in the treatment of senile dementia of the Alzheimer type. *Alzheimer Dis Assoc Disord* 1999; 13: 20–5.

Nourhashémi F, Andrieu S, Sastres N, et al. Descriptive analysis of emergency hospital admissions of patients with Alzheimer disease. *Alzheimer Dis Assoc Disord* 2001; 15: 21–5.

Olde Rikkert MGM, Dekkers W, Scheltens Ph, Verhey F. Memantine in Alzheimers disease. *Alzheimer Dis Assoc Disord* 2004; 18: 47–8.

Pinner G, Bouman W. Dementia: To tell or not to tell: on disclosing the diagnosis of dementia. *Int Psychogeriatr* 2002; 14: 127–37.

Post SG. Slowing the progression of Alzheimer diseases: Ethical issues. *Alzheimer Dis Assoc Disord* 1997; 11: S34–6.

Post SG, Whitehouse PJ. Emerging antidementia drugs: A preliminary ethical view. *J Am Geriatr Soc* 1998; 46: 784–7.

Purtilo RB, Have ten HAMJ, eds. *Ethical foundations of palliative care for Alzheimer Disease*. Baltimore: John Hopkins University Press; 2004.

Thorpe J, Widman LP, Wallin A, Beiwanger J, Blumenthal HT. Co-morbidity of other chronic age-dependent diseases in dementia. *Aging Clin Exp Res* 1994; 6: 159–66.

Wind AW, Gusseklo J, Vernooij-Dassen MJF, Bouma M, Moomsma LJ, Boukes FS. NHG standard dementia. *Huisarts Wetensch* 2003; 46: 754–68. [In Dutch.]

Further reading

Holstein J, Chatellier G, Moulias R. Prevalence of associated diseases in different types of dementia among elderly institutionalised patients: Analysis of 3447 records. *J Am Geriatr Soc* 1994; 42: 972–7.

Morrison RS, Siu AI. Survival in end-stage dementia following acute illness. *JAMA* 2000; 284: 47–52.

Tolson D, Smith M, Knight P. An investigation of the components of best nursing practice in the care of acutely ill hospitalized older patients with coincidental dementia: A multi-method design. *J Adv Nurs* 1999; 30: 1127–36.

chapter 48

Towards a more adequate moral framework: Elements of an 'ethic of care' in nursing home care for people with dementia

Cees MPM Hertogh

Modern healthcare ethics has its roots in the movement for patient rights and the process of patient emancipation that started in the 1970s. Its core concepts are the principles of respect for autonomy and the right to free and uncoerced self-determination. In the Netherlands, these rights and the correlated duties of healthcare professionals are embedded in the Medical Treatment Act (WGBO) and related legislation such as the Special Admissions to Psychiatric Hospitals Act (BOPZ) that stipulates the rights of patients admitted against their will to psychiatric hospitals and psychogeriatric (wards of) nursing homes. This emancipatory process and the subsequent 'juridification' of the relation between patients and healthcare professionals thoroughly influenced the healthcare system and certainly changed the role of the physician: from a paternalistic figure who knows what is best for his patients, the physician has become a careful deliberator who informs about the pros and cons of treatment options, thus letting patients decide for themselves what is best. Hence, there is an emphasis in the contemporary training of medical students not only on technical skills but also on communicative skills.

This specific morality also bears on the nursing home setting and the professionals working there are bound by the same legal rules. Certainly, in some relevant aspects, nursing home residents have benefited from this development. Professionals have become more aware of the intrusiveness of many institutional house rules, and long-term care facilities are encouraged to develop a policy of scrupulous and restrictive use of fixation, sedation, isolation and related interventions directed towards dealing with so-called problem behaviour or challenging behaviour. Also, more attention is paid nowadays to rights and rules of privacy.

On the other hand, a strict application of this ethic – developed mainly in the realm of acute care medicine – to the practice of long-term care reveals some serious shortcomings. More specifically, it fails to offer moral guidance to those caregivers who have to offer 'good care' to such vulnerable care recipients as people with dementia. There are three related reasons for this failure and all three pertain to the central focus on autonomy.

First of all, to have one's autonomy respected, an individual must have decisional capacity. Most demented residents lack this capacity and thus cannot be involved in important decisions regarding their care and treatment. According to the current ethic, care-providers therefore have to resort to proxy decision-making. But in day-to-day practice and communication, this approach provides no relevant support, since people with dementia continue to express wishes and preferences. Questions they ask like: 'Where am I?', 'Where is my home?' and 'Where are my parents?' cannot be disposed of as being merely symptoms of dementia and it does not help to view them as signs of incompetence. They are serious questions that express the tragedy of the dementia process but that also have a probing ethical meaning. People with dementia are entitled to a reliable and trustworthy answer to these kind of questions but the prevailing right-based ethics has nothing to offer in this respect.

Secondly, respect for autonomy implies that great store is set on the principle of non-interference, thus bestowing individuals with a purely negative freedom. Already in the 1970s, the psychiatrist Appelbaum warned that a strong reading of the principle of respect for autonomy would result in 'a right to rot' and in the Netherlands the strict application of the BOPZ Act has indeed resulted in a growing group of social outcasts, termed 'the languished and the depraved': chronic psychotic patients without disease insight who refuse treatment and who tramp around in our cities. A parallel problem arises in the field of long-term care for people with dementia. Here, too, caregivers feel that a strict obedience to the principle of respect for autonomy in a way alienates them from their nuclear responsibilities. As George Agich (2003) has put it, at best the development of efforts to secure the rights of long-term care recipients in the name of respect for autonomy helps marginally to improve their care, at worst these efforts work out in 'a right to be left alone' and fail to ennoble the elders.

Finally, by articulating the values of independence and self-sufficiency so strongly, the autonomy-based ethic puts a bad light on care and being dependent on care. In our modern Western society, with its powerful and almost omnipotent medicine, care-receiving is viewed by many as a necessary evil that is acceptable and endurable as a temporary situation in order to get well again but which is problematic when dependency on care amounts to a permanent state. By specifically neglecting the real interdependency of human life, the current ethic, in a way, is accessory to this negative value judgement and even, to some extent, gives support to the suggestion that a life in dependency is not really worth living any more. This does not do justice to people with dementia or to their caregivers and results in a devaluation of the caring practice.

For all these reasons, there is a need for an alternative moral framework that is more adequate to the realities of long-term care for people with dementia. A promising new approach is to be found in the so-called 'ethic of care', which proposes a more relational view on autonomy. The focus here is on care as a human practice, defined as: 'everything we do to maintain, continue and repair our "world" so that we can live in it as good as possible' (Tronto, 1993). According to the ethic of care, being vulnerable and dependent on others are not just the characteristics of a specific group of people, they typify the situation of all people. Of course, the extent and nature of dependency will vary, but people are always involved in care in all phases of their lives, whether as care receiver or caregiver. By emphasizing that care relationships are essential to human existence, the ethic of care not only allows criticism of a society that is too unilaterally orientated towards the maxims of individual autonomy and independence but also makes the case for a (political) change in which the provision of care is recognized as a vital activity. Central to the ethic of care is not the principle of negative freedom or non-interference but the perspective of taking the other's needs as the starting point for what must be done. In addition to central values such as *attentiveness* to the needs of others and *responsibility* in fulfilling these needs, the ethic of care set great store in the *competency* of the caregiver and his alertness to the *responsivity* of the care receiver to the care delivered to him.

Although the perspective of the ethic of care is primarily political, the values it articulates fit in closely with the internal morality of long-term care practice and are in keeping with the current focus of dementia care on the experiential world of people with dementia. In the Netherlands and Belgium, this approach is known as 'perception-based' care; in the United Kingdom, terms such as **'person-focused'** or **'person-centred'** care are used to indicate a similar approach. Central to this focus on personhood is the (re)discovery of the psychology of dementia: the recognition that people with dementia are to be seen as active agents. Contrary to earlier assumptions and prevailing prejudices, dementia patients are actively trying to make sense of their world, to cope with the threats of the disease to their sense of self and to resolve the emotional challenges posed by the dementia process. However, due to the progressive nature of the disease process and the resulting weakening of their capacities, these coping efforts in the end cannot but fail, thus resulting in strange, maladaptive behaviour, often termed 'problem' behaviour by an environment that lacks understanding and sympathy.

These insights have put an end to the therapeutic nihilism that character-ized the field of dementia care for so many years and have resulted in what has been termed 'a new culture of dementia care'. Caregivers are now encour-aged to move beyond a simply custodial approach to caring and focus on the residual abilities and subjective experience rather than on the functional deficits of people with dementia. In a certain sense, this shift from 'patholo-gy to people' can very well be typified as an emancipatory process, but under the recognition that this emancipation of the person with dementia follows a different pattern from that of the emancipation of the competent patient and hence involves an orientation on other moral values. Central to an 'ethic of psychogeriatric care' based on this newly developed concept of care for people with dementia are the two values of *safety* and *self-esteem* (Hertogh, 2004).

Promoting self-esteem

On an experiential and psychological level, dementia is not only or primarily a memory disorder: it is first and foremost a 'disease of the self'. For that reason Oliver Sacks has made a plea for a new discipline, called 'the neurology of identity', because 'in the higher regions of neurology and in psychology the study of disease and of identity cannot be disjoined.' Indeed, coping with dementia – certainly in the earlier stages of the disease – amounts to a considerable extent of performing 'identity work': to try to hold on to a sense of self and to uphold a positive self-image. The self of the dementia sufferer, however, is not only undermined from the inside, through neurological impairment, but also through the loss of social roles and through negative social interaction that undermines the patient's feelings of dignity and self-esteem. Tom Kitwood (1997) has coined the term 'malignant social psychology' to identify these kinds of degrading interactions and opposed them with so-called 'positive person work': meaningful interactions that can enhance and strengthen a patient's personhood. Examples are validation (acknowledging the reality of a person's emotions and feeling) and facilitation (enabling a person to do what otherwise he would not be able to do).

Other important treatment approaches in this respect are life review, reminiscence and – more generally – allowing or supporting people with dementia to construct a narrative that helps them to shape their world, although this narrative may have little bearing on reality and is regularly construed on confabulations. But what is of importance here is not primarily the truthfulness of such narrative, but how the past is used to find meaning and footing in the present. Thus, there are many ways through which caregivers can promote self-esteem of dementia sufferers. Respect for autonomy and freedom of choice can also be of significance here, but such respect cannot be a goal in itself, amounting to a simple negative freedom. Instead, caregivers should exert themselves in affording people with dementia meaningful choices, choices that allow them to enhance their self-esteem and personhood.

Offering safety and security

Fear and anxiety are among the basic constituents of the emotional world of the dementia sufferer. The loss of control and recognition and the progressive threatening of their identity creates feelings of insecurity and results in the experience of being in an unsafe, foreign and frightening world. Good care for people with dementia requires from caregivers that they are attentive to these feelings, but also that preventative efforts are made to spare demented patients from being confronted with an environment that arouses fear. This implies first of all 'an ethic of space': nursing homes and other residential settings for people with dementia should be devised and furnished in such a way that they offer a safe and prosthetic environment for their residents. The word 'safety' here has a double meaning; it refers to the organization of the physical environment, which should be safe in an ergonomic sense, but it also refers to the psychological sense of providing a homelike atmosphere, a safe haven where people can feel 'at home' and secure. For many people, privacy is a fundamental value when it comes to living and living arrangements, and the families of people with dementia often attach great worth to a private room or apartment for their dear one in choosing the appropriate nursing home. But from a perception-orientated approach to caregiving in dementia, it is not privacy, but security, that comes first. Privacy here has no value in itself, but is of value in so far as it serves self-esteem and does not undermine security. Thus, words like 'home' and feeling 'at home' fundamentally have no topographical meaning but refer to an inner state of mind.

This brings us to a second and equally important aspect of the value of safety. For safety and security are also the values that typify the attitude of the good carer and that are central characteristics of the care relation. Just as children will look to their parents for reassurance when confronted with a fearful event, so people with dementia will equally seek safety and security with their carers. In this connection, Miesen (1993) has shown convincingly that the search for their deceased parents and the vivid conviction that they are still alive is a specific expression of the demented patient's need for attachment relationships. In addition, Kitwood (1997) and other specialists in dementia care have pointed to the important parallel between the mother–child relationship and the care relation in psychogeriatric (nursing home) care. They refer to concepts like 'holding', which illustrate the need for an empathetic caregiver who provides a safe psychological space and who functions as a 'container' for the overwhelming and fearful emotions of the person with dementia.

It should be clear that to care in such a way for people with dementia not only requires specific skills and expertise but also a willingness to become engaged and attached. The standard is not to hold patients at a clinical objective distance but to become involved in an empathetic relationship. Thus, interpersonal communication is not an 'extra' that can be offered when the 'real work' is done, or that can be sacrificed in times of shortage: the bringing together of functional caring and empathetic treatment is exactly what defines the specific *competency* needed for caregiving in dementia.

However, in order to enable care staff to deliver high-quality care according to these standards, it is also necessary that attention be paid to their own needs and experiences. Demented patients are vulnerable, but so are their caregivers. Their work is demanding and burdensome, specifically because of their emotional attachment to the people they care for, their vulnerability for the often challenging behaviour of demented persons, the frequent losses they have to deal with and – not to be underestimated – the lack of prestige and societal recognition for their work and for dementia care in general. The ethic of care insists that caring should not be restricted to a dyadic relationship: even child-rearing is never the sole responsibility of the (birth-) mother, nor can it be. Thus, caring for people with dementia equally requires a 'care for the carers' that focuses not only on promoting skills and competence but also on offering emotional and moral support to those who are engaged most directly and on a day-to-day basis with the needs of people with dementia. The provision of this type of 'care for carers' is an important responsibility of the organization and should be a central element of its quality policy.

References

Agich GJ. *Dependence and autonomy in old age*. Cambridge: Cambridge University Press; 2003.

Hertogh CMPM. Between autonomy and security. Ethical questions in the care of elderly persons with dementia in nursing homes. In: Jones GGM, Miesen BML, eds. *Caregiving in dementia, Vol. 3*. New York: Brunner/Routledge; 2004: 375–90.

Kitwood T. *Dementia reconsidered: The person comes first*. Buckingham: Open University Press; 1997.

Miesen BML. Alzheimer's disease, the phenomenon of parent fixation and Bowlby's attachment theory. *Int J Geriatr Psychiatry* 1993; 8: 147–53.

Tronto J. *Moral boundaries. A political argument for an ethic of care*. New York: Routledge; 1993.

Index

Milton Keynes UK
Ingram Content Group UK Ltd.
UKHW031126141024
449569UK00006B/418